Care of the Elderly

Previous Anglo-American conferences:

1971: **Medical Care**

SBN 9501555 1 9

1973: **Drug Abuse**

ISBN 0 9501555 5 1

1974: **Continuing Medical Education**

ISBN 0 9501555 7 8

Reports of these conferences may be obtained from The Publications Department, Royal Society of Medicine, Chandos House, 2 Queen Anne Street, London, W1M 0BR, or through any bookseller

1976: **Sexually Transmitted Diseases**

ISBN 0 12 164150 3

Published by Academic Press Inc (London) Ltd

Care of the Elderly:

Meeting the Challenge of Dependency

Proceedings of a Conference
sponsored jointly by the
Institute of Medicine, National Academy
of Medicine, Washington, DC,
the Royal Society of Medicine and the
Royal Society of Medicine Foundation Inc
held at
the National Academy of Sciences
Washington, DC, USA
17–19 May 1976

Edited by
A N EXTON-SMITH and J GRIMLEY EVANS

1977

ACADEMIC PRESS London
GRUNE & STRATTON New York

ACADEMIC PRESS INC. (LONDON) LTD
24/28 Oval Road
London NW1

U.S. Edition published by
GRUNE & STRATTON INC.
111 Fifth Avenue
New York
New York 10003

Library of Congress Catalog Card Number: 77 71797
ISBN (Academic Press): 0 12 244950
ISBN (Grune & Stratton): 0 8089 1055 8

Printed in Great Britain at
The Spottiswoode Ballantyne Press by
William Clowes & Sons Limited
London, Colchester and Beccles

Preface

The increasing number and proportion of old people in Western populations and the difficulties associated with providing appropriate health and social care are currently matters of public concern and debate. In their attempts to cope with these problems, the United States and the United Kingdom have over the last twenty-five years followed different traditions and policies. None the less, because of their common cultural heritage there is essentially agreement throughout the two nations on the basic social and personal values which determine the objectives of health and social care. This agreement on objectives with experience of different methods of trying to attain them provides the background to the Anglo-American Conference.

Those attending the Conference came from many disciplines including medicine, gerontology, sociology, economics, nursing, administration and public policy. The specific purposes of the Conference were threefold:

(1) To delineate the special problems of those among the elderly who require or are at risk of requiring supportive health, personal and social services.
(2) To compare approaches in the United Kingdom and the United States toward care of the elderly and the prevention and minimization of dependency.
(3) To assess critically the social policy implications of current or anticipated social responses to the special problems of the dependent elderly.

The structure of the Conference took the form of five sessions, each comprising invited papers on specified topics followed by prepared commentaries and informal discussion. This format has been followed in this report of the proceedings.

The Conference was held at the National Academy of Sciences, Washington, DC, and was organized by the Institute of Medicine in association with the Royal Society of Medicine and the Royal Society of Medicine Foundation Inc.

The Institute of Medicine was created in 1970 by the National Academy of Sciences to enlist distinguished members of the medical and other professions in the voluntary examination of policy matters pertaining to the health of the public. It is now a national resource independent of government or any specific interest groups for impartial and informed analysis, advice and judgment on the problems of health and medicine.

The Royal Society of Medicine was founded in 1805 as the Medical and Chirurgical Society of London. It has one of the most comprehensive medical libraries in the world and publishes a monthly journal of its proceedings which range over the whole field of clinical and pre-clinical medicine. It has a distinguished record in fostering contacts between medical workers in different lands and organizes international conferences and symposia each year.

The Royal Society of Medicine Foundation Inc is a tax-exempt New York corporation established to provide a link between the medical professions in the United States and the United Kingdom. The Foundation sponsors young American doctors as travelling Fellows to the United Kingdom, and participates in the organization of Anglo-American Conferences.

A N Exton-Smith
J Grimley Evans

Members of the Conference Committee

Michael R Pollard Karl D Yordy	*Institute of Medicine*
A N Exton-Smith J Grimley Evans Sir John Stallworthy	*Royal Society of Medicine*
Alexander G Bearn Harry J Robinson	*Royal Society of Medicine Foundation Inc*

This project was supported in part by a grant, No. 90-A-777, from the Administration on Aging, Office of Human Development, Department of Health, Education and Welfare, Washington, D.C. 20201; and by a contract, No. 263-76-C0423, from the National Institute on Aging, National Institutes of Health, Bethesda, Maryland 20014.

Contents

Editors' Note: American spelling has been used in all the papers contributed by American members of the Conference, and English spelling in the papers from British speakers.

Index of Contributors

Introductory Remarks

Dr David A Hamburg

President, Institute of Medicine

Ladies and gentlemen, welcome to the National Academy of Sciences for the Anglo-American Conference on Care of the Elderly. This occasion is the culmination of almost a year of collaborative planning and preparation of the three sponsors; the Institute of Medicine, Royal Society of Medicine, and the Royal Society of Medicine Foundation. Coming as it does during the celebration of the American Bicentennial, I think it is particularly appropriate that we have joined together once again, belatedly, to explore an issue of vital concern to both the United States and the United Kingdom, and the concern for which there are no ready or easy solutions.

The Institute of Medicine, as a part of the National Academy of Sciences, was founded in 1970 for the express purpose of bringing together individuals renowned for exceptional contributions to health and medicine in order that they might confront the most difficult, even the intractable, problems in the health field. This confrontation with such tough issues as assessing the quality of medical care, determining the costs of education in the health professions, exploring the implications of increased regulation in the health care system, to name only a few, has evidenced a willingness to cut across the traditional boundaries that have so long and unwisely separated the professional groups.

The products of the Institute's work incorporate a diversity of views. There is no party line. These studies have striven for a consistently high quality. In this framework we are very pleased to join in the sponsorship of the present conference. I hope that all of us here today will engage with the significant issues presented and will participate actively, so that we can pool our information and ideas. Clearly, many of you here in the audience could just as well be on the program. There is a great pool of information and ideas on this subject present at the meeting. We are not here as partisans for any particular causes or interests, but rather as concerned individuals trying to reach a better understanding of the factors involved in the physical dependency of old people.

I will just take a moment or two to outline briefly the structure of the conference and to make some announcements. Today we will hear from a group of speakers who will define the nature and origin of physical and social dependency among the elderly by setting it in its biological and psychosocial context. Margot Jefferys and Robert Ball will initiate this examination by respectively describing the parameters of the problem in the United Kingdom and the United States. We will then hear papers dealing with changes in functional capacities associated with age. The afternoon session will consist of presentations about mental health problems of the elderly followed by a panel commentary.

We have scheduled two open discussion sessions, one just prior to the mid-day recess and the other immediately after the panel commentary this afternoon. During the discussion periods we hope you will take an active part. You may proceed to the microphones located along the aisles and stand there until recognized by the moderator. Please identify yourself. Since we would like to facilitate participation by all, I would ask you to try to formulate your questions in advance and to be as concise as you can about the points you wish to make or the questions you wish to raise.

Tomorrow the speakers and panelists on the program will describe and analyze various responses to the onset of dependence among the elderly. In the morning we will hear presentations on institutional care, community-based and home care, the integration of health and social services, and the role of the physician. Papers presented during the afternoon session will review recent research findings that bear on the appropriateness of different responses to problems of the elderly. We will then also consider various categories of manpower capable of delivering needed services.

On Wednesday we will turn to the implications for public policy and the options available for future action. This task is the most difficult one before us and a crucial task. It is one thing for us to recognize, describe or conduct research on a social problem; it is another to relate the outcomes of those activities to the realities of the environment in which public policy-makers must function. The two speakers on Wednesday, Congressman Conable and Sir George Godber, are particularly well suited by their experience and interests to consider policy options.

As we go along I hope it will be possible to distill from the papers presented those elements that are especially relevant to building future policies. Let us hope that these few days can truly make a useful contribution toward relieving one of the great social problems of our time.

I can't conclude these introductory remarks without expressing a deep sense of appreciation that I and the rest of us at the Institute of Medicine feel about the help we have had in preparing this undertaking. We are very grateful to the Administration on Aging within the Department of Health, Education and Welfare, the National Institute on Aging, and the Florence V Burden Foundation for the support they have provided for this conference. I would also like to take this opportunity to thank those members of the Institute of Medicine who played a vital role as advisors in preparation for the conference, especially Robert Ball, Ewald Busse, John Cassel, Carl Eisdorfer, Melvin Glasser, and Anne Somers. Michael Pollard and Jana Surdi of the IOM staff have done so much to make this meeting possible.

Finally, a very warm welcome to our guests from Britain who have much to teach us on this subject, and our gratitude to the members and staff of the Royal Society of Medicine who helped us prepare the meeting.

Now, it gives me great pleasure to introduce an old friend and distinguished Briton who has joined us here and who has helped us so much in the preparation of this meeting, Sir Gordon Wolstenholme, President of the Royal Society of Medicine.

Sir Gordon Wolstenholme

President, Royal Society of Medicine

Dr Hamburg, ladies and gentlemen. I would like to echo all the thanks that you have expressed to the many people who have contributed to the inception and the organization of this meeting. On behalf of the British here, I would like particularly to thank you, sir, and the Institute for acting as hosts on what we hope will be an auspicious occasion.

I hardly need to point out that for an individual to come here on his own initiative is nowadays a luxurious extravagance. But it is indeed a privilege for all of us from Britain to join in celebrating this birthday of so great a nation, and we do this with a sense that we have been here before.

It may be worth mentioning to the non-British members of this audience that the Royal Society of Medicine, under its first name of the Medical and Chirurgical Society of London, was created in 1805, but it was formed by a breakaway group from the Medical Society of London which was formed in 1773. There was a breakaway because they had a president who one year after he was elected to the presidency changed the rules so that he would be elected indefinitely thereafter, and he went on for 22 years until 26 very distinguished gentlemen, many of them well known in this part of the world, decided they had had enough and went elsewhere. This is not an unknown phenomenon in modern times.

The Royal Society of Medicine now has over 18 000 members. About one-quarter of these are in North America, in this country and in Canada, and there is a very substantial number of those who are members of the Medical Society of the District of Columbia. So, in one sense we are on our home ground.

Because of this international membership and because those of us here are not only doctors but also members of other professions which contribute to health services, we do feel that we are paying a tribute to America which is both international and from the whole range of our British health services.

I have a daughter whom, when she was about 6, I wanted to impress, and I pointed out a gentleman who was in the same room who was 100 years old. I failed; her reply was: "When will he be 200?" I think this is an occasion not only for looking back, but very much for looking forward. We are all aware in this hall what a great contribution has been made to the care of the elderly through many aspects of deep concern for our ever-increasing elderly population. But we also in this room are deeply aware that concern is not enough and that research into the facts on which we can more appropriately base that concern and care is now all-important.

I therefore look upon this meeting and this programme as a very considerable contribution to the future of the care of the elderly and a great stimulus to each of us personally. Once again, I would like to express on behalf of my British colleagues, which I hope they will permit me to do, our very warm thanks for being your guests on this occasion.

Statements of the Problem: United Kingdom and United States

The Elderly in the United Kingdom

Margot Jefferys
Department of Sociology,
Bedford College, University of London,
London NW1

I take my role in this seminar to be that of scene setting. I am here to draw attention to the main factors in present-day Britain which have influenced our approach to the care of the elderly. I shall also set out some of the reasons why we are not satisfied with our present provision and the general direction in which we think solutions should be sought. Subsequent speakers will deal in detail with particular aspects of the care of the elderly. I will not encroach on their ground. My data come, in the main, from the 1971 Census, from a General Household Survey conducted in 1972 by the Office of Population Censuses and Surveys, and from Annual Reports of the Department of Health and Social Security.

Who are the Elderly in Britain?

The process of aging is, by definition, a continuous one and one which, in physiological and psychological terms, is not identical in any two individuals. Nevertheless, the number of years an individual has lived has increasingly become a way of identifying a person as elderly or aged irrespective of his physical or mental state, as well as a means of legitimating his or her rights to various statutory benefits. Equally important, it is also a signal for employers legitimately to dispense with a person's services, and hence for a substantial and usually unwelcome change in the place he occupies in the economy. Instead of a current contributor to the gross national product (a role from which he derives some status), he is likely to become abruptly only a consumer of that product. Not everyone who is a consumer only is stigmatized in our society where the ownership of property attracts deference irrespective of contribution to the economy; but for most working people status derives from being a job holder rather than a pension drawer.

In Britain, for various historical reasons which are fascinating but too long to detail, the age at which men and women are entitled to draw retirement pensions in their own right differs by five years. Although they lived longer than men even at the beginning of this century, women were then presumed to be frailer than men. In 1924 when old age contributory (now retirement) pensions were introduced, women were allowed to draw them at 60 whereas men drew theirs at 65. Since then, the rationale for this sex discrimination has only once been seriously examined as far as I know (Committee on the Economic and Financial Problems of the Provision of Old Age 1954). Perhaps it survives today because women are not sure whether the discrimination is favourable or unfavourable to them. For every "objective" argument in its favour there are many against it.

Since 1924, then, 65 for men and 60 for women have become the ages used for a variety of social and economic administrative purposes and increasingly for medical ones too. While recognizing the arbitrariness of such criteria, I shall, when I consider the elderly, be talking primarily about the 65 and overs, although sometimes I shall take women of 60–64 into account as well simply because it is not always possible to exclude them from statistical data much of which relate to persons of pensionable age.

(*a*) *Numbers, Age and Sex*

In common with all industrial societies, Britain has seen a dramatic growth in the relative, as well as the absolute, numbers of individuals of advanced age in the course of the first three-quarters of the twentieth century. In 1901, there were one and a half million people aged 65 or more in a population of just over 37 million. In 1971 the respective figures were 7.1 million and 54 million. In percentage terms, the over 65s had increased threefold from 4.0% to 13.3%, while the population was not quite half as much again in the same period (DHSS 1974).

As I have implied, these figures are not unusual in western industrialized countries. They, like Britain, have experienced similar increases in their populations of advanced age as a result of a decrease in mortality in child and early adulthood and a consequent increase in life expectancy at birth. Britain's elderly population in relative terms, however, is greater than that of the United States today for three reasons (Shanas *et al.* 1968). First, the population of the latter was growing through the early years of the twentieth century through net immigration as well as by natural growth, the two growth rates being related to one another since immigrants are preponderantly young adults likely to contribute to the birth rate and hence to the numbers of young people. Second, the United States experienced a more pronounced "baby boom" in the years immediately following World War II than did Britain. Third, as a consequence of differences in Britain in the emigration rates of the two sexes and in their mortality rates during the 1914–18 war the reproductive rate for every female was less in Britain than in the USA. In short, differences in the late nineteenth and early twentieth century histories of our two countries and not those in our current health service provision, account in the main for the contemporary differences in the relative number of elderly people in our societies.

In common with other industrial societies the majority — roughly two out of every three of the over 65s and three out of four of the over 80s — are women (OPCS 1972). Life expectancy at birth has increased for both sexes over the past century and males now outnumber females in every age group from birth to 45. But after that male mortality rates greatly exceed female ones; women survivors at age 50 can expect to live to 78.4 years while men can only expect to reach 73.1. Even at 85 British women on average live one year longer (5.1) than their male contemporaries (DHSS 1974).

Disparities in the survival of the sexes are paralleled by disparities in their marital status. While nearly three-quarters (72.7%) of men aged 65 and more are married, this is true of only a little more than a third (35.9%) of the women. Women are more than twice as likely as men to be single (12.0% compared to 5.5%) and widowed, divorced or separated (52.1% and 21.9%) (DHSS 1974). I am, I think, correct in saying that Britain has more single women amongst its very elderly survivors than has the USA, due to the particularly drastic effect on the cohort now over 75 of the two factors already mentioned, namely differential sex migration in the early 1900s and the greater relative slaughter of British than of American young men in the 1914–18 war.

The population projectionists forecast a continued growth in the British population aged 65 and over, but at a diminishing rate (Government Actuaries Department 1975). If their predictions are correct (and they are better for obvious reasons in forecasting total numbers of elderly in the next three decades than they are the total numbers of new born), the total numbers in the age bracket 65–74 will only increase slightly between 1971 and 1991 (i.e. by less than 1%), but there will be an increase of over a third in the numbers aged 75–84 and of nearly a half (46.24%) in those aged 85 and over. Moreover, if there is any reduction in the mortality rate of middle-aged men — and there is ample room for such an improvement — the increase will be even greater.

So much then for some bare facts about the elderly. It is the rapidly increasing numbers of the very old in our society, at a time when the rate of growth in the economy has slowed down together with our apparent willingness as a society to transfer more of our total national resources from one segment of the population (basically the higher income earners) to another (basically the non-earners) through the mechanism of fiscal policy, which lies behind the increasing pessimism, if not panic, of those who want the old generally to be able to live secure, tranquil and dignified lives. To many the current problems seem bleak, the future still bleaker.

What evidence do we have about the quality of life of our elderly people today? Are there many who live in conditions which as one of the rich nations of the world we should not tolerate? In so far as there are too many in preventable conditions of squalor, loneliness, psychic or physical pain, why are they not prevented? These are questions to which I now want to turn, inevitably selectively.

The Conditions of the Elderly in Britain Today

Critical to an appraisal of the conditions of any group of people is knowledge of their housing conditions, i.e. where and how they are accommodated. In the popular imagination a high proportion of the elderly population in Britain lives in hospitals or residential institutions. In practice, however, 95 out of every 100 people of pensionable age in Britain in 1971 lived in private households (OPCS 1974*a*). Less than 3% lived in hospitals and less than 3% in residential homes or hotels.

Nevertheless, 5% represents not far short of half a million individuals (442 355) of whom slightly more than a third were in local authority or voluntary association homes for the elderly, slightly less than a third in non-psychiatric hospitals, a sixth in psychiatric hospitals and the remainder in hotels or private residential establishments.

(*a*) *The Elderly in Hospitals*

We have good reason to believe that there are few people of any age or social class who would choose voluntarily to live in an institutional setting in preference to a household alone or with their kith and kin. It is true that we tend to generalize pejoratively about institutions. We impute to them certain Goffmanesque characteristics (Goffman 1961) and with some justification. The inmates of our asylums, whether they are children or adults, enjoy little independence of action. Their activities are monitored and restricted by others. In Victorian England the asylums used to house the poor, whether sick, aged or able-bodied, were not intended to be pleasant places; they were cold and bleak (emotionally as well as physically) because a prevailing belief of the upright, industrious middle class was that that was the appropriate way to discourage idleness and prevent pauperism. Unfortunately many of the buildings which the Victorians erected to house the sick-poor and the mad are still in use today as psychiatric or long-stay geriatric hospitals. It is true that many of the old workhouses have now been demolished. Few of the residential homes administered by local authorities or voluntary associations for the elderly who are frail but do not require regular nursing now house more than 100: they are more likely to have from 20 to 50 places in them (DHSS 1975*a*).

However, there are still many grim forbidding structures in the hospital sector. They have proved difficult to modernize and as a nation we have not felt able or willing to give the necessary priority in the use of limited resources to their replacement. I am sure they contribute to the depressing image of geriatric care which is apparently shared by many members of the caring professions as well as by the general public including the elderly. A further tragedy is that not all of those who live permanently in these prison-like buildings require skilled nursing or medical care. They are there either because they lack the social competence or the will to live independently outside or because suitable "sheltered housing" or a place in a local authority or voluntary association's residential home is not available to them.

We have real cause for concern about the general quality of life of the elderly who live out their days in many geriatric and psychiatric hospitals. Several independent enquiries (South East Thames Regional Health Authority 1976) following allegations of cruelty or neglect made by a small number of nursing staff and patients' relatives have substantiated the accusations. They have shown that the physical and psychosocial environments of many patients are harsh and humiliating. Nursing staff, apathetic or demoralized, lacking guidance from physicians and administrators have sometimes taken to persecuting those in their charge. Lay members of health authorities have too readily been brushed aside and satisfied by somewhat complacent statements from doctors and administrators, aware of the difficulties under which their staffs labour and perhaps sharing with the latter the view that work with the elderly is "nonrewarding".

Nationally, and in particular since 1960, we have agreed that our first objective should be to reduce the number of individuals who live permanently in institutions of all kinds and particularly in hospitals. To this end the stated objective has been "community care", and there are some successes to record as others contributing to this symposium will indicate. At the same time we have committed ourselves at least in principle to trying to improve the conditions of those who will have to remain in long-term hospital settings. The Hospital Advisory Service, set up in 1969, to listen, observe and advise the care givers at all levels has undoubtedly helped to improve conditions for patients and staff;

and some of the limited new money available annually to the hospital sector has gone to replacing sub-standard provision.

We have to face it, however, that improving significantly the quality of life for elderly patients who through mental or physical infirmity and social circumstances need nursing and constant surveillance which cannot be provided in their own homes is likely to prove one of the most difficult of our objectives to achieve. In my view we have made relatively little progress since the heady, optimistic days of the 1950s when we thought our greater enlightenment would quickly eliminate custodial and authoritarian methods of dealing with the aged sick. Subsequent experience has indicated that we were over-optimistic, that there was more obduracy in the situation than we had anticipated. Things have had a way of reverting back to older established practices when a charismatic innovator moves on or loses his initial enthusiasm and energy (Brown 1973).

(*b*) *The Elderly in Residential Homes*

The situation in residential homes run by local authorities and voluntary associations is I believe better than that in our long-stay hospitals. The wind of change has blown through many of them with good effect since Peter Townsend's study, "The Last Refuge", published in 1962. The National Corporation for the Care of Old People, a voluntary body, has done much to encourage research, experiment and innovation in both voluntary and statutory homes and to educate through the dissemination of practical information. Physical amenities have been improved. The multiple-bedded dormitory, if not entirely a thing of the past, is much less in evidence today. More emphasis is given to the suitability of staff who work in the homes and attention is increasingly paid to their education. The homes are encouraged to open themselves to the surrounding community.

One of the major problems which we have not solved arises through the uneven distribution of homes throughout the country, a distribution which bears little relationship to the geographical distribution of the elderly in need of the minimal surveillance provided by most homes. The legacy of past benefactors and municipal provision is a poor guide to present needs. In some areas residential provision meets all locally generated needs and has surplus accommodation to offer. In others there is a dire shortage. This can raise real problems when, ideally, most elderly people want to remain in frequent contact with their younger kith and kin.

Another frequent problem for elderly people in residential homes is a lack of security. Such has been the shortage of places that many local authorities and voluntary organizations have felt compelled to let someone else have the place made vacant when an elderly person has had to be admitted to hospital for prolonged treatment following, for example, a stroke or a fractured femur. The knowledge that they have no place to which, by right, they can return can hardly reduce anxiety or speed recovery; it may also be a cause of anticipatory concern and as such mar or prevent a full adjustment to life in a residential institution after the independence of one's own home. This problem will remain with us as long as accommodation in hospitals and homes falls far short of the demand for it. Indeed, it is likely to grow with the parallel growth in the proportion of those occupying residential homes who are very old and very frail.

(*c*) *The Elderly in Their Own Homes*

Now how about the 95% of elderly people who live in private households? What do we know about the quality of their lives?

Just under half the people of pensionable age live with one other person — usually their spouse; a quarter are in households of three or more people, including most frequently someone of working age; a quarter, and the proportion increases with increasing age, live alone (OPCS 1974*a*).

Those who live alone are the most likely to lack modern domestic facilities. For example, nearly one in five (19.2%) of those of pensionable age living alone have no inside toilet and nearly the same proportion no fixed bath. One in six have no tapped hot water supply. Such figures reflect not only the fact that the elderly are more likely to live in remote rural areas: they are also more likely to live in the decaying centres of cities.

In Britain as a whole rather over half of all the units of accommodation inhabited by private households is owner occupied. A third is rented from local authorities and most of the remainder from private landlords. The elderly are slightly less likely to be owner occupiers (45%) and a good deal less likely to be local authority tenants (20%). They are thus more dependent on private landlords who own the least satisfactory as well as the most luxurious property. It is in the former rather than the latter that the elderly are likely to be housed. Indeed, both because they have had much less priority in rehousing than have young couples with children and because they are often reluctant to move away from the house or district in which they have lived for years, they are often the last denizens of slum clearance areas in the twilight zones of city centres. It was estimated in 1972 that the median length of housing residence was 6 to 10 years; but for those aged 65–79 the median was between 11–20, and for those over 80 it was 21–30 years (OPCS 1975).

In Britain we are prone to think that if we were able to improve the standard of housing for elderly people many of the problems which they face in maintaining their social independence, their capacity to cope and their morale, would be solved. The difficulty of coping with the activities of daily living in inconvenient, insanitary and hypothermia-inducing surroundings is often the straw which breaks the camel's back and induces the elderly or their relatives to seek residential accommodation or deters the latter from welcoming back to the community an elderly person who has been admitted to hospital with an acute episode of pneumonia or a fractured neck of the femur. The single greatest housing need is for more purpose-built sheltered accommodation, where the elderly alone or in couples can continue to look after themselves in comfortable, functionally appropriate surroundings, secure in the knowledge that if they fall sick or have an accident someone will come quickly to their rescue. Here we have made only little progress and it would be unrealistic to think that our current economic circumstances will allow us to make many inroads into the backlog of deferred rehousing schemes for the elderly, let alone meet the increasing demand occasioned by the increasing numbers of elderly people.

(*d*) *Employment and Income*

In 1972, only one in seven of those of pensionable age was economically active, a reflection of the dramatic effect which reaching pensionable age has on employment status among men and unmarried women (OPCS 1975). It is probable, however, that these figures underestimate considerably the numbers who continue to earn, perhaps erratically, in part-time, casual employment. A man or woman over pensionable age but not yet 70 is not entitled to draw his full state pension if he or she earns more than a token sum weekly; it is thus possible that some informants may wish to conceal from interviewers employed by a government agency the fact that they are working.

This General Household Survey had another interesting finding to report. It found that the over 65s who worked expressed much greater satisfaction with their work than did younger workers, and were less likely to take time off work for either sickness or personal reasons. This is support, if support is needed, for the existence of a negative association between work satisfaction and work absence even if it does not tell us whether liking for work is the causative element in the association or whether we need to search back to the factors which have induced a liking for work, among which may be such attributes as psychic and physical energy. These in themselves may be determinants of who continues to work in their seventh and eighth decades when there are so many pressures to retire.

I do not need to point out, especially to the present audience, that retirement is for many people not the peaceful, welcome retreat to pleasant pastures from the hurly-burly of unmitigated toil. Work provides most people with a source of legitimate income and hence with self-respect. For many it also provides companionship, supportive routinized rituals and intrinsic interest or challenge. At one time shortly after the war when we were able to offer employment to all who wanted work, it looked as though we might be able to smooth out the sudden transition from full-time work to total economic inactivity through part-time employment. Now when the labour market is no longer able to absorb men and women of working age (and the numbers of the latter seeking work are increasing dramatically), the prospect for the elderly and the handicapped of all ages in inevitably bleaker. It would be a brave person who would predict any radical increase in remunerative employment for the elderly in Britain in the next decade. We can, however, hope for an increase in the proportion of elderly people engaged in purposeful voluntary activities of many kinds.

The median income of the elderly is considerably less than that of younger persons. In 1972, for example, the OPCS calculated that the median income of a person aged 65 and over living alone was between £7.50 and £10.00 per week (OPCS 1975). For a person aged 65 or more living with one other person it was more — between £12.50 and £15.00. But these compared with the national median income per head of between £20.00 and £25.00. The main reason for the lower income of the elderly is, of course, the dependency of most of them on state-supported retirement benefits. Incidentally a fifth of all those with retirement pensions also obtained regularly a means-tested supplementary pension (DHSS 1975*b*). Indeed it is clear that the contributory retirement pension, despite a greater improvement in its real value over the past 25 years (roughly it doubled) compared with that of the average gross earnings of manual workers (which increased by roughly three-quarters), was not great enough to ensure even a minimally acceptable standard of living.

Once again, many of us have been convinced by the evidence of several nationally and locally conducted surveys (Townsend and Wedderburn 1965) that the bare subsistence income of many of the elderly is a substantial contributory factor to their poor health. Low incomes contribute particularly to poor nutritional standards; they have also been a factor in deaths from hypothermia — a particular hazard for the very poor at a time of soaring costs for house warming. Our method of trying to counteract the effects of low income — by categorical means-tested allowances of various kinds — is a clumsy one, administratively expensive and often ineffective because it stigmatizes or is too dependent on self-referral. Yet while we, as a nation, are unwilling to allow the state to transfer a larger part of our national income to the aged in the form of social security benefits as of right, we are forced to adopt unsatisfactory, inefficient and piecemeal devices to salve our consciences.

(*e*) *Health of the Elderly — Subjective and Objective Measures*

This is not the place for a discourse on the legitimacy of various ways of measuring the health of a population. By most measures which I presume we would all accept as related to health, however idiosyncratic our own definition of that concept may be, the elderly are less well than the young. Let me take a selection of the available recent statistics for illustrative purposes.

In the General Household Survey (OPCS 1975) 20% of all the adult informants reported a long-standing illness or disability; but among those aged 65–74 the proportion was 48% and in the 75 and over age group 62%. In an earlier study Harris found that nearly two-thirds of the impaired were over 65 while the age group itself only constituted 12% of the population (Harris 1971). The severely handicapped were even more concentrated in this age group; 85% of bedfast or chairbound people were found to be over 65. Even so, we need to keep a sense of proportion. Less than a quarter (23.8%) of the impaired over 75 were rated on certain objective measures of coping ability as very severely or severely handicapped (Harris 1971). Put in another way, only a little more than a third of the over 65s who lived in private households (OPCS 1975) regarded themselves as restricted or limited in what they could do compared with others of their age.

The measures I have discussed so far are based mainly on self-assessment and relate primarily to physical disorders. They are confirmed, however, by certain other measures which are sometimes wrongly presumed to be "harder", that is, more reliable. If we assume that hospitalization and general practice consultation rates are related to sickness experience, even while recognizing that the relationship can be and is distorted by many other factors, the over 75s constitute 10% of all hospital discharges and deaths in a year while they are less than 5% of the population (4.7%). The women in the group occupy nearly a third of all the occupied female beds because their mean duration of stay (at 50.7 days compared with 14.3 for women of all age groups) is long (DHSS and OPCS 1974).

Not unexpectedly, 70% of the beds allocated to geriatric departments of district general and long-stay hospitals are occupied by men and women of 75 or more. In addition, 50% of the beds in general practitioner units on any given day are occupied by the over 75s and if the age group 65 and over is included the figure reaches 73%. Even more startling perhaps is the fact that the over 65s occupy nearly half the general medicals beds (49%), 42% of those in chest units, 40% of those in urology and in radiotherapy, 39% in dermatology, 37% in general surgery and in orthopaedic surgery and 31% in rheumatology. (These figures exclude maternity and psychiatric beds in general as well as special hospitals) (DHSS and OPCS 1974).

Yet another source of information indicates that the over 65s and particularly the over 75s are much more likely to use general practitioner services than younger people (OPCS 1974*b*). While a third of the over 65s did not consult their general practitioners at all over the year, the average number of consultations of women aged 75 and over was 4.46 compared with 3.43 for women of all ages. The disparity for men was even greater, 4.51 for the over 75s compared with 2.56 for men of all ages. Moreover, nearly two-thirds (64.4%) of the general practitioner consultations with women over 75 took place in the patients' homes compared with about one in six for women patients of all ages.

Turning to measures of mental illness, the picture of the concentration of ill health among the elderly is also there, but with a difference. Women of 65 and over at any one time occupy 62% of all the beds for female patients in psychiatric hospitals and men of the same age 39% of the beds for their sex. On the other hand people of this age are not very much more likely than younger people to consult their general practitioner for mental disorder (OPCS 1974*b*). It would seem that either mental illness, when it occurs, takes a more serious form among the elderly and particularly amongst women than it does among younger age groups or that, when it occurs amongst the elderly, it is more difficult for others to tolerate in a community setting. I suspect that both explanations are right but that we have not done the studies which would allow us to assess the relative contribution of both to the greater tendency to hospitalize the very old than the young.

There is one statistic, however, which suggests that some progress may have been made in the last decade towards reducing the amount of hospitalization of elderly folk with mental disorder. First admission rates for the age group 75 and over fell by a quarter between 1964 and 1972 and for the 65–74s by a third (DHSS 1974). We do not know for certain what this is due to. What Dr Arie has to say later may indicate that it is cooperation between the psychogeriatric service, the general practitioner, the social service department and the family which achieves this kind of containment and prevents the hospitalization which we all know can in itself often exacerbate the mental distress and disturbance which first occasioned the request for hospitalization.

Services for the Care of the Elderly: Present and Future

This inevitably partial and selective review of the conditions of the elderly in Britain today has indicated that this age group includes more seriously disadvantaged people than does any other. Two questions must now be asked. First, are the resources which we currently devote to the care of the elderly, and this includes the resources they already possess without state intervention as well as those we deliberately transfer to them from other sections of the community, sufficient to achieve the levels of physical, mental and social well-being which we believe are technically feasible? Second, are we using the resources we do devote to them in the most effective way?

Of course these questions are to a degree rhetorical. I feel sure none of the British contingent at this seminar would answer either of them in the affirmative, although some might feel that the resources are so meagre that their time and that of all those who care for elderly people should be primarily devoted to the essentially *political* task of obtaining a larger share of the cake for geriatrics, while others might concentrate on advocating the need to use existing resources in a more effective way. I posed the questions, however, in order to consider what would be involved in extorting more resources for the care of the elderly from the rest of the community, and in re-allocating existing resources to better effect.

With the major exception of social security benefits the elderly were not until recently formally distinguished administratively from younger people in terms of securing their access to and use of health and social services. It is a moot point whether they would have a larger share of scarce resources if they were. Like everyone else in Britain the elderly still have no conditions to fulfil other than residence in the country to be accepted on a general practitioner's list for free advice and service and the same is true of admission to hospital as an in-patient, day patient or out-patient. Like other citizens they may apply for a chiropodist, home nurse, or home help, or for a health visitor or social worker visit. If they are disabled or chronically sick they, like younger people, may apply for free or subsidized meals-on-wheels or help with house alterations or with the installation of such amenities as a radio, television or telephone, and they will be subjected to the same means test. In practice nearly all the services I have mentioned are used much more frequently by the old than by the young, but still perhaps not with great enough frequency either because the old are too proud or too ignorant to apply or because the facilities are in short supply.

However, in recent years a number of distinctions have been made between the elderly and the rest of the community with a view to securing or increasing the former's share of resources. For example, someone of pensionable age is able to obtain doctor-prescribed drugs and appliances free without means test while the rest of the community pays a small sum towards their cost. The general practitioner is also encouraged to take or keep elderly patients, who use more of his time especially on home visits, by paying him a larger per capita sum for each person of 65 or over. It does not follow, of course, that he uses the extra money for increased services to the elderly since it is not given on a fee for service basis; but figures already given indicate that the general practitioner at least sees the elderly more frequently. We can say little about the quality of his services or indeed the services provided by others in meeting the medical needs of any age group.

Other forms of distinction are also emerging in many areas which do not have the sanction of national legislation. For example, most of the metropolitan areas provide free or subsidized passes for pensioners on their public transport outside rush hours. Many provide day centres or luncheon clubs which are almost exclusively used by the elderly.

Perhaps the most important development of all, however, has been the development within the National Health Service of the specialty of geriatric medicine and the growth of departments around the consultants and junior medical staff. This has been accompanied by the formation of a professional society, membership of which is restricted to medically qualified people working in geriatrics and, with the encouragement of this society and a voluntary funding agency, of a new research body, the British Council for Ageing.

This development has not taken place without controversy. We can ignore that part of the opposition which appears to flow from fear of the new specialty's threat to its own income and prestige: but those in and outside medicine who argue that the split between the general physician and the geriatric physician can result in a deleterious labelling of the old and their increasing isolation in the least salubrious facilities have clearly a *bona fides* point of view. If those with most prestige in the hospital can restrict the use of their wards to the young, acutely ill on the grounds that elderly people are the geriatric department's responsibility, the elderly may well suffer by being given low priority in the use of resources from which they could benefit. On the other hand, it can be argued that general physicians have often failed to study the psycho-social as well as the physical aspects of ageing to the detriment of the elderly who will benefit from the growth of a specialty concerned particularly with them. As someone fast approaching pensionable age I can see the force of both arguments. I feel that the label "geriatric" is somehow derogatory and I wish to postpone the time when it is applied to me. On the other hand, I want in my old age if I need medical and social care to be treated by those who will allow me to maintain my dignity and will not imply that I am blocking a bed which could be better occupied by a young person presenting a really worth-while medical challenge. If geriatric departments succeed in obtaining more of the limited resources available to the hospital sector, and if they are able to train and instil enthusiasm into a growing proportion of our young doctors and nurses, then the outlook for me and my generation of oldies may be better than that of the present 80-year-olds.

It could be further argued that it is the elderly with the likelihood of a multiplicity of social as well as medical needs who are most likely to be the victims of the administrative division of responsibility between health authority and local authority. A combined health and welfare service for elderly people alone, responsible for supplying the full range of their hospital, residential and domiciliary health and social care needs, might be the most logical step to take in securing a larger share of scarce resources for the elderly, but it would conflict with current social work wisdom which holds that services should be delivered by generically trained non-specialized workers on a family basis. Furthermore, the recent reorganization of both our health services' administrative structures and our local government boundaries appears to have done little so far to coordinate or improve services for the elderly. It is perhaps unfair, however, to judge those concerned with the services at present since their energies have been largely consumed in setting up the organization and its planning and monitoring machinery; and this at a time of national stringency, which has exacerbated latent conflict between the Government and sections of the medical profession, itself deeply divided on many issues.

This brings me to what must be my final point. The services which any of us receive from others reflect to a great extent our value in their eyes. The rich and the powerful may or may not be liked by those who serve them; but their riches and their power are likely to earn them a consideration that few of us show to those who lack these assets. (Some of course are powerful by virtue of their personal attractiveness rather than their possessions, which can include past reputation as well as current material wealth.)

In short, the services which those who have riches in the form of material wealth, a revered reputation or a lovable nature now receive in their old age are I believe considerable and on the whole satisfactory. Most such people live graciously and contentedly outside institutions. As their biologically determined dependency increases they are usually cared for by relatives, neighbours and friends, a general practitioner, perhaps a district nurse and a home help. Their eccentricities are tolerated and their wisdom valued. Only if they lose their wealth or their lovability — and possibly their families and their sphincter control — will they be accorded less value and the quality of the service they receive deteriorate.

But many of those who become old are poor in material possessions and lacking in personal attractiveness. They are not valued greatly by the rest of us and in this respect the attitude of professional carers is little different from that of society at large.

If I am right in this very general and possibly tendentious proposition it would seem to argue that we will not materially improve our services to the elderly unless we change the value we attach to the old. They are not valued in general it seems to me unless they are wealthy or attractive. It is because the old are so often pauperized by forced retirement and subsistence level pensions that old age itself becomes a devalued state. It is my belief, therefore, that if as a society we were able to even out the distribution of resources so as to ensure that a reasonable level of income and wealth is possessed by all, those reaching an age where they might well wish to retire, perhaps 10 years or so beyond the present statutory minimum pensionable age, would not be begrudged the resources spent on them.

I would like the lead to come from the care givers. Indeed in some ways the caring professions have not been giving sufficient of a lead. Boldness and enthusiasm, even aggression, may be the characteristics which we most need in the care providers, as well as tender loving care, if we are materially to improve the services for the elderly. We have a long haul in front of us — a tremendous task of understanding and changing those things about ourselves which prevent us from providing the elderly with services to which they are entitled and which our society is rich enough to give them.

References

Brown, G. W. (1973). *Social Science and Medicine* **7**, 407–424

Committee on the Economic and Financial Problems of the Provision of Old Age (1954). "Old Age" (Phillips Committee). Cmd. 9333. HMSO, London

Department of Health and Social Security (DHSS) (1974). "Health and Personal Social Services Statistics for England." HMSO, London. (1975*a*). "Census of Residential Accommodation 1970." HMSO, London. (1975*b*), "Annual Report for 1974." HMSO, London

Department of Health and Social Security (DHSS) and Office of Population Censuses and Surveys (OPCS) (1974). "Report on Hospital In-Patient Enquiry for the year 1972." HMSO, London

Goffman, E. (1961). "Asylums". Anchor Books, New York

Government Actuary's Department (1975). "Population Projection for the United Kingdom." HMSO, London

Harris, A. I. (1971). "Handicapped and Impaired in Great Britain", Vol. 1. HMSO, London

Office of Population Censuses and Surveys (OPCS) (1972). "Census 1971: Preliminary Age and Sex Tables for Great Britain." HMSO, London. (1974*a*). "Census 1971 for Great Britain: Persons of Pensionable Age." HMSO, London. (1974*b*). "Morbidity Statistics from General Practice in 1972." HMSO, London. (1975). "General Household Survey for 1972." HMSO, London

South East Thames Regional Health Authority (1976). "Report of a Committee of Inquiry into St Augustine's Hospital, Chartham, Canterbury." Limited mimeo edition, Croydon

Shanas, E., Townsend, P., Wedderburn, D., Friis, H., Milhoj, P. and Stenhouwer, J. (1968). "Old People in Three Industrial Societies". Routledge and Kegan Paul, London; Atherton Press, New York

Townsend, P. (1962). "The Last Refuge." Routledge and Kegan Paul, London

Townsend, P. and Wedderburn, D. (1965). "The Aged in the Welfare State". Bell, London

United States Policy toward the Elderly

Robert M Ball
Senior Scholar, Institute of Medicine

Introduction

This conference will be concerned primarily with the care of those among the elderly who have such physical or mental limitations that they need help from family, friends, or social agencies to perform the ordinary tasks of daily living. Out of a population of 23 million persons over 65 in the United States today, they number between 3 and 4 million. About 1.2 million, 5% of the population 65 and over, are in long-term care institutions, with over 1 million in that unique American institution, the nursing home.[1]

The number who have such a limitation and who are living in their own homes or with relatives is more difficult to determine, but the approximate size of the group is clear. In the Health Survey for 1973, 9% of the persons 65 and over and not living in institutions classified themselves as in poor health as compared to others of the same age. Adding those self-classified as in poor health to those in institutions gives us 14%, or 3.2 million when applied to the population 65 and over today. If instead of this approach, we add to the 5% in institutions the 5.2% of the non-institutionalized persons over 65 who in 1972 were bedfast or homebound, and the 6.7% who could not leave the house without help, we get 16,9%, or 3.9 million of the population

[1] Except as otherwise noted, the data in this paper are from "Health, United States 1975," National Center for Health Statistics, DHEW Publication No. (HRA) 76-1232, and "Social and Economic Characteristics of the Older Population, 1974," Bureau of the Census, "Current Population Reports, Special Studies," Series P-23, No. 57.

over 65 today. A range of 14 to 17% as the proportion of the elderly who need help to perform the tasks of daily living is slightly larger but generally consistent with other estimates based on earlier surveys.[2] We cannot, of course, be precise. A few people in long-term care institutions may not need the degree of help specified and some not in institutions may be incorrectly classified. However, it seems plausible that the size of the group of primary concern to this conference is from 3 to 4 million persons, 14 to 17% of the 23 million people 65 or over in the United States today.

Federal Policy

For good or ill, the policies of the federal government toward the elderly have been focused primarily on making life better for the 19–20 million elderly who are not — at least not yet — in the unfortunate position of the other 3 to 4 million. US policy for the elderly has been primarily an income policy. Our emphasis has been on retirement, widows' and widowers' benefits under a nearly universal social security system (9 out of 10 jobs are covered under social security), the establishment of a federal minimum income floor for all the elderly under Supplemental Security Income, the promotion of private pension plan supplementation to social security through tax incentives, and the establishment of quite generous career pensions for the military and employees of government at all jurisdictional levels.

Even our national health insurance plan for the elderly and disabled, Medicare, conceptually has been an extension of retirement insurance, protecting the retiree against the cost of episodic illness on the rationale that such costs are unbudgetable and cannot reasonably be met by a regular monthly pension. The Medicare plan has not been designed to cover the cost of long-term care for the chronically ill. Its coverage of nursing home care is only for post-hospitalization for the same condition as treated in the hospital, and lasts for only 20 days without copayments and an additional 80 days with copayments. Medicare is the primary source of payment for only about 1% of the nursing home residents who have been in a home for more than 30 days. We have chosen to finance long-term nursing home care on a means-tested basis, through the state-operated, but partly federally financed, programs of Medicaid and public assistance. Together, these programs are the primary source of financing for 60% of the nursing home residents who have been in a home for more than 30 days. In almost all other such long-term cases, the patient or his family are the primary source of financing.

[2] See the discussion in "Reflections on the Sick Aged and the Helping System," Odin W. Anderson, prepared for the Conference on Social Policy, Social Ethics, and the Aging Society, May 30–June 1, 1975, to be published by the Committee on Human Development, University of Chicago.

In the design of Medicare, there are two exceptions to its orientation toward episodes of acute illness: physicians' services are paid for wherever performed, in a nursing home or other long-term facility, as well as elsewhere, and perhaps most importantly for the future, Medicare fostered the development of the home health agency and is the major source of support for such agencies today.

These two exceptions have worked to the very considerable benefit of the chronically ill. Most nursing home patients, thanks to Medicare and Medicaid, are visited frequently by physicians. According to the Nursing Home Survey of 1973–74, three-fourths of the nursing home patients had been visited by a physician within 2 months of the survey, 60% within a month, even though of those who had been in the home for a year or more 9% had not been examined by a physician for at least a year prior to the survey.

The number of home health agencies approved for reimbursement under Medicare has increased greatly from the beginning of the program in 1966, going from 1275 and 2311 in 1970. Since 1970, the number has stayed about the same, with some 2200 approved today. Of the 2200, 1270 are operated by state and local health agencies, 541 are private, voluntary visiting nurse services, 244 are hospital based, and 187 have a variety of sponsorship. All of the agencies provide nursing care, 1600 provide physical therapy, 1500 home health aid services, 480 occupational therapy, 682 speech therapy, and 518 medical social services.

It needs to be remembered that these agencies are *medical* agencies. The services are prescribed by doctors, and if all a person needs is help with household tasks, or shopping, or home repairs, or transportation, Medicare does not pay the bill. Thus, even in the major area where Medicare has supported efforts to keep the chronically ill at home and avoid institutionalization, it is limited by being a medical program, when what is needed is an integrated medical and social agency. Yet this can be changed. We do have this one nationally financed program of services for the elderly in their own homes, and there is no logical reason why we cannot add a variety of social services for inclusion in federal reimbursement, starting perhaps with homemaker services.

But, as I said, the home health agency is something of an exception from the general emphasis in Medicare. The primary object of Medicare is to protect the elderly and disabled against the cost of short-term hospital stays and other costs associated with episodic illness, not to pay for long-term care or support services for the chronically ill in their own homes.

Although not designed primarily for the 3 to 4 million elderly people who are the focus of this conference, income provisions and the

Medicare program are of great importance to them as well as to the 19–20 million elderly who can live independently. An adequate pension and a general health insurance program like Medicare, while not enough to meet the special needs of the chronically ill, will make it much easier for us to build special programs for the chronically ill in the future, particularly programs designed as an alternative to institutional living. So in spite of the emphasis of this conference on the special needs of the chronically ill, it is perhaps reasonable first, as general background, to address US income policy toward the elderly. Here we can be quite optimistic.

Income Programs for the Elderly

The income programs of the federal government for the retired elderly are being increasingly successful. One may say with considerable confidence that for those retiring in the future the great majority will have reasonably adequate incomes measured against their level of living while working, *as long as they do not require the special services needed by the very old and those with severe chronic disabilities.*

The percentage of the elderly population below the government-defined, rock-bottom, low-income level has been more than cut in half in just 15 years, from 35% in 1959 to 16% in 1974. And the mechanism now exists at the federal level to reduce that 16% to zero. All we have to do is raise the income standards of the Supplemental Security Income program to the poverty level, and poverty among the elderly would be abolished, at least statistically. State supplementation would still be required where living costs were above average and to cover emergencies, or where a state wished to guarantee a level of living above the bare-bones standard. It would cost from $3 billion to $3.5 billion a year — not at all a staggering amount as we return to a full-employment economy — to raise the standard to the poverty level for both the elderly and the disabled. Over time, very gradually, the proportion of persons needing Supplemental Security Income under the improved standards should decline as social security is improved.

But the arrangements that we have created to provide the elderly with a secure income go considerably beyond the goal of the abolition of poverty. Income security, after all, is not a matter for most people of having enough to meet a budgetary minimum defined in subsistence terms. Security for most means having an income which makes it possible for the individual to maintain a level of living near that attained while working. The wage replacement ratio needed to accomplish this objective will differ among retirees. Some differences between the money income needs of retired people and workers are nearly universal: for example, differences in tax treatment, the absence of expenses of working, and the ability to partly substitute one's own labor for purchased goods and services. Other differences exist for a high proportion of the elderly, but are not universal: for example, lower housing costs because of home ownership (77% of elderly couples own their own homes, 80% mortgage free), fewer people in a family dependent on retirement income than on the previous work income, and a decreased need to buy home furnishings and durable consumer goods. Other differences exist only for a minority of the retired elderly, and are, therefore, not useful in helping to determine a reasonable ratio of retired income to previous earnings. For example, for the large majority who have very little, if anything, in the way of earnings, it is not significant that 10% or so of elderly people work regularly and have substantial earnings. Taking the proper items into account, it is likely that, for most people, retirement income of from two-thirds to three-fourths of previous gross income will produce for the elderly who are in good health an ability to live independently at a level roughly comparable to what they had attained while working. Of course, the benefits then must be kept up to date at least with the cost of living, as now provided by social security and most government career plans, but not pension plans in private industry.

I don't believe the country as whole is yet fully aware of how far we have advanced toward this goal for those now retiring and those who will retire in the future. Because social security benefits are inadequate for so many people now receiving them, and because for so long the amounts payable have been so low, it is no wonder that the public generally has not yet caught up with the fact that for those who retire in the future, social security will be a much more nearly adequate program than it is for those now drawing benefits.

The ratio of social security benefits to previous earnings will more than anything else determine the income security of older people. Even in the long run, probably 40% of retired persons over 65 will be dependent on social security alone for a regular retirement income. About 10% will find that social security is not enough and will need help in addition from the needs-tested Supplemental Security Income program. Another 45% will be getting both social security and retirement protection through either private pensions or government career plans. Perhaps 5%, under present policy, will get only a government career pension.

Since private pensions and government career pensions are more likely to supplement the social security benefits of higher-paid workers than of those with average wages and below, it is particularly important that social security alone be adequate to maintain at least previous levels of living for those earning low wages. For married workers who work regularly under social security and work until age 65, the present formula now achieves this goal for both the low-wage earner and the worker who earns the median wage for men. For those workers retiring at age 65 next month who have been earning the federal minimum wage, a husband and wife will get about 90% of the earnings in the year before retirement and the single worker something over 60% of the earnings in the year before retirement. The dollar figures are about $3900 and $2600 a year.

For a husband and wife, with the worker earning the median wage for male workers, benefits will be about two-thirds of the earnings in the year before retirement; for the single worker, 45% of earnings in the year before retirement. The dollar figures are about $5700 and $3800 a year.

At maximum earnings, the dollar figures are about $7000 a year for the couple and $4600 a year for the single worker, with the couple getting almost 50%, and the single worker about 33% of earnings in the year before retirement. But it should be remembered that a high proportion of those earning above the median wage will have supplementary retirement protection and that in total their retirement pay, too, will approach the two-thirds to three-fourths level for a couple.

Most importantly, the 1972 amendments provided for keeping social security protection up to date with wages and prices.

Now, the future for the retired aged is not quite as good as this sounds. More than half the retirees claim benefits before age 65, and thus get actuarially reduced benefits which, for those retiring at the earliest possible age of 62 are 20% lower than the figures given. And, if workers are out of a job, or for any reasons are not covered under social security for a total of more than 5 years during their working career, their benefits will also be less than indicated. But all in all, the retirement income position of the elderly in the future, certainly as compared with the past, looks encouraging. The biggest remaining need is for improved benefits for the single worker, particularly single women workers, and for widows.

In the last 10 years we have also greatly improved protection for the elderly against medical bills. Although we may be correctly concerned with how much Medicare has cost, from the standpoint of the elderly it has done a good job in meeting a very high proportion of the cost of short-term care in general hospitals, for after the payment of a little over $100 as a deductible, the full costs of care are paid for up to a 60-day stay. The major benefit improvement needed in hospital insurance under Medicare is to cover without coinsurance the few cases where long stays in general hospitals, or a series of shorter stays within the same year, are required. There are not many cases involved, but the few there are should be protected, and without the patient having to pay part of the cost, as is now the case.

Protection against the cost of physician care covered under the supplementary medical insurance part of Medicare is much less satisfactory. The retired person has to pay a monthly premium for this protection, there is a $60 annual deductible before any bills are paid by the plan, and there is 20% coinsurance. Actually, the individual may be called upon to pay much more than 20%, because a physician who wants to take a chance on collecting his own bills, rather than being reimbursed directly by Medicare, is allowed to charge the patient more than the fee on which Medicare reimbursement is based. Under these circumstances, the plan pays the patient, not the doctor, but the physician can bill for any amount he pleases. Thus, many elderly people under Medicare are now paying not 20% of their physicians' bills after a deductible, but 30 or 40%. This procedure can and should be changed.

I would also propose that the supplementary medical insurance program be combined with hospital insurance and that the combined protection be financed partly by a contribution paid by the worker and his employer throughout his working career, and partly by a government contribution. Thus, the worker would have paid-up protection for physician coverage in retirement, just as he does now for hospital coverage, without paying a premium after he is retired. This proposal was endorsed by the 1971 Advisory Council on Social Security.

Medicare needs to be broadened to cover additional health costs. Prescription drugs, for example, are now covered only while an individual is in a hospital or receiving covered care in a nursing home. For many elderly people with chronic illnesses, the regular drug bill — $30, $40 or even $50 a month, month after month — may be a very serious drain on income. The cost of prescription drugs for at least chronic illness should be covered now.

With all their limitations, Medicare and the income-tested Medicaid programs have done much to equalize the availability of services among the elderly regardless of income. Between 1964 and 1973, the rate of hospitalization increased by almost 40% for the elderly poor and by 16% for the aged who were not poor. The rate which was higher for the not poor in 1964 was higher for the poor in 1973. In 1964, the elderly poor averaged 6 physicians' visits per person per year, as compared with 7.3 for those who were not poor. By 1973, the gap had been decreased to 6.5 for the poor and 6.9 for those who were not poor.

Medicaid, as well as Medicare, has been an important program for the elderly, filling in for lower-income people the coinsurance and deductibles of Medicare and supplying for the low-income elderly in many states additional services not covered under Medicare, including those which are of particular importance to the chronically ill. As I have already indicated, Medicaid, not Medicare, is the major program that pays for long-term nursing care. Perhaps it should continue to be so. I, for one, would certainly have concern about extending Medicare to cover long-term nursing care as a matter of right and without regard to income, unless such an extension were to be accompanied by universally available and effective support services designed to keep people out of institutions. It seems to me quite possible that an extension of Medicare to cover the cost of long-term nursing home care might lead, under present circumstances, to over-institutionalization. I can easily imagine that some of the elderly now being cared for at home might be transfered to nursing homes if such care were paid for under the contributory insurance program without regard to need. It is doubtful whether such a transfer on a large scale would be a net gain from the standpoint of elderly persons.

A main difficulty with Medicaid is that its scope depends on state initiative and the availability of state funds, and today the level of service is being cut back in state after state. Perhaps the best thing that could happen with this program in the near future would be for Medicare to take over some of its functions by extension of coverage and leave to Medicaid the long-term care function, at least until we have in place community services that would help provide for many a reasonable alternative to the nursing home.

But in spite of these needs for reform in the Supplemental Security income program, the cash benefit social security program, and Medicare and Medicaid, we will do quite well even under present policy for the retired elderly who can continue to function independently without special help. Let me turn, then, to focussing narrowly on the group the rest of the conference will be concerned with — the 3 to 4 million who need help to perform the tasks of daily living.

The Chronically Ill and the Very Old

First of all, it seems to me remarkable, although perhaps only a coincidence, that in both Britain and the US the proportion of the elderly population in long-term care institutions is not strikingly different, perhaps 3–4% in Britain and 5% in the US. Yet Britain has assiduously pursued a general policy of discouraging institutionalization and has made generally available support services to make it possible for people to remain at home whereas, in the United States, I can detect no general policy on this point.

The United States has a variety of important and helpful demonstrations and experiments in support services, and, in some places good, comprehensive services are available to substantial numbers of people, but, except for home health services under Medicare, we have not, as a matter of government policy, undertaken to make generally available the social and health services that are intended to make it possible for the very old and the chronically ill to remain at home if they wish. In the United States, the availability of meals-on-wheels, friendly visiting and telephone services, homemaker and handiman services, the provision of out-patient mental health services, rehabilitation, counseling, transportation services, day-care centers, all support services depend on the happenstance of where you live. More often than not, comprehensive services are not available.

Yet we have only 5% of the elderly population in long-term care institutions. Perhaps in the absence of a deliberate policy of adequate institutional care and promoting its acceptance — for example, as in Sweden, which, as Sir George Godber indicates in his paper, has three times as many elderly in institutions as does Britain — the elderly themselves and their families and friends make do with what they have as long as they can, to some extent regardless of how much help they get from outside. Certainly in the United States the typically unsatisfactory nature of long-term care arrangements and their cost create a strong incentive to remain at home if at all possible. Few families can afford the average cost of $6000 a year per person, and there is considerable reluctance on the part of many to turn to public assistance or Medicaid.

This is far from an argument against making it more satisfactory to stay at home if that is one's choice, but the fact that the proportion of elderly in the UK and the United States is not widely different may indicate that reducing the proportion of older people who are institutionalized is very difficult to accomplish, particularly as the elderly population itself ages. Clearly there is some irreducible minimum percentage of the population which should be in long-care institutions; if not 5%, then 4% or 3%. It behooves us then not just to attack institutionalization, but to improve the institutions. Our need for such an improvement in the United States is well documented by both federal and state investigations. We have some good nursing homes, but we also have many that are a disgrace.

From 1963 to 1973, nursing home beds in the United States more than doubled, going from 569 000 beds to 1 328 000, reflecting the growth in — and the aging of — the older population, the shift from state and county mental hospitals (between 1964 and 1973 the resident patient rates in state and county mental hospitals per 100 000 persons 65 and over dropped from 805 to 331)[3] the advent of Medicaid, and perhaps to some small extent the advent of Medicare. Medicare, however, has approved for reimbursement only 3960 skilled nursing homes to give the relatively intensive post-hospital care required under the Medicare program out of a total of about 15 000 nursing homes (or nearly 22 000 if personal care homes and domiciliary care homes are included).

Because of the 1973–74 Nursing Home Survey, we have much better

[3] National Institute of Mental Health, Statistical Note 112, March 1975.

information about nursing home residents than ever before, and, I must say, that the characteristics of that population do not give one much reason to hope for returning large numbers of elderly nursing home residents to living in the community. It is quite possible, however, that with proper support services a sizeable percentage might have chosen to remain longer in their own homes, or in the homes of friends and relatives.

The percentage of those over 65 in institutions varies greatly by age. Only 2.1% of those 65 to 74 are in institutions, and 7.1% of those 75 to 84; but 19.3% of those 85 and over are in institutions, mostly nursing homes. First of all, then, nursing home residents are very old. Seventy-four per cent are 75 or older, and 38% are 85 and older. Women outnumber men in nursing homes 7 to 3, and 64% are widows; for the group over age 85, 80% are widows.

The most common primary diagnosis among the residents was hardening of the arteries (22.5%), followed by ill-defined conditions such as "senility" and "old age" (13.6%), strokes (10.5%), and mental disorders (9.6%). Few are completely blind (2.8%), completely deaf (1.0%), or unable to talk (3%), but many have serious impairments of sight, hearing, and speech. Over one-fourth cannot read ordinary print even with glasses, about 30% cannot hear a conversation on an ordinary telephone, and 22.8% have impaired speech.

About 41% of the nursing home residents received intensive nursing care — full bed bath, catheterization, intravenous injections, enemas, blood pressure readings, etc.; about 10% limited nursing care services, such as hypodermic injections; and practically all the rest received personal nursing care such as a rubdown or massage, or assistance in personal hygiene or eating. Few receive therapy services — 15% recreational therapy, 10% physical therapy, and 6% occupational therapy. Eight per cent received professional counseling.

What of the Future?

I would like to turn now to the question of whether we can continue the policy of adequate retirement income for the elderly that we have adopted, improve the protection where it is needed, expand and improve Medicare and Medicaid, and at the same time improve the general quality of institutional services for the elderly and add the broad range of community services needed for the non-institutionalized elderly who cannot live entirely independently. Have we serious problems in meeting the needs of the elderly because of the growth in both the number and proportion of persons over 65?

The conclusions to be drawn from the demographic facts presented in Professor Jefferys' excellent paper also apply generally to the United States. The demography of all western industrialized countries is similar. We share the fact that the over-65 population is itself aging, increasingly female, and non-married, and the fact that an increasing proportion will need special care because of disabling conditions.

I would add from demography only a few points that are, perhaps of special importance to the United States. While the growth of the population 65 and over since 1900 has been very large and quite steady — rising from 3.1 million in 1900 to 23 million today, an average increase of more than 30% every 10 years — future growth will not be a straight-line projection of the past. After 1980, the rate of increase begins to drop sharply, so that it takes three decades for another 30% increase, with the population over 65 reaching a total of about 30 million people between 2005 and 2010. Then, as the generation born in the post-war "baby-boom" reaches retirement age, the numbers will shoot up from 30 million to 50 million in about 20 years. And this is quite certain. This group has already been born, and its size has been estimated on the assumption of only modest improvements in mortality rates.[4]

By the measures of either the percentage of the total population or the ratio of those over 65 to the population of usual working age, the increase in the number of elderly during the next thirty years does not, in itself, present substantial difficulty. As a percentage of the entire population, those over 65 have gone from 4.1% in 1900 to 10.5% today and will rise to an expected 11.9% in 2010. For every 100 persons aged 18 to 64, there were 7 above 65 in 1900, 18 today, and there will be about 19 thirty years from now.

Although during the next 30 years the *total* population over 65 does not increase at a rate to cause concern, shifts within the over 65 group are significant. The increasing proportion of the very old among the over 65 group continues the trend of the past, and the ratio of females to males continues to increase.

By 2010, those over 80 will make up about 25% of those over 65 as compared to 20% today, while those 65 through 69 will have dropped from 36% to 31%. Later on the proportions will reserve as the baby-boom generation begins to reach 65 and increases first the proportion in the 65 through 69 age bracket.

The comparatively few males among the elderly is well known, but the size of the sex differential is worth noting. Today in the 65 and over group there are 69.3 males per 100 females, and among those 75 and over, 58.4 males per 100 females. Thus it follows that elderly men usually live with a spouse, whereas elderly women are very often living alone, without the kind of support and help that one elderly person can give another. The gap between the number of males and females

[4] The population figures in this paper are from "Demographic Aspects of Aging and the Older Population in the United States", by Jacob S. Siegel with the assistance of Mark D. Herrenbruck, Donald S. Akers, Jeffrey S. Passel, Bureau of the Census, "Current Population Reports, Special Studies," Series P-23, No. 59. May, 1976.

will continue to widen. By 2010, it is expected that the ratio of males to females will have dropped to 65.5 men per 100 women over 65, and 51.8 over 75.

Although the changes are not major, overall, up to about 2005 or 2010, beginning then we will have over the next 20 years this one-time, tremendous increase in the total number over 65, followed by a leveling off in the number of the elderly as we approach a relatively stationary population. By 2030, assuming a continuation of fertility rates that do not exceed the replacement rate of 2.1 children per woman, the 50 million people over 65 will probably be at least 17% of the total population, and there will be around 30 people in this age group (as compared with 19 in 2010) for every 100 persons in the age group 18 to 64.

The sudden jump in the ratio of those over 65 to those of usual working age could have a serious impact on the relative cost of caring for the elderly, since the support of those who are retired must come from the goods and services produced by those at work. There are some mitigating factors: the lower fertility rates that produce the problem in the first place will mean that there are fewer children to support, so that the total number of non-workers — the elderly plus children — will be about the same proportion of the 18–64 age group as today, and then, too, with fewer children, a higher proportion of women will work, so that more people in the 18–64 age group will be producers. But I would not want to count on these factors to completely offset the sudden growth in the proportion of the elderly. Fewer children might make it *possible* for the working population to do more for the elderly, but they might not want to. They might want more for themselves while at work and for their children even if there are fewer of them.

I believe, if we want to continue retirement plans that replace wages to the extent we have promised, improve health insurance and long-term institutional care for the elderly, and add the services needed to allow people to be cared for outside institutions if they prefer, we had better give high priority over the next thirty years — before the crunch comes — to reversing the trend toward earlier and earlier retirement.

It is one thing to be able to support such programs under conditions of a rapidly increasing population over 65 if most people work up to 65 or later. It is something else again if people generally stop working at 60 or younger.

I believe older people would welcome increased employment opportunities, and, if we pursue a policy of full employment, such opportunities should become available as the 18 to 64 age group stops growing, under conditions of zero population growth, while the number of the elderly greatly increases. What we need to avoid is acceptance of the notion that people ought to stop work at 65 or earlier. As a society we need to avoid extending compulsory retirement age policies and making retirement benefits available at earlier and earlier ages. We need, instead, to be in a position to respond to the need for more older workers that is very likely to develop in the next century.

Conclusion

Taking all this into account, what should our national policy be toward the chronically ill and the very old? How can we organize to provide the combined social and health services to make it possible for people to function in their own homes as long as they can and wish to? How do we organize to support residential centers for those who would choose this arrangement in later life? And how do we protect the individuality, humanity, independence, and dignity of those who have no other recourse but prolonged institutionalization?

It is not my task at this conference to answer these questions but rather to place the problem of the chronically ill and the very old in the larger context of our policy toward the elderly in general, and to highlight the neglect. I will say, though, that it is past time that we made these questions a matter of central concern.

Whatever we propose to do that is generally effective will cost money. And to do it well, on a national basis, may cost lots of money, easily, I would say, in the neighborhood of $6 billion to $7 billion. It has become fashionable today to point out that problems are not solved by "throwing money at them", but I submit that they are not solved without money — the wise and judicious use of money.

A final question: Will the increasing drain on resources necessary for adequate care of those of advanced age and with chronic illnesses lead to tension among the generations? Will the middle-aged and the young resent the cost needed for the care of the very old? Perhaps, but perhaps not. No one stays young, or even middle-aged. We are all moving in the same direction. Life is a continuum, and a cross-section analysis, so often seen in economics, pitting the wage earner against the retired elderly is not a very useful abstraction. Planning social arrangements like pensions and the care of the very old and chronically ill are of great importance to all of us, not only because such arrangements relieve us of an immediate burden that can become overwhelming for an individual family, but because such institutions shape our own future. There is no real dichotomy of interest between the wage earner and the elderly retired. The issue is how much should be given up in earlier life to provide for later life, not only for someone else, but in support of social arrangements that we will want for ourselves if we survive to become a part of the group that needs special care.

Functional Consequences of Aging

Physiological Changes and Disease[1]

Ewald W Busse
Medical and Allied Health Education,
Duke University Medical Center,
Durham, North Carolina 27710

Definitions

All people, animals, plants, as well as non-living matter, become older and undergo changes with the passage of time. The biological term *aging* is a word that when applied to living organisms includes changes that take place gradually and end with death. Such changes may be observed as a decline in body efficiency, a maladaptive change in structure, and a stoppage or reversal of growth. *Primary aging* (senescence) refers to numerous biological processes that are inherent in the organism and are inevitably detrimental, and although time related are to varying degrees influenced by the social and physical environment. The terms *growth* and *development* usually represent biological processes which are the opposite of aging; that is, they are processes moving towards maximum functional efficiency and often size. *Secondary aging* (senile changes or senility) refers to disabilities resulting from trauma and disease.

The bodies of humans and higher animals all consist of three biological components. Two are cellular and one is non-cellular. There are cells capable of reproducing themselves throughout the animal's or the person's life span. Skin cells and white blood cells are examples of such cells that have this capacity to reproduce. There are other cells that cannot reproduce, and when lost, cannot be replaced. Such cells are the neurons of the brain and of the nervous system. The third biological component is non-cellular; that is, it is the material that occupies the space between cells. Aging is different in each of these components of the body. Consequently, biochemists, molecular biologists, and cell biologists have described numerous aging processes and have advanced a number of theories. Some of the theories are

[1] This paper is based in part on research supported by grant #AG-00364, National Institute on Aging, USPHS (formerly #HD-00668, National Institute of Child Health and Human Development, USPHS).

overlapping, and some of the aging processes can be found in more than one component of the body. Some are restricted in that they are found only in non-cellular material, others in only certain organelles or in types of cells. Scientists working at this level are frequently concerned with mutations, alterations in genetic coding, defects in information processes, deliberate biological programming, etc. Physiological changes are equally complex as physiology is concerned with the functional capacity and the integration of numerous organs and systems. My remarks will be largely concerned with those alterations in human functioning often referred to as symptoms or signs that are manifestations of physiologic aging.

Appearance as a Sign of Age

Observing the bodily appearance of humans and the manner in which they think and behave often makes it possible for us to judge the chronologic age of an individual. Age changes can be camouflaged or hidden by clothing, cosmetics, and the continuing use of behavioral patterns characteristic of a younger age. But in addition, individual age changes vary widely from one person to another; for example, the young person who is prematurely gray haired or balding. Graying of the hair and other changes such as the arcus senilis (ring around the margin of the iris) are largely hereditarily determined and are related to the immune system in the body. Numerous changes come about in the skin, and as one would expect each of the components and activity of skin are affected. For example, there are changes in sweat, excretion of sebaceous material, the number and reproductive capacity of skin cells, and the interstitial material. Furthermore, skin normally shows considerable racial differences as to pigmentation and thickness. Dark-complected individuals have a certain degree of natural protection. Hence, their skin does not show the damage of exposure to ultraviolet sunlight over many years.

Aging and Perception

At approximately the age of 40 years in most normal persons in western societies there begins a decline in both hearing and vision. It has been claimed that these changes do not occur in some primitive societies, and there is little doubt that high noise levels are detrimental to the hearing of Americans. The visual age change is called presbyopia, and the hearing alteration is referred to as presbycusis. With advancing age hearing is characterized by an inability to distinguish high frequency sounds. This type of hearing loss is probably a primary aging process, as it occurs in individuals who have not been exposed to high noise levels. Hearing is particularly important to maintaining personality integration and adaptation; therefore, I am very concerned with the detrimental effect of high noise levels in our society. Sound and noise are quantified on a scale known as decibels. The decibel scale is not one of equalized units. It is a logarithmic scale. Every upward step of ten decibels represents a hundredfold multiplication of sound energy. Thus a sound of 60 dB is 100 times more powerful than one at 50 dB. Soft speech is at 30 dB; conversational speech, approximately 60 dB; the noise of a subway, 90 dB; and the blast of an automobile, 120. There is no doubt that noise is adversely affecting the functioning capacity of many Americans, particularly the elderly.

The visual change is more familiar because we are all aware of the high number of people who require glasses for reading and close work after the age of 40. Presbyopia is the result of the loss of the ability of the lens to accommodate for near and distant vision and can be corrected by the use of appropriate lens. In addition, in advanced years vision is affected by the slowing of adaptation to darkness and an increased requirement for illumination. The level at which light is perceived is particularly altered in older people. Older people often require a brighter light to do certain tasks.

Taste and smell are also altered by age. Old people have lost approximately 50% of their taste buds, and 40% have markedly diminished capacity to detect odors (Rockstein *et al.* 1973). This loss of sensitivity to taste and smell is age related. From middle adulthood on, taste buds are lost. Taste buds which are primarily located on the tongue atrophy from the front of the tongue posteriorly. The first to go are the taste buds that detect sweet and salty, leaving those devoted to the detection of bitter and sour tastes. This loss results in some older people complaining that all food tastes bitter or sour. Food preference is a very complex matter (Schiffman 1974), and it includes not only smell and taste but also temperature, consistency, texture, and appearance. Ability to identify foods does decline significantly with advancing age.

Musculo–Skeletal Changes

The cells that make up voluntary muscles diminish in number with age, and approximately one-half are left at the age of 80 years. As muscle cells disappear, they are replaced by fat and fibrous connective tissues. Despite continuing physical exercise, there is a reduction in the muscle strength as a person gets older.

Metabolism and Drugs

Drugs are metabolized differently in older people than they are in younger people. The term metabolism is employed to designate the sum of all chemical reactions that take place in a living organism

(Timiras 1972). How the drug is handled within the body has a number of metabolic dimensions including absorption, distribution, destruction, excretion, kinetics of drug binding, and alterations in biological rhythms (Reinberg 1974). All these and other changes seem to decline as the result of the aging processes as well as from the insults of disease and trauma. Some of the major aging changes are the loss or decline of efficiency of renal function, a redistribution of body content with a decline in protein and an increase in fat, a decline in basic metabolic rate, and the dropping out of non-replaceable cells. The loss of brain cells probably makes the brain more sensitive to certain drugs, while the increase in fat content is important as drugs are frequently stored in fat. Striated musculature diminishes to about one-half by approximately 80 years of age. As these muscle cells disappear, they are replaced by fats and fibrous connective tissue; hence, the drug storage capacity increases. It is estimated that the basic metabolic rate through the adult years declines 16% from age 30 to 70 years, while the caloric requirement because of decreased metabolism and exercise drops approximately one-third.

Aging in the Central Nervous System

One of the earliest observations that continues to be of great significance is the gradual loss of neurons, particularly those in the brain. There are numerous other changes within the central nervous system including the accumulation of pigments within nerve cells and a decline in the weight of the brain. A number of factors contribute to this weight change. Evidence is accumulating that the neuronal loss is not evenly distributed throughout the brain. The counting of neurons in more circumscribed areas has revealed that variation occurs in the cortex and in the brain stem (Brody 1973). Age changes are complicated by the recent work demonstrating that there are alterations within the synapsis of the brain, and a decline in dendrites further disrupts the neuronal networks (Scheibel *et al.* 1975, Bondareff and Geinisman 1976).

In addition to these identifiable anatomical changes, electrophysiological measurements clearly reflect age changes.

Electroencephalographic Changes

A common characteristic of EEG changes is the progressive slowing of the dominant frequency involving the alpha frequency and the appearance of slow waves in the theta or delta range. A slight slowing of the alpha index is not pathognomonic for any particular brain disorder. However, moderate to severe slowing is characteristically found in brain disorders whether they are classified as degenerative or vascular in origin. Elderly subjects in good health are found to have a mean occipital frequency which is almost a full cycle slower than that found in healthy young adults. Furthermore, about 7% of the EEGs in the elderly subjects were dominated by slow waves in the theta range, that is, 6 to 8 per second (Wang and Busse 1969). Since a good correlation has been demonstrated between EEG frequency and cerebral oxygen consumption or blood flow, the slowing of the dominant frequency in the majority of elderly people may indicate a depression of cerebral metabolism.

Residents of institutions for the aged are found to have EEG slowing that correlates with measures of psychological impairment. Unfortunately, this correlation is not nearly as clear in subjects remaining in the community. It is possible that those who live in the community are actually adjusting at a borderline level and may be vulnerable to stress which would precipitate the appearance of organic brain disease. Throughout adult life fast waves are more frequent in women than in men and tend to increase in females. Fast activity is present in 23% of females age 60–79 years but in only 4% of elderly males.

Focal abnormalities of EEG, predominantly over the temporal areas of the brain, and maximally on the left, have been repeatedly observed in 30 to 40% of apparently healthy elderly people. This finding was first reported by Busse *et al.* in 1955. Since that date the observation of the frequent occurrence of a left-temporal focus in old people has been reported by other investigators. A study of healthy volunteers between the ages of 20 and 60 reveals that only 3% of normal adults under the age of 40 years have temporal lobe EEG changes. This increases so that in the 20 years between 40 and 60, 20% of the subjects show temporal lobe irregularities. After age 60, the severity of the focal disturbance tends to stabilize, but new foci are more likely to appear in women, hence a higher percentage of women have the change as compared to men (Busse 1973).

The exact origin of these foci as well as their significance is still not clear. The localized EEG abnormality is usually episodic in nature and is composed of high-voltage waves in the delta and theta range, occasionally accompanied by focal short waves. The disturbance is found in the waking record, is maximum in the drowsy state, and disappears in sleep (Busse and Obrist 1963). In 75–80% of the cases the abnormality is at a maximum or completely confined to the left side of the brain. It is not related to handedness, and although it is evidently episodic in nature, it is unrelated to seizures. Numerous attempts have been made to relate temporal foci to localized cerebro-vascular insufficiency and transient ischemic attacks. No consistent relationship has been established. Furthermore, the focal disturbances in senescent EEGs have not been consistently correlated with any particular psychological function or measure.

Averaged Evoked Potential (AEP)

This particular method of studying the physiological changes in the brain is an EEG derived bioelectric response of the central nervous system elicited by a brief stimulus. The phenomenon is usually referred to as the averaged evoked potential (AEP) and sometimes it is called the cerebral evoked response (CER). I prefer the latter. The characteristics of this bioelectric measure are influenced by the type of stimulus and the area of the central nervous system being affected; consequently, studies differentiate accordingly. Visual stimulus or visual evoked response may be referred to as VER; auditory stimulus, AER; somatosensory evoked response as SER.

These complicated studies have been made possible only by the utilization of computer capabilities. For those who are interested in having a more detailed and yet understandable review of the origin and the composition of these interesting responses, I suggest the publication of Beck and Dustman (1975). The measured response is usually divided into two parts, an early and a late component, and at least eight subcomponents are also observed for age changes. It does appear that this type of research will be extremely useful in understanding the physiological basis for learning, memory, and the value of pharmacological agents in improving the functioning of the brain. At the present time, one aspect of AEP seems to have received particular attention, and this is the so-called late positive component (LPC). Furthermore, it appears that the visual stimulation results in a response that is most sensitive to age changes (Marsh 1976).

Sleep

During the past decade considerable advancement has been made in our understanding of the physiological changes during sleep although the functions of sleep in a large degree remain a mystery. Four major stages of sleep have been identified. Stage one commonly known as rapid eye movement sleep (REM) after its initial appearance in a night of sleep is the stage that is most likely to be associated with dreams. Four to five REM episodes occur during a night's sleep, and these REM periods become progressively longer during the sleep period. Sleep patterns and sleep requirements change throughout the life span (Williams *et al.* 1974). In advanced age, the REM periods become more equal in duration and stage four, the deepest stage of sleep, virtually disappears.

Elderly people require a longer period to fall asleep, their sleep is lighter, and they experience more frequent awakenings. It is important that people in the latter part of their life span recognize that the process of going to sleep lengthens and that they as part of their normal aging changes will be aware of more frequent awakenings. Throughout adult life women sleep differently than men. Women spend more time in bed, sleep more, and awaken during the night less often than do men.

A variety of sleep complaints occur in the elderly, and these are reflected in their utilization of sleeping pills. In one study of apparently well-adjusted community subjects over the age of 60, up to 40% occasionally used sleeping pills, and 10% habitually took medication to induce or assure sleep. In elderly subjects who were free of physical pain, those who used sleeping pills excessively were found to have many other neurotic complaints and to be poorly adjusted socially (Busse *et al.* 1955). Recent studies indicate that sleep changes are more pronounced in persons with organic brain disease (Feinberg *et al.* 1969).

Why Do Women Live Longer Than Men?

Since 1900, the percentage of the United States population age 65 and over has more than doubled, from 4.1% in 1900 to an estimated 10.3% in 1975, while the actual number of aged persons has increased sevenfold from 3 000 000 to over 21 000 000 (8.9 million males and 12.8 million females) (Neugarten 1975). There has also been a clear reversal in life expectancy trends for men and women. In 1900, in the United States there were 98 old women to every 100 old men. Women have had longer life expectancies from 1900 onward (Riley and Foner 1968). During the period 1900 to 1902 life expectancy for white females below age 20 was lower than for males of a like age but slightly higher for females through the adult years.

In 1964, the longevity of the young female had improved remarkably and had considerably surpassed that of the young male. Apparently this was not the result of selective immigration, that is, more men than women coming into the country, but a shift in health as related to sex.

Women are outliving men. In fact, there are about 138.5 older women per 100 older men. Life expectancy for women is still increasing faster than for men. During the next 20 years, although it is unlikely that the percentage of older people in the population will increase significantly, their actual number will go over 27 000 000 (US Department of Labor, Bureau of Census 1971). Assuming that the current life expectancy trends continue, by the year 2000, the ratio of elderly women to men will be approximately 149 women to 100 men.

In the United States the high mortality of males as compared to females appears to be a complex interaction between genetically determined physiological differences, socioeconomic factors and cultural values, and expectations and environmental conditions that may be more dangerous to the man than to the woman.

Waldron (1976) presents data to indicate that 40% of the excess male mortality is due to arteriosclerotic heart disease. An additional one-third is due to the male having a higher rate of suicide, fatal motor accidents and other accidents, cirrhosis of the liver, carcinoma of the lung, and emphysema. Thus these conditions account for 75% of the causes of the male mortality. It is clear that cultural behavioral patterns which are more prevalent among men than women contribute to arteriosclerotic heart disease, as well as habits of excess smoking and drinking and a higher risk behavior found so often in men as compared to women.

Genetic factors undoubtedly play a role, but the interaction of such factors with the environment must be kept in mind. It is true that in many species males have a higher mortality rate than females, particularly in insects and in other Arthropoda. However, a higher female mortality appears to be just as common in many birds and mammals. For example, in mallard ducks it appears that the female mallard suffers a much higher natural mortality than the male (Donnelly 1974).

Human males do have a higher fetal mortality as well as a higher mortality during the first year of life. Prior to the development of the fetus there are male/female differences, as the male-producing Y-carrier sperm is smaller with a head resembling an arrowhead and having a longer tail and is much speedier in its movements. The X-carrying female-producing sperm has a larger round head, a shorter tail, and moves at a comparatively sluggish pace. The difference in speed of motility is believed to account for the greater number of male fetuses as opposed to female fetuses (Rosenfeld 1974).

The genetic difference between the male and female cannot be ignored as the female does have the advantage of having two X chromosomes, one in effect backing up the other. The egg or ova of the human female is always an X chromosome. Therefore, when it unites with a female-producing sperm, an XX chromosome combination results. A Y sperm produces an XY or a male fetus. It is also likely that sex hormones play a role, but no consistent information regarding the impact of male/female hormones upon longevity is available at this time. More is known about the detrimental effects of hormones than the positive ones as sex hormones are implicated in atherosclerosis, carcinoma, and high blood pressure.

References

Beck, E. C. and Dustman, R. E. (1975). *In* "Brain Function and Malnutrition". Eds. J. W. Prescott, M. S. Read and D. B. Coursin. John Wiley, New York: pp 187–206

Bondareff, W. and Geinisman, Y. (1976). *American Journal of Anatomy* (in press)

Brody, H. (1973). *In* "Development and Aging in the Nervous System". Ed. M. Rockstein. Academic Press, New York: pp 121–133

Busse, E. W. (1973). *Clinical Electroencephalography* **4**, 152–163

Busse, E. W., Barnes, R. H., Silverman, A. J., Thaler, M. B. and Frost, L. L. (1955). *American Journal of Psychiatry* **111**, 896–901

Busse, E. W. and Obrist, W. D. (1963). *Postgraduate Medicine* **34**, 179–183

Donnelly, J. (1974). *Wild Life in North Carolina.* December, 18–19

Feinberg, L., Braun, M. and Schulman, E. (1969). *Electroencephalography and Clinical Neurophysiology* **27**, 128–141

Marsh, G. R. (1976). *Annual Review of Experimental Aging Research* (in press)

Neugarten, B. L. (1975). *Gerontologist* **15**, 9

Reinberg, A. (1974). *In* "Chronobiological Aspects of Endocrinology". Eds. J. Aschoff, F. Ceresa and F. Halberg. Schattlauer Verlag, Stuttgart and New York: pp 305–333

Riley, M. W. and Foner, A. (1968). "Aging and Society". Russell Sage Foundation, New York: p 28

Rockstein, M., Schiffman, S. and Wilkie, F. L. (1973). *In* "Mental Illness in Later Life". Eds. E. W. Busse and E. Pfeiffer. American Psychiatric Association, Washington: p 269

Rosenfeld, A. (1974). "If Oedipus' Parents had only Known". *Saturday Review World.* September 7, 49–52

Scheibel, M. E., Lindsay, R. D., Tomiyasu, U. and Scheibel, A. B. (1975). *Experimental Neurology* **47**, 392

Schiffman, S. (1974). *Annals of the New York Academy of Sciences* **237**, 164–183

Timiras, P. A. (1972). "Developmental Physiology and Aging". Macmillan, New York

US Department of Labor, Bureau of Census (1971). "Statistical Abstract of the US", Table 6; p 81

Waldron, I. (1976). *Journal of Human Stress* **2**, 2–19

Wang, H. S. and Busse, E. W. (1969). *Journal of Gerontology* **23**, 419–426

Williams, R., Karacan, I. and Hursch, C. (1974). "EEG of Human Sleep — Clinical Implications". John Wiley, New York

Clinical Manifestations

A N Exton-Smith
Department of Geriatrics,
St Pancras Hospital, London NW1,
and University College Hospital,
Medical School, London WC1

In man and higher vertebrates aging takes the form of morphological and functional involution affecting most of the organs and leads to a gradual decline in the performances of the individual. This decline in function can also be viewed as a decreased adaptation of the individual to his environment and this in turn is reflected in an increased mortality.

Benjamin Gompertz in 1825 was first to point out that the mortality of humans after middle age is a logarithmic function of age. During the period from about 35 to 90 years an individual's probability of dying doubles in about 8 years. Following this period, in extreme old age, there is a slight decline in the rate of increase in mortality. This probably represents the continued survival of the biological elite — individuals with certain characteristics which enable them to outlive their former contemporaries.

Differential aging in bodily systems leads to variations in the rate of decline in function in these systems. Whatever be the relative importance of vitality in each subsystem the integrity of function in the nervous system must exert a dominant role. Not only does it influence function in other systems, but the maintenance of acquired skills and the retention of intellectual powers enable the individual to make satisfactory adjustments to environmental hazards. All functions in the nervous system show a progressive decline throughout adult life. It is well known that degeneration of fibres takes place in nerve tracts and that cell loss occurs in cerebral tissues with increasing age; more recently an age-related decline in function in the autonomic nervous system has been recognized. The insidious and progressive changes are reflected in the organism by a steady decrease in the adaptability of the individual and by a parallel increase in the susceptibility to environmental stresses. Homeostasis is still maintained, but with increasing difficulty as the years pass.

The manner in which an age-related decline in function leads to the appearance of clinical manifestations will be examined by reference to three phenomena: impairment of thermoregulatory capacity due to autonomic dysfunction, falls associated with postural imbalance, and the liability to fractures at certain sites due to changes in the quantity and quality of bone. These conditions become increasingly common with advancing years and in the very old they are associated with considerable incapacity and a high mortality.

Temperature Regulation and the Thermal Environment

Heat-waves and severe cold weather each lead to a considerable increase in mortality amongst the elderly population. It is now believed that the number of deaths from all causes provides a more valid measure of the effects of extremes of temperature than the numbers revealed by death certification as due to heat illness or hypothermia. The excess mortality of the elderly during heat-waves is due mainly to the increased number of deaths from ischaemic heart disease and cerebrovascular accidents (Ellis 1972, Ellis *et al.* 1975). Similarly during the winter months periods of severe cold lasting two or more days are associated with highly significant changes in the death rates from myocardial infarction and cerebrovascular accidents in persons over the age of 60 (Bull 1969, Bull and Morton 1975*a*, *b*).

Mortality During Heat-Waves

The adverse effects of extremely high climatic temperature on the elderly population have been observed mainly in the United States and Australia. There was a considerable increase in mortality in persons over the age of 65 on the days following the hottest periods in two heat-waves of only moderate severity in New York City in 1972 and 1973 (Ellis *et al.* 1975). In a study conducted in a large home for the aged in Sydney (Macpherson *et al.* 1967) it was found that mortality was lowest when the afternoon temperature was between 21 and 26°C, but it was 13% above the daily average when it ranged between 27 and 32°C. This effect of temperature became most marked in persons over the age of 70 years.

Impairment of thermoregulatory function in old age is believed to be one of the factors responsible for this differential in mortality. Foster and his co-workers (1976) have shown a failure of sweat response to thermal stimulation and to the intradermal injection of acetylcholine in over half the old people tested. This lack of response was more often seen in the limbs than on the trunk.

Studies of Accidental Hypothermia

In the United Kingdom the adverse effects of cold exposure leading to accidental hypothermia are of greater importance than those caused by high environmental temperatures. The prevalence of hypothermia in hospital admissions has been investigated in two studies of the Royal College of Physicians conducted during the winter months of 1965 and 1975. In the second study 3.6% of all old people admitted to hospital were found to be hypothermic (deep body temperature below 35.0°C) and there was found to be a significant correlation between a low deep body temperature and cold exposure immediately prior to admission (Goldman *et al.* 1977).

Until recently surveys of accidental hypothermia have been confined to old people admitted to hospital, (for example, Duguid *et al.* 1961, Rosin and Exton-Smith 1964) and a low reading rectal thermometer has been used to measure deep body temperature. The development of the Uritemp technique by Fox and his colleagues (1971) has enabled the studies to be extended to old people living at home. The effects of low environmental temperatures were investigated in the National

Study of Body Temperatures in the Elderly sponsored by the Nuffield Foundation (Fox *et al.* 1973). A random sample of 1000 people over the age of 65 in Great Britain living in their own homes was surveyed in the first three months of 1972. The room temperatures were generally low and in 754 cases (75%) they were at or below 18.3°C, the minimum level recommended by the Parker–Morris Report on Council housing. The results and correlations are summarised in Fig 1.

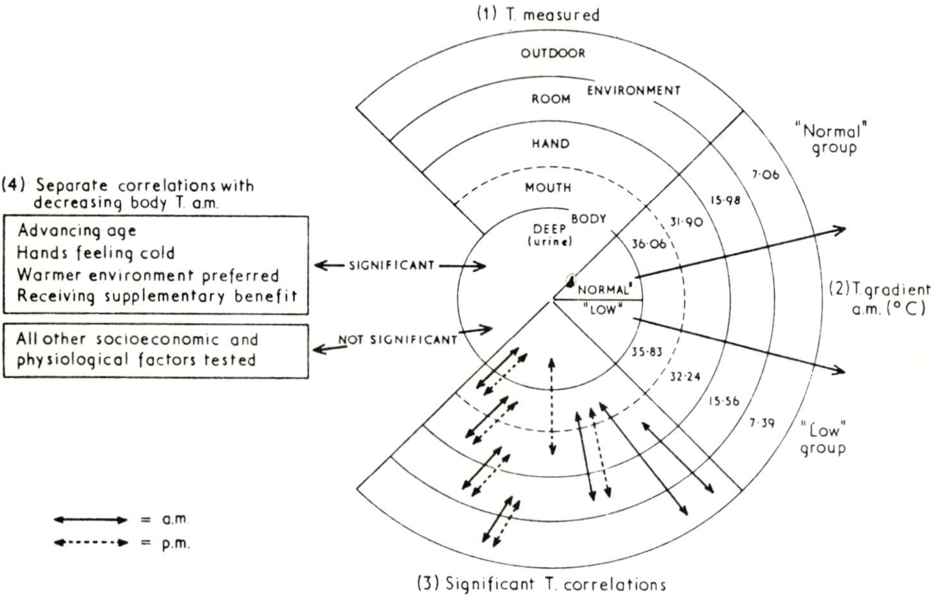

Fig. 1 *Body and environmental temperature (T) and socio-economic factors: National Survey*
(*1*) *Temperatures forming gradient between body core and external environment.*
(*2*) *Comparison of mean (a.m.) temperatures (°C) for the "low" and "normal" groups.*
(*3*) *Significant correlations (a.m., p.m.) between temperatures.*
(*4*) *Important significant correlations with certain physiological and socio-economic factors.*
Reproduced from Fox et al. (1973) British Medical Journal **i**, 200, *by courtesy of the Editor.*

Significant correlations with a decreasing deep body temperature were found to be: advancing age, the complaint of hands feeling cold, the preference for a warmer environment and the receipt of supplementary benefits (which was used as a crude index of poverty). Ten per cent of the subjects were found to be potentially hypothermic with deep body temperatures of less than 35.5°C. These subjects are referred to as the "low" temperature group and were compared with a "normal" group whose core temperatures were 36.0°C and above. There was a significant difference in the core to periphery temperature gradients for the two groups (2.9°C for the low group and 4.6°C for the normal group). It was suggested that a combination of living in cold rooms, diminished bodily heat production and impairment of thermoregulatory function was responsible for the lowering of deep body temperature in the low temperature group.

This hypothesis was confirmed by the results of a more intensive study carried out on a subgroup of an additional 1000 old people living in the London Borough of Camden. Following the temperature measurements made at home 153 subjects (15%) participated in an intensive study aimed at investigating the relationship between low environmental temperatures, clinical disorders and thermoregulatory function.

Clinical Conditions

Medical examination revealed a high incidence of pathological conditions; two-thirds of the subjects suffered from disease resulting in physical and mental disability. Four aspects, which are concerned with the problem of hypothermia, will be mentioned. The incidence of these disorders was: Restriction of mobility 28%, Nocturia 69%, Insomnia 45% and Postural Hypotension 14%.

Restriction of mobility directly reduces heat production by limitation of bodily heat production; for those living alone it can lead to social isolation which is in turn associated with a number of unmet needs. *Nocturia*, with its necessity for getting out of bed, is a potential cause of falls at night and of hypothermia during the winter months. *Insomnia* is particularly common in the elderly population, but more important 28% take hypnotics regularly; these drugs may depress body temperature, impair psychomotor performance up to 12–15 hours later and may increase the liability to fall. The finding that 14% of the elderly population suffer from *postural hypotension* is similar to that reported by others, for example, Rodstein and Zeman (1957) 11%, Johnson *et al.* (1965) 17% and Caird *et al.* (1973) 24%. This widespread occurrence of postural hypotension in the elderly population is important because it is an indication of impairment of autonomic function which may also involve thermoregulation, and it is associated with an increase in sway and liability to fall with consequent risk of cold exposure.

Thermoregulatory Function

Autonomic control. The 153 old people who participated in the Camden Study were tested using a specially designed air-conditioned bed (Fox *et al.* 1967). The responses in terms of skin and deep body temperatures, peripheral blood flow, heart rate, sweating and metabolic rate were measured. The test procedure was as follows:

(1) A period of 14 minutes with air temperature neutral at 30°C
(2) A period of cooling with air temperature lowered to 15°C for 16 minutes
(3) A period of warming with air temperature at 45°C for 46 minutes or until the subject sweated.

Complete records of the temperature measurements of the subjects at home, the results of medical examination and tests of thermoregulatory function were available in 144 subjects. Abnormalities of autonomic function were found to be very common:

(1) 56% of the men and 45% of the women had abnormal peripheral blood flow patterns; these were found to be rare in young control subjects
(2) 42% of the men and 62% of the women failed to sweat on warming
(3) The shivering reaction was observed in only 28 of the 144 (20%) of the old people tested

When the results of the tests were related to the temperature measurements made at home it was found that in 12 subjects who had deep body temperatures below 35.5°C (low temperature group) 9 had abnormal blood flow patterns, 8 failed to sweat on warming and 7 had postural hypotension. In only one case was there no evidence of autonomic dysfunction; she had true hypothermia (with a deep body temperature of 34.4°C) which was probably accounted for by the limitation in mobility and an extremely low room temperature (10.5°C). By contrast, evidence of autonomic dysfunction (abnormal blood flow responses, absence of sweating and postural hypotension) was much less frequently seen in 93 subjects who had a normal deep body temperature (36.0°C and above).

Thermal perception. Tests of thermal perception were carried out on a small group of subjects during the survey (Cowburn and Fox 1974). The subjects were asked to discriminate between the temperatures of two plates accurately controlled by Peltier junctions. A marked falling off in sensitivity was found in subjects over the age of 65 years. Whereas young subjects could distinguish temperature differences of 0.5°C, many old people could not discriminate between temperature differences of 5°C or more. It seems likely that a lessened sensitivity to cold is one of the reasons for the relatively large numbers of old people who appear to be able to tolerate cold conditions without discomfort. Nevertheless, such individuals may be at risk of over-taxing the heat conserving capacity of a failing thermoregulatory system.

Liability to Fall and Postural Imbalance

Sheldon (1948, 1960) drew attention to the rising incidence of falls with advancing age. He emphasized the association of falls with vertigo, the liability to trip, difficulty in recovering balance and the sudden loss of postural control (drop attacks). The incidence of falls has been investigated in 963 people over the age of 65 who participated in a Nutrition Survey sponsored by the Department of Health and Social Security (*see* Fig 2).

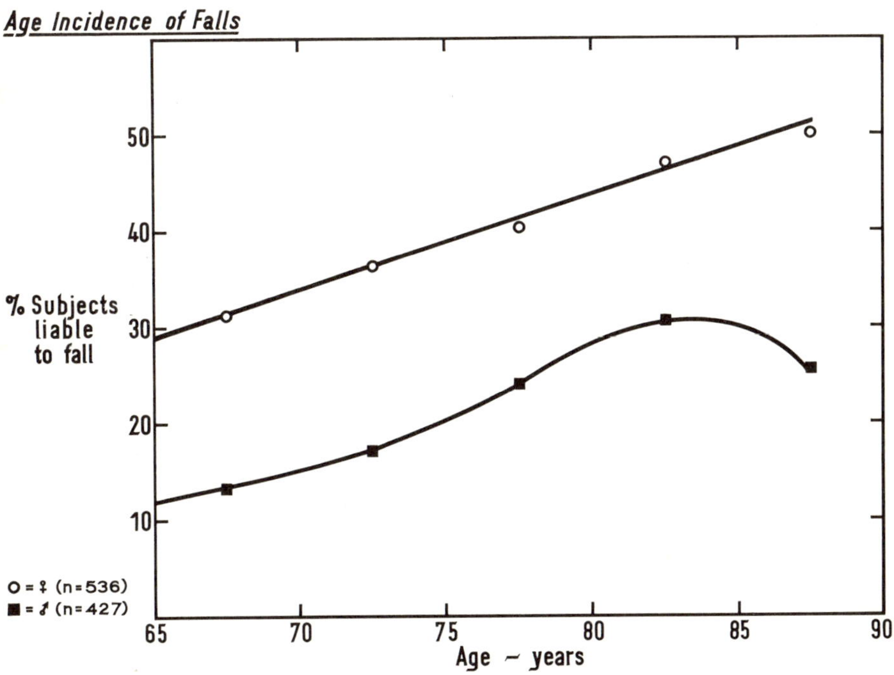

Fig. 2. *Age incidence of falls in elderly men and women*

In women, the proportion who fall increases linearly with age from about 30% in the 65–69 year age group to over 50% in those over the age of 85. For men, the proportion who fall increases from 13% in the 65–69 age group to reach a peak of 31% in the 80–84 age group; thereafter in those over the age of 85 there is a slight decrease. The lower incidence of falls in very old men is a characteristic of the biological elite whose physical fitness enables them to outlive their former contemporaries.

The single most important cause of falls is tripping which occurs rather more frequently in people age 65–74 than in those aged 75 and over. The frequency of the major causes of falls in elderly women is shown in Table 1.

Table 1
Causes of falls (Females)

Cause	*Age*	
	65–74 ($n = 77$)	75 and over ($n = 113$)
Giddiness	6%	16%
Loss of balance	10%	9%
Drop attacks	14%	12%
Tripping	37%	22%

Drop attacks occur in 12–14% of subjects, and giddiness as a cause of falls increases two-and-a-half fold between the younger and older age group. The pattern of causes of falls is similar in the two sexes, although drop attacks are much less frequent in men. Thus tripping occurs more often in the younger people who in general are more active and therefore more likely to trip. Whereas giddiness has a higher incidence in very old people who usually have changes in the nervous system, including labyrinthine disturbances.

Sheldon (1963) investigated the control of sway in relation to age. The striking feature of his tracings was the number of small movements maintaining the upright posture and these he considered to be of random origin. Sway is marked in childhood; during middle life sway is at a minimum due to the accurate control of movements which is again diminished in old age. He suggested that the investigation of sway might be a promising approach to the study of control of posture in old age and its relationship to falls.

We have carried out such a study relating causes of falls to the control of sway (Overstall *et al.* 1975). Sway was measured in the anterior–posterior direction using the ataxiameter described by Wright (1971). It was found that sway is more marked in women than in men at all ages ($P < 0.01$). It seems likely that the greater sway in women corresponds with their greater liability to sustain falls. When the falls were due to drop attacks or to loss of balance the amount of sway was significantly greater than that occurring in old people of similar age who were not liable to fall (*see* Table 2).

Thus these falls are associated with a decline in the efficiency of physiological mechanisms controlling posture. On the other hand, in

Table 2
Average sway in elderly females

Non-Fallers	*Tripping*	*Drop attacks*	*Giddiness or loss of balance*
3.66	3.69 N.S.●	4.60 $P < 0.01$●	4.73 $P < 0.05$●

●Difference between means compared with "non-fallers"

those old people whose falls are due to tripping the amount of sway was similar to that occurring in old people not liable to fall. The physiological defect is therefore different in tripping and environmental factors may also be of greater importance.

Fractures and Age-Related Disorders of Bone

Apart from accidental hypothermia, fractures constitute the major consequence of falls in the elderly. Not only does the liability to fall increase with age, but there is also an age-related increase in the risk of sustaining a fracture following a fall (*see* Table 3). Each of these liabilities is greater in women than in men.

Table 3
Falls resulting in fractures

	Number with falls	*Number* (%) *sustaining fractures*
Men		
65–74	44	10 (18%)
75 and over	87	26 (30%)
Women		
65–74	77	21 (27%)
75 and over	113	46 (40%)

The incidence of certain fractures increases exponentially with age. Thus after the age of 60 for femoral neck fractures the rates approximately double every 5 years in women and every 7 years in men (Knowelden *et al.* 1964). For the female population the cumulative risk of sustaining a femoral neck fracture by the age of 90 is 25%.

The factors responsible for the age-related increase in fracture rate have been analysed in a series of 384 cases of fracture of the femoral neck investigated by the author in collaboration with Professor J

Brocklehurst in London and Manchester. The two main components were found to be:

1. *An increase in the liability to fall.* Apart from the rise in the incidence of falls with age, which is more marked in women than in men, the fracture series had a higher incidence of falls during the year prior to the fracture compared with the age-matched general population. The difference was most striking in the older age groups; thus for persons aged 85 and over 70.1% of the fracture series had a previous history of falls compared with 45.8% in the control series without fracture ($P < 0.01$).

2. *A decrease in the quantity and quality of bone.* The quantity of bone in the second metacarpal in patients in the femoral neck fracture series was calculated from measurements made on hand radiographs using the technique described by Exton-Smith *et al.* (1969*a*).

When the individual values for the metacarpal cortical ratio in the femoral neck fracture cases were plotted on the percentile ranking curves which have been constructed for the general population (Exton-Smith *et al.* 1969*b*, Gryfe *et al.* 1971) it was found that for both male and female patients the mean values were lower than the corresponding 50th percentiles for the general population. That is, the fracture patients have generally a diminished amount of bone compared with age-matched individuals without fractures. Nevertheless there is a wide scatter of values and many are in the higher percentile ranges.

Newton-John and Morgan (1968) considered that the rising incidence of femoral neck fractures with age could be accounted for on the basis of osteoporosis which they attributed to senescence rather than to disease and to an inferior skeletal status at maturity. From their model of metacarpal bone loss in women they plotted the frequency with which the amount of bone in individuals within the general population fell below a limiting value 2.5 SD below the mean amount of bone at the age of 30. The resultant frequency distribution is an exponential curve which parallels closely the increasing rate of femoral neck fracture with age. Our results, however, do not support this hypothesis since many femoral neck fracture patients have been shown to have a bone mass well above the limiting value. It is therefore unlikely that there is for the whole population a single critical level of bone mass below which fractures will occur. But it is possible that there is a critical level for each individual; the loss of bone occurring immediately after the menopause in women, and the loss due to "aging" and in some cases to pathological processes in both sexes could account for the weakening of the femoral neck compared with its former strength during the period of maximal skeletal development. Longitudinal studies have shown that loss of bone with aging is a universal phenomenon, affecting all individuals (Garn *et al.* 1967, Exton-Smith 1970). Such studies need to be extended by the measurement of quantity of bone at frequent intervals after the age of 40 in order to determine whether people who subsequently develop fractures are those individuals who have lost bone excessively or whether they represent a selected group whose skeletal status in earlier years was inferior to that of the general population. Solomon (1973) concluded that normal healthy individuals, who still manifest the progressive loss of bone with age, seldom develop osteoporosis so profound that it would account for the marked increase in femoral neck fractures with age.

Another important factor in the pathogenesis of fracture of the neck of the femur is an alteration in the quality of bone. Biopsy specimens were obtained from the iliac crest of patients with femoral neck fractures and the histology was compared with that found in specimens from subjects of similar age without fractures. Estimation of the amount of osteoid by an automated image analysis technique (Quantimet) showed that the mean value for the trabecular osteoid area in the fracture group was 4.0% compared with 1.0% in the control group (Faccini *et al.* 1976). Measurement by the use of the eyepiece graticule stereological method of the proportion of trabecular surface covered by osteoid also revealed a striking difference; the mean value for the fracture group was 24.5% compared with 7.9% for the control group. These findings are in agreement with those of the investigators in Leeds (Aaron, Gallagher, Anderson, Stasiak, Longton, Nordin and Nicholson 1974) who found histological evidence of osteomalacia in one-third of their patients with femoral neck fractures. The rising incidence of osteomalacia with age has been attributed to many factors: a fall in the dietary intake of vitamin D (Exton-Smith 1971), a reduction in exposure to sunlight (Stamp and Round 1974), an increase in physiological requirement for vitamin D (Dent 1970) and impaired conversion of 25 hydroxycholecalciferol to the active 1,25-dihydroxycholecalciferol due to decline in renal function in old age (Fraser and Kodicek 1970, Lund *et al.* 1975). The etiology is often multifactorial, but the major contribution of exposure to sunlight has been shown by the seasonal variation in the serum 25-hydroxycholecalciferol levels which correlated with exposure to sunlight as measured by a "sunshine score" (Stephen and Dattani 1976) and by the seasonal change in the proportion of osteoid covered surface in patients with femoral neck fractures (Aaron, Gallagher and Nordin 1974).

Conclusions

The relationships between clinical manifestations and decline in physiological function due to aging in the systems we have discussed can be compared:

(1) The thermoregulatory system is involved in the process of aging like other bodily systems and there is a reduced efficiency in response to cold and thermal stimuli. These physiological

disturbances are extremely common in old people and those individuals with more serious degrees of autonomic dysfunction are likely to respond to even moderate cold stress by a fall in deep body temperature.

(2) Impairment of physiological mechanisms maintaining postural balance can be demonstrated by an increase in sway with age and is related to an increased liability to fall. Pathological changes in the nervous system further impair postural balance in subjects with falls due to certain causes, e.g. drop attacks.

(3) Loss of bone with age is a universal phenomenon affecting all individuals after maturity. It is unlikely that this factor alone can account for the rising incidence of osteoporosis and of certain fractures with age. In nearly all instances pathological processes leading to an accelerated rate of bone loss or to an alteration in the quality of bone contribute to skeletal failure.

Thus in each of the examples considered aging exerts a variable contribution to the decline in physiological functions which lead to clinical manifestations. In each case decline in function cannot usually be identified by medical examination alone and often impaired homeostasis (for example in thermoregulation) can only be demonstrated by measuring physiological performances when systems are subjected to stressful stimuli.

Much of our present knowledge on aging in bodily systems is based on cross-sectional studies in which physiological performances in groups of individuals of different ages are compared. Longitudinal studies are required, to differentiate the decline in function due to physiological aging from that associated with disease and for the investigation of the differential rates of aging in various bodily systems. Moreover such studies are essential to determine whether our fate in old age is related to environmental influences or to the levels of physiological performance in childhood and adult life.

References

Aaron, J. E., Gallagher, J. C., Anderson, J., Stasiak, L., Longton, E. B., Nordin, B. E. C. and Nicholson, M. (1974). *Lancet* **i**, 229

Aaron, J. E., Gallagher, J. C. and Nordin, B. E. C. (1974). *Lancet* **ii**, 84

Bull, G. M. (1969). *Gerontologia clinica* **11**, 193

Bull, G. M. and Morton, J. (1975*a*). *Age and Ageing* **4**, 19

Bull, G. M. and Morton, J. (1975*b*). *Age and Ageing* **4**, 232

Caird, F. I., Andrews, G. I. and Kennedy, R. D. (1973). *British Heart Journal* **35**, 527

Cowburn, E. J. and Fox, R. H. (1974). *Journal of Physiology* **239**, 77P

Dent, C. E. (1970). *Proceedings of the Royal Society of Medicine* **63**, 401

Duguid, H., Simpson, R. G. and Stowers, J. M. (1961). *Lancet* **ii**, 1213

Ellis, F. P. (1972). *Environmental Research* **5**, 1

Ellis, F. P., Nelson, F. and Pincus, L. (1975). *Environmental Research* **10**, 1
Exton-Smith, A. N. (1970). *Experimental Gerontology* **5**, 273
Exton-Smith, A. N. (1971). *British Journal of Hospital Medicine* **5**, 639
Exton-Smith, A. N., Millard, P. H., Payne, P. R. and Wheeler, E. F. (1969*a*). *Lancet* **ii**, 1153
Exton-Smith, A. N., Millard, P. H., Payne, P. R. and Wheeler, E. F. (1969*b*). *Lancet* **ii**, 1154
Faccini, J. M., Exton-Smith, A. N. and Boyde, A. (1976). *Lancet* **i**, 1089
Foster, K. G., Ellis, F. P., Doré, C., Exton-Smith, A. N. and Weiner, J. S. (1976). *Age and Ageing* **5**, 91
Fox, R. H., Hackett, A. J. and Turk, J. (1967). *Journal of Physiology* **194**, 55P
Fox, R. H., Woodward, P. M., Exton-Smith, A. N., Green, M. R., Donnison, D. V. and Wicks, M. H. (1973). *British Medical Journal* **i**, 200
Fox, R. H., Woodward, P. M., Fry, A. J., Collins, J. C. and MacDonald, I. C. (1971). *Lancet* **i**, 424
Fraser, D. R. and Kodicek, E. (1970). *Nature (London)* **288**, 764
Garn, S. M., Rohmann, C. G. and Wagner, B. (1967). *Federation Proceedings* **26**, 1729
Goldman, A., Exton-Smith, A. N., Francis, G. and O'Brien, A. (1977). *Journal of the Royal College of Physicians* (in press)
Gryfe, C. I., Exton-Smith, A. N., Payne, P. R. and Wheeler, E. F. (1971). *Lancet* **i**, 523
Johnson, R. H., Crampton-Smith, A., Spalding, J. M. K. and Wollner, L. (1965). *Lancet* **i**, 731
Knowelden, J., Buhr, A. J. and Dunbar, O. (1964). *British Journal of Preventive and Social Medicine* **18**, 130
Lund, B., Hjorth, L., Kjaer, I., Reimann, I., Friss, T., Anderson, R. B. and Sorenson, O. H. (1975). *Lancet* **ii**, 1168
Macpherson, R. K., Ofner, F. and Welch, J. A. (1967). *British Journal of Preventive and Social Medicine* **21**, 17
Newton-John, H. F. and Morgan, D. B. (1968). *Lancet* **i**, 232
Overstall, P., Imms, F., Exton-Smith, A. N. and Thornton, C. (1975). Paper given to the British Geriatrics Society, London
Rodstein, M. and Zeman, F. D. (1957). *Journal of Chronic Diseases* **6**, 581
Rosin, A. J. and Exton-Smith, A. N. (1964). *British Medical Journal* **i**, 16
Royal College of Physicians (1966). Report of Committee on Accidental Hypothermia, London
Sheldon, J. H. (1948). "The Social Medicine of Old Age". Nuffield Foundation, London
Sheldon, J. H. (1960). *British Medical Journal* **ii**, 1685
Sheldon, J. H. (1963). *Gerontologia clinica* **3**, 129
Solomon, L. (1973). *South African Journal of Surgery* **11**, 269
Stamp, T. C. B. and Round, J. M. (1974). *Nature (London)* **274**, 563
Stephen, J. M. L. and Dattani, J. (1976). *Transactions of the Royal Society of Tropical Medicine and Hygiene* **70**, 278
Wright, B. M. (1971). *Journal of Physiology* **218**, 27

Discussion

Dr Hamburg We will open this afternoon Session with discussion by any of the participants on the papers presented this morning.

Dr Alexander Bearn (New York) As people are still assembling, I wonder whether I could ask a rather trivial question. I was very interested in whether male sperm move more rapidly than female. I know this is often stated in textbooks, and I was just wondering how robust the data were and whether this referred to animals other than man.

Dr Busse I can very much appreciate his concern about this, because I too am aware that the literature reports really quite different information. I simply took what I thought was the consensus of the people that work in the same medical school that I am in. They confirmed their belief that the sperm speed is different, as is the shape of the head, which you are probably quite cognizant of. There are some who say that the male sperm has a sharper head, while the female has a round head, which is supposed to have something to do with penetration.

Dr Monica Blumenthal (University of Michigan) I just wanted to comment about how budgets for old people are calculated. In American policy, the notion prevails that two people require more money than one person. For older people, who are often somewhat disabled, what is not counted in the budgets at all is the value of household work and personal services. But it may turn out that people living in pairs have a proper sort of fit between disabilities; one person can do something for the other person and the favor can be returned. If one member in that pair disappears, somebody else has to provide that service. That isn't added into the budget in any kind of way, and I contend it may be entirely possible that it takes considerably more money for one person to exist than for two people. It would like to hear a few comments about that.

Mr Ball The point is absolutely correct about the backup arrangements that two people can work out. I have seen some very touching situations of two elderly people, husband and wife, whose disabilities do fit and it works extremely well. One of the most disturbing things about the greater longevity of women is the fact that at the upper ages such a high proportion are widows.

It has seemed to me that the Social Security formula of giving a couple one-and-a-half times that given to the single worker is undoubtedly too high, even without regard to talking about those with disability or very advanced age. My own view is that about one-and-a-third might be a better ratio — and I rush on to add that I am not for reducing what the couple gets as a proportion of earnings. I would propose holding the replacement rate to wages for the couple where it is today; you could do that by dropping the ratio from one-and-a-half to one-and-a-third and at the same time raising the benefits for the worker by 12½%. That would increase the money going to single workers, particularly single women workers and widows, who are the worst off. It also would add greatly to the equity of the program by giving more to a couple, both of whom work, as compared with the amount given when only one member of the couple works.

I took the opportunity of a question to go on to some other things that I wanted to comment on.

Mr Nelson Cruikshank (National Council of Senior Citizens) Mention the type of Consumer Price Index for older people that is being worked on.

Mr Ball I am not sure how it will come out, but there is work going on to determine whether elderly people and poor people are being short-changed by the use of the general CPI. The question is whether benefits tied to a CPI that is applicable to the whole population, which is now the case, is the best way to automatically keep up Social Security and income tested benefits, or whether a specially designed index would be more accurate in reflecting the actual market basket for older people and poor people.

Ms Hannah Lipsky (Mt Sinai Hospital Medical Center) I have a question for Mr Ball. It has to do with the health problems of the aged poor, which I think are really just an inherited problem from being poor all along. I thought there was a notable lack of comment here about a national health program that would cover the total age spectrum and would then perhaps counteract any generation problem.

Mr Ball I am personally strongly in favor of a comprehensive national health insurance program. But I don't believe it is desirable to wait for that before moving ahead to improve the national health insurance program that we have. I would reluctantly have to guess that we are five years away from an operating comprehensive national health insurance system. When a new administration comes into office, it takes from a year to two years to develop the specific legislation to be presented to the Congress and a year or two to pass it in both houses, and a couple of years to implement it. I did not mean to imply, by emphasizing what I think ought to be done in Medicare, that I wasn't even more in favor of a general comprehensive plan.

I am for moving right ahead and trying to make Medicare closer to a model that we could use for general health insurance and fix up some of the things about it that are really quite bad; particularly the supplementary program.

Dr Robin Bennett (Pasadena, California) May I ask one question, sir? I am one of the aged, you know, and I came all the way, 3000 miles, to learn something about keeping my life longer, extending it. I am amazed at your optimism, sir, that in the year 2005, the elderly would have more equity in living, when we hear so often, that the Social Security service will be bankrupt in 1985 or something like that. Please address yourself to that.

Mr Ball I guess that does have a lot to do with the health of the elderly, too, so it is very pertinent to this. Let me just say categorically, first, before I expand a little, that the system is certainly not bankrupt in the sense of there being any doubt that it will pay off the benefits that have been promised. On the other hand, the Social Security system will need more income than is provided by the contribution rates in present law. You do not have to take my word for it, obviously, but just think of what is involved. Would a congressman repudiate the pledges that have been made to all his constituents? Everybody, practically, is under the program. And if you can think of one congressman doing it, can you think of a majority doing it? No. The money will be provided.

Between now and the end of the century, the problem is quite easily manageable in traditional terms. The system needs 10 to 15% more income than present law provides. That is the equivalent of a little over 1% of payroll. It could be handled by about a 0.6 increase on the employee and a like amount on the employer. I don't want to do it that way, personally. I am for raising the earnings base. But all I am saying is it could be done within the traditional self-financed system.

In the next century there is a potential problem of an increased number of the elderly relative to those of normal working age, but I very much believe that we will be helped by two possibilities. One is almost a certainty: a much greater proportion of women working, more paying in as compared with taking out. The other possibility, which I think we have to really think about, is to have more elderly people participating in work. They should have the choice, and many certainly will want to work beyond 60 and beyond 65. To the extent that they do, that means more paying in and less paying out.

Should there develop in the next century a problem because of an increasing proportion of aged — the number of aged is quite certain to increase, but the proportion depends on future fertility rates — we need to think about more older people working. If we don't have enough working, then personally I would favor at that point the introduction of some general revenue financing into Social Security on the rationale that out of general revenue's more progressive taxation you would pay for some of the social aspects of the program; the weighted benefit formula, the fact that those with dependents get more for their money, and that sort of thing.

Dr Pearl German (Johns Hopkins University) I would be eager for Professor Exton-Smith's opinion. In some of the studies that we have been doing on delivery of ambulatory health care to the elderly, we have been particularly interested in the potential for health education among this population. I was wondering if Professor Exton-Smith's experience makes him believe that the elderly would be amenable to programs aimed directly at them rather than having their environment manipulated.

Professor Exton-Smith Yes, I am quite sure that in some of these areas one could do a lot to prevent some of the increase in morbidity and mortality to which I have referred. This applies perhaps particularly to falls, and as we have heard, the problem of impaired dark adaptation leads to an increase in the rate of falling at night. If one can make elderly people aware of the difficulties, I think one could prevent many of the falls which occur at night. But in the case of fractures, it is often too late by the time people reach old age to prevent a greater risk of fracturing of bone because of the reduced strength of bone. There may be an opportunity of trying to prevent Colles' fracture, with a peak incidence between 40 and 60, in post-menopausal women by estrogen administration. There are some quite encouraging effects of this in experiments done in the United States and in our own country. It would take rather longer to see if this therapeutic regime had any effect on fractured neck of the femur, which only begins to rise in incidence about the age of 60 onwards.

There are some encouraging results from experiments on improving nutrition in elderly people by means of talks given at Clubs and Day Centres. Similar measures might be used in informing old people about the risks of hypothermia in winter. The importance of adequate heating of corridors and bedrooms, especially on the top floor of the dwelling, should be emphasized and there is a need for more information on fuel allowance to which many old people are entitled but do not claim. In some cases it would be necessary for health visitors and social workers to visit the houses of elderly individuals who are especially at risk on account of physical frailty and social isolation.

Mental Health Problems: United States and United Kingdom

Mental Health Problems in the Aged

Carl Eisdorfer
Department of Psychiatry and Behavioral Sciences, University of Washington, Seattle

There seems relatively little disagreement that to deal effectively with problems it is valuable to start from a valid base of knowledge. Since the data base in mental health, certainly no less than in any other aspects of health, is often characterized by the substitution of idiom for ideas and demagoguery for data, it has been a matter of some controversy as to whether we should invest our resources in efforts to deliver more services to people or spend more time to understand the problem in order to improve the quality of services to be delivered. Certainly some balance between these strategies is in order. The good news is that the knowledge base in psychiatry and behavioral sciences has been increasing quite profoundly over the past several decades and aspects of this improved understanding have specific relevance to older persons.

The mythology of aging has carried with it the stereotype of the helpless, hopeless, incompetent and dependent oldster. Among the various problems cognitive loss has been a significant concern in aging (Botwinick and Storandt 1974), yet a life span developmental psychology is emerging with far improved conceptualization and models of data analysis. Cross-sectional research models which yielded spurious patterns of decline and deterioration have given way to paradigms of longitudinal and cross-sequential research which give us much greater insight into the focal areas characterized by life long stability, as well as highlighting those areas of decline (Jarvik *et al.* 1973). Such broad concepts as intelligence and cognition in the aged are being redefined in the light of new data and more precise concepts such as crystallized and fluid intelligence are emerging. Associated processes are being related to the activity of dominant and non-dominant cerebral hemispheres which at least potentially can be studied separately. Improved understanding of patterns of response and learning strategies in older cohorts have brought with them conjectures about educational interventions (Labouvie-Vief and Gonda 1976) for improved performance as well as retention in the verbal as well as non-verbal spheres. All of these bring with them the hope of significant new therapeutic modes for preventing or coping with at least some of the problems of cognitive change as these relate to the mental health of the aged.

Personality change in aging is a well accepted belief, yet the last decade has also witnessed recognition of the need for a theory of life span personality development to contrast with theories which focus almost exclusively on the preadolescent state. If, as now seems clear, learning persists into advancing years, and physical as well as social environments change, then the adapting human is making shifts to accommodate to such changes. In fact, the research of Lowenthal (1975), Neugarten (1972) and others is addressing these issues. While the infants and the young have perhaps the most to learn about the world, and certainly the most rapid somatic changes with which to cope, analogies between the aged and adolescent periods of life, so far as accelerated physical, environmental and social change rates are involved, are valid to contemplate. Expectations and role changes among the aged are mediated by predictable events such as retirement, but also by "accidental" or non-planned stressors such as the death of loved ones and the acute onset of physical disease (Eisdorfer and Wilkie 1976).

Losses are in the main traumatic and lead to predictable consequences such as grief, sadness and, in many cases, depression. For children significant personal losses can be quite devastating, leading them to long term, maladaptive coping styles, as well as to residual affective change (Bowlby 1973). For older persons who have a history of successfully coping with such events, anticipated or "on time" losses may be of less permanent consequence (Neugarten 1972), but we have yet to assess the impact of persistent or accumulated multiple losses (Eisdorfer and Wilkie 1976). In recent months a patient was reported to me with "a shoulder syndrome" which was necessitating that he leave his well-loved home and children in the northwest to retire in Florida. The syndrome was not an orthopedic one, but rather was consequent on his having served as pallbearer to 17 of his friends and relatives over a period of less than two years. His reaction was to withdraw physically from a situation with which he felt unable to cope at close range. We have reason to believe that the older individual remains quite plastic, but exactly how adaptive can someone be in the 7th or

8th decade of life, particularly as this involves making new relationships and dealing with grief at a time of limited physical, economic and perhaps social resources. Is depletion of energy a cause or an effect of psychological rigidity where it occurs?

The impact of lengthening leisure time on more complex social patterns as they emerge is being assayed but the work ethic is still strong among our aged cohort who consequently need to feel useful and to have a sense of personal worth.

A new problem may be emerging as successive cohorts of aged are involved in divorce and multiple marriages, including remarriages in later life, with the consequent complications of parent–child or –stepchild interactions. Much more careful scrutiny of family patterns in aging is needed. For the practitioner, such pragmatic issues as the impact on parents and children of parental remarriage in late life, interpersonal crises around potential redistribution of inheritance and even such things as choice of grave site could lead to significant interpersonal consequences easily rivaling those of the decision to institutionalize or not to institutionalize an aged parent.

Friends and families are among the most significant mental health resources and those without a family or confidante are at heightened risk for mental health problems and institutionalization (Lowenthal 1975; Gottesman and Brody 1975).

Labeling and role theory bring the hope of improving our understanding of later personality in the adapted as well as the maladapted older person, particularly as we appreciate more concerning expectancies and attitudes of young and old toward old age. The aged have more negative attitudes toward older persons and the concept of being superfluous is a source of concern (Eisdorfer 1975). A knowledge of physical environmental impact on behavior, particularly in institutional settings, is also emerging from the laboratory. Environmental barriers which constrict behavior and result in reduction of sensory or social contact may also yield problems, as does change in the neighborhood over time (Rosow 1967).

To shift from the behavioral to the more biological, it should be appreciated that over the past decade or two, advances in neuroanatomy and psychopharmacology have become of considerable potential import to mental health care. Anatomically our improved understanding of the basis for most Senile Dementia, now felt to be primary neuronal degeneration of the Alzheimer's variant, suggests the relevance of a disease model for certain aspects of true cognitive loss. We are also distinguishing between vascular and non-vascular dementia when possible, and defining other causes of cognitive change, particularly acute brain syndromes and clinical depression which may present as pseudodementia (Libow 1973). The important interaction between physical and behavioral manifestations of disease in the elderly constitutes a particular problem. Too often older patients may be poorly evaluated and the metabolic basis of behavioral disturbance, or the psychological basis of apparent medical difficulty overlooked.

Advances in pharmacokinetics have brought a variety of new insights into metabolism as well as an improved technology for studying serum or red cell levels of drugs and sensitivity to drug effects. In the clinical field, particularly through advances in anti-depressant medication, we have improved our potential for dealing with some segments of the most prevalent mental health problem manifested by older persons (Gurland 1976). Most psychopharmacologic research is still done on young subjects and in most instances the pharmacokinetics of individual agents in older persons have yet to be worked out. Altered protein to fat or water balance, absorption difficulties, reduced or increased receptor sensitivity, long-term adaptation or hyper-reactivity to drugs, as well as tissue destruction, are age-related phenomena which create challenging problems, over and above the issue of drug interactions and effects on concurrent diseases or conditions.

Considerable criticism of many of the existing clinical psychological tests of older persons has emerged (Eisdorfer 1969). It is clear that in parallel with the developments in cognitive and personality structure, we need a more definitive clinical psychology and psychiatry of aging. This is on the horizon and portends improved measurement and screening for the practitioner.

In summary, there is considerable reason to believe that the past few decades have brought with them an improved data base in aging and mental health and the promise of more definitive information to come. We now know too that subsets or combinations of behavioral, interpersonal, environmental and biological therapies are effective in dealing with mental health problems of aging and there is reason for optimism in dealing with problems in many instances previously felt to be intractable. Indeed, we may even be able to think in terms of preventing certain aspects of decline and of changing the course of behavior by improved socialization, and changes in expectancy and opportunities of the aged, as well as improved physical care of the individual. In a recent review (Eisdorfer and Stotsky 1975) the range of effective therapies was impressive.

So much for the good news.

The problems in mental health service delivery in the US are well documented. We are all aware of the profound demographic changes which have occurred this century. Concurrent with the two-and-a-half fold increase in the population of the United States since the year 1900, we have seen a roughly seven-fold increase in the number of persons aged over 65. Older Americans now number approximately 21 million and the projections are for the proportion and number of aged to continue to increase, so that by the turn of the century, between 12 and 13% of the population or approximately 29 million Americans will be aged 65 and older. Of more consequence to me is the even more rapid relative population increase in persons aged 75 and older, for whom data indicate the greatest risks of psychiatric disability (Kay 1972; Dohrenwend and Dohrenwend 1969).

In view of the rather dramatic recent changes in the delivery of mental health services in the US generally, service delivery to the aged has to be appreciated in historic context. If we look at the data between 1955 and 1968, it is quite clear that the risk for psychiatric institutional care increased monotonically with age past adolescence. In 1955, the resident patient rate in State and County mental hospitals in the US was 246 per 100 000 population for those aged 25–34 and 1419.8 per 100 000 for those 75 and above. By 1968, the rates had approximately halved for each group, 157.8 per 100 000 at age 25–34, 734.9 per 100 000 at age 75 and over. For rate of first admission reflecting so-called new or newly identified disorders, again the aged showed the highest rate in 1962, although the curve in this case is not monotonic (Kramer *et al.* 1973).

It should be recognized, however, that the drop in psychiatric inpatient care episodes in State and County hospitals was associated with a substantial increase in the total number of other types of patient care episodes. For the young and adults, this meant that more and more care was being delivered in general hospitals in the community and in the community mental health centers. There is a clear age patterning, however. Outpatient clinics provide services predominantly to persons under 35 years of age and mental hospitals to persons 35 years and older. High rates of patient care episodes in mental hospitals for the oldest age group were attributable to two factors, the large number of patients in the population who had grown old in hospital, and high admission rates for mental disorders of older age.

Between 1962 and 1969 alone, the rate of first admissions to State and County mental hospitals in the United States, among the aged, dropped more than 30%. During this period there was no substantial change in rate of first admissions for other population groups. These trends are continuing and superficially this appears to be a good sign. It is important to note, however, that during this period of declining enrollment in State hospitals, there has been a substantial increase in nursing home beds in the United States. This trend, which may be largely a US phenomenon, has resulted in a current bed capacity of over 1.2 million units, 90% of which are occupied by persons over age 65. It is important to note that approximately 25 to 30% of these patients are estimated to be primarily psychiatric patients, although there is much data to support the contention that a majority of patients have significant psychiatric problems and estimates of beyond 80% have also been made (Special Committee on Aging 1975). The current estimate (Levine and Willner 1976), is that expenditures for direct mental health care in nursing homes exceeded 4.2 billions of dollars in 1974. During this period of time community-based mental health care contributed 2% of its services to the aged, although community mental health centers reportedly provided as much as 4% of their services to the aged. In a recent estimate of the persons in need of services, for all ages and including those 65 years and over, projections by the National Institutes of Mental Health indicate that between 80–85% of those aged persons needing services will not receive services by 1980 (Kramer *et al.* 1973). In this regard, however, it should be noted that in the most recent change in legislation, community mental health centers which are federally funded are now obligated to provide services to the aged as well as to children. The impact of this new regulation is not yet known, but there is clearly much more activity going on in community mental health centers at this time.

In long-term care, the role of mental health services has been minimal and at least one study (Epstein and Simon 1968) would indicate that patients fared better in the State hospital environment than in nursing homes. The emphasis in nursing homes has traditionally been on custodial care or drug therapies. This is not surprising in view of the lack of expertise in psychiatry and psychology, psychiatric nursing and social work which characterized most such facilities (Special Committee on Aging 1975) and the fact that historically most of these institutions emerged from a custodial care rather than a health-oriented or therapeutic tradition.

There are some bright signs on the horizon. Recent emphasis on the creation of day care facilities and the provision of community-based services for the aged in collaboration with mental health centers carry the promise of re-orienting the current pattern of mental health care. Indeed, some long-term care institutions are attempting to develop improved alternatives within the institution.

Attempts to improve the provision of mental health care to the aged, however, appear to be fraught with some difficulties which I will briefly review with you in the hope that by understanding these barriers we may be able to develop improved methods for achieving our goals. At the outset I would contend that at this time we have in the United States a number of problems in delivering mental health services. One of the most impressive is a professional versus social dilemma involving tolerance of deviance versus early intervention in aberrant behavior. The right to treatment which has become a salient legal issue subsumes the right to refuse treatment and only apparent danger to oneself or others constitutes a basis for legally compulsory intervention. A second issue of consequence resides in the geographic locus of the problem. Aged individuals may be adapted at home but in an acute medical setting where they may be cared for at a time of crisis, they will exhibit behavior felt to require custodial management. The reverse of this is also an issue in that there is a hidden population of aged who could profit from care, but who are not ambulatory, are poor, frail and under-use community facilities. Extensive outreach programming might identify these people and bring them into treatment. Improving mental health care of the aged brings with it some additional special problems. As indicated earlier, we still have a relatively poor data base, with a paucity of clinical guidelines and inadequate norms for most clinical psychological tests. Thus practitioners tend to be shy of becoming involved. Furthermore, our professions too have had a bias. We have postulated the drying up of energy, the inability to teach older persons, and the poor therapeutic risk of the aged. This therapeutic nihilism also involved us in the conception that all of the aged had incurable brain damage and we focused more on pathology than upon individual adaptive capacity.

The multiple problems of older persons, typically a mixture of physical and psychological as well as social-environmental problems, are a challenge often obligating us to go beyond single professional boundaries. This, of course, leads to one of the more complicated problems in service delivery, that is, who owns the patient? We run into narrow professional rivalries, and perhaps of more difficulty, we exhibit quite different conceptualizations of "the problem". Society at large has not been of much help. Quite the contrary, the old are often seen as superfluous, with a life expectancy that is too short for therapeutic investment. Older people do not seem pretty to our youth-oriented culture and the conception that all older people are brain damaged, impotent and incompetent does not induce much enthusiasm for professional involvement. In the end, we often find ourselves pitting the needs of the aged against the "investment" in children and it becomes a political ploy to play the interest of one group off against the other. Older people typically do not like the stigma of mental health care, nor do they like mental health professionals. This response is, of course, often reciprocated, particularly since most mental health professionals have had relatively little experience in dealing with aged patients except for brief diagnostic interviews. There are many primary care physicians who do not like to send their patients to mental health professionals, and the children of the older patients, now playing the role of the parent-surrogate, have little enthusiasm for labeling their elderly mother or father as having some deviant psychologic process.

As we know, dealing with death and the dying person have been difficult for health professionals. The aged are closer to death than the young, and perhaps this creates an aura which keeps us away.

In this conception there are some consequences such as a poor understanding of the nature of the aging process and what declines are to be expected and what are pathologic. The training of health care professionals and mental health professionals comes in for much fault in this regard. In this regard, too, the aged certainly accept as "normal" a goodly amount of what we would label pathology. We have a bias toward acute care and cure and this complicates our attitudes toward all long-term illness, certainly toward much of the illness exhibited by the aged. "Rehabilitating" does not have quite the same status as "therapizing."

In closing, we do have good news and bad news. Gerontology, now only about three decades old as a defined science in much of the world, recognizes that aging is the end result of a bio-psycho-social process which has genetic and physical-environmental limitations. The improved data base and increasing concern with the somatic psychological and social integrity of individuals is beginning to give us a clearer understanding of the adaptational difficulties and assets in aging. What many of us believe and needs to be said, is that the health and mental health of the nation will never be any better than the care we provide to the most deprived constituency. Since most of us are striving enthusiastically to join the distinguished group of people we call the aged, in a sense we are only working for ourselves.

The dramatic changes in demography we are currently witnessing are primarily the result of improving survival in early life. In the US life expectancy at birth has increased by approximately 20 years during this century but during this same 75-year period, life expectancy at age 65 has changed by only slightly over two years (Siegel 1975). An increased life span for older persons, given the current state of knowledge and system of care, would be at best a mixed blessing. The challenge is great. We can afford to waste little time in meeting it.

References

Bowlby, J. (1973). "Attachment and Loss". Vol. 2: "Separation, Anxiety and Anger". Hogarth Press and the Institute of Psycho-analysis, London

Botwinick, J. and Storandt, M. (1974). "Memory, Related Functions and Age". Charles C. Thomas, Springfield, Ill.

Dohrenwend, B. P. and Dohrenwend, B. S. (1969). "Social Status and Psychological Disorder: A Causal Inquiry." Wiley, New York

Eisdorfer, C. (1969). *In* "Behaviour and Adaptation in Later Life." Eds. E. W. Busse and E. Pfeiffer. Little Brown, Boston: pp 327–350

Eisdorfer, C. (1975). *The Centre Magazine* 8, 2, 12–19

Eisdorfer, C. and Stotsky, B. A. (1976). *In* "Handbook of the Psychology of Aging". Eds. J. Birren and W. Schaie. Van Nostrand Reinhold, New York (in press)

Eisdorfer, C. and Wilkie, F. (1976). *In* "Handbook of the Psychology of Aging". Eds. J. Birren and W. Schaie. Van Nostrand Reinhold, New York (in press)

Epstein, L. and Simon, A. (1968). *American Journal of Psychiatry* **124**, 955–961

Gottesman, L. and Brody, E. (1975). *In* "Long-term Care: A Handbook for Researchers, Planners and Providers". Ed. S. Sherwood. Spectrum, New York: pp 455–510

Gurland, B. J. (1976). *Journal of Gerontology* **31**, 283–292

Jarvik, L., Eisdorfer, C. and Blum, J. (Eds.) (1973). "Intellectual Functioning in Adults." Springer, New York

Kay, D. W. K. (1972). *In* "Aging and the Brain: Advances in Behavioural Biology". Vol. 3. Ed. C. M. Gaitz. Plenum, New York: pp 15–27

Kramer, M., Taube, C. A. and Redick, R. W. (1973). *In* "The Psychology of Adult Development and Aging". Eds. C. Eisdorfer and M. P. Lawton. American Psychological Association, Washington, DC: pp 428–509

Labouvie-Vief, G. and Gonda, J. N. (1976). *Journal of Gerontology* **31**, 327–332

Levine, D. S. and Willner, S. G. (1976). "The Cost of Mental Illness 1974." Mental Health Statistical Note No. 125. DHEW Publication No. (ADM) 76–158; pp 1–7

Libow, L. S. (1973). *Journal of the American Geriatrics Society* **21**, 112

Lowenthal, M. F. (1975). *Gerontologist* **15**, 6–12

Neugarten, B. L. (1972). *Gerontologist* **12**, 9–15

Rosow, I. (1967). "Social Integration of the Aged." Free Press, New York

Siegel, J. S. (1975). *In* "Epidemiology of Aging". Eds. H. Ostfeld and D. C. Gibson. DHEW Publication No. (NIH) 75–711; pp 17–82

Special Committee on Aging (1975). Nursing Homes in the US: Failure in Public Policy, Introductory Report. US Senate, Washington DC

Issues in the Psychiatric Care of the Elderly

Tom Arie
Goodmayes Hospital,
Ilford, London

Old people with mental disorders, and particularly brain failure, are top consumers of health and social services in all developed countries (World Health Organization 1972). This paper is about "the psychogeriatric problem", its size, shape and composition, the issues which it raises, and some of the approaches which are being made, or which could be made, towards meeting more effectively the needs of these old people — and scarcely less important, of those who look after them.

The psychiatry of old age stands in the setting of social and demographic change which Margot Jefferys has set out for us this morning. In summary, since the turn of the century people aged 65 years and over in England and Wales have increased from 1 in 20 of the population to 1 in 7. They include the great cohort of late Victorian births, and their numbers will continue to rise for more than a decade. Among them it is the very old that are at the centre of our problem, and it is they whose numbers have increased most rapidly, and will continue to increase when the increase of the elderly as a whole has levelled off; most of them are women. The over 75s are now more than 35% of all old people, and by the end of the century they will be nearly 45%.

A falling birth rate will increase still further the proportion of the population which is elderly, and if the attack on killing diseases of middle age achieves much success there will be still more old people. The consequences for society and for health services in particular derive both from the increased numbers and the increased proportion; more and more old people, now the largest group of the poor in our country (Atkinson 1973, Office of Population Censuses and Surveys 1973), are supported by relatively fewer workers. The fact that more middle-aged married women are going out to work (Central Statistical Office 1974) has helped to expand the pool of workers, but obviously this is a two-edged development in regard to the care of the elderly.

Issues of the status and integration of the elderly in modern industrial societies are matters which others will discuss (Shanas *et al.* 1968). Of particular relevance for health services is that these old people and, much more so, their families have greatly increased expectations of well-being, and at the same time medicine has a much greater capacity to help them, and not least in the field of mental disorders.

And yet only 5.7% of old people in England and Wales are in institutional care or other "non-private households" — and this figure from the 1971 Census includes people who are only temporarily in hospital; the proportion rises steadily with age to around 15% in the over 80s. Of those who are not in private households around one half are in hospitals, and of those who are in hospitals one third are in psychiatric units. The lines of division between these sectors of care are ones which give rise to almost as many questions as the line of division between domiciliary and institutional care itself.

The 2.6% of the elderly who are in hospitals account for approximately one half of all beds in British hospitals (Department of Health and Social Security (DHSS) 1973, 1974). A consequence of the contrast between the relatively tiny proportion of old people who are in institutional care, and the fact that the elderly are the main users of institutional care of almost every sort, is that the relationship between those in hospitals or residential care and those at home is one of high-ratio gearing; a shift in the direction of institutional care such as may have little effect on the overall number of old people remaining at home could generate tremendous pressures and could easily bring the institutional sector to its knees. Considerations such as this underlie the friction, anxiety and buck-passing which is so common in the care of the elderly; psychiatrists, long accustomed to thinking in terms of psychodynamics, need, I think, to add another dimension to their explanations of human behaviour by considering the figures that underlie it, or what one might call the "arithmodynamics".

Epidemiology of Mental Disorders in Old Age

In the 1960s the prevalence of dementia in old people living at home in Newcastle (where of course the bulk of British epidemiological work in this field has been done) was 6.2%, a figure which excluded "mild" cases; the prevalence rose to over 20% in the very old (Kay *et al.* 1964*a*, Kay *et al.* 1970). Six out of seven of the demented live at home, and yet dementia is the prime determinant of breakdown leading to institutional care. When two cohorts of old people living at home in Newcastle were followed up over 2½ to 4 years, the demented proved to have been by far the heaviest users of hospitals and residential homes. By comparison with a matched group of "normal" patients, the demented were 2½ times as likely to be admitted to hospitals or homes, and their aggregate stay was four times as long in hospital and ten times as long in homes — despite their much shorter life expectation. Successive surveys of old people in communal residential homes reveal dementia in about one half (Kay *et al.* 1962, Carstairs and Morrison 1971, DHSS 1976), and growing pressure by an ageing population on such accommodation means that priority will more and more have to go to those with failing brains.

In this there is one of the now familiar vicious circles of social medicine — Tudor Hart has called it "The Inverse Care Law" (Hart 1971). For whilst dementia is the disability most likely to lead to breakdown, it is also the condition least often known to exist by general practitioners: Williamson and his colleagues found in Edinburgh that 80% of old people with moderate or severe dementia who were living at home were unknown by their doctors to be demented (Williamson *et al.* 1964). The establishment of routine programmes of surveillance is thus high among the priorities in this field; the logistics are manageable, and the key staff need not of course be doctors (Harwin 1973). In the absence of such programmes it is little wonder that dementia presents to caring services largely as a series of crises.

The functional disorders of old age offer rewarding therapeutic opportunities with outcomes often comparable with the most gratifying in medicine. In Newcastle around 12% of old people had neurotic or character disorders and a further 2% or so had major functional psychoses. Of the affective and neurotic group some 40% were severe, and in 5% they had arisen for the first time in late life (Kay *et al.* 1964*a*).

Suicide, which becomes more common with increasing age, is a particular hazard; in the elderly it is mostly due to depression, a highly treatable disorder (Post 1972) and one which in the elderly carries a much higher risk of suicide than in younger people (Barraclough 1971).

The Newcastle data suggest a prevalence of hardcore psychiatric morbidity, most of it "functional", of some 25% among the elderly living at home. Yet referral to psychiatrists for neurotic disorder shows a rapid falling-off after middle age, despite the fact that the rate at which people consult their family doctors for such problems remains remarkably steady throughout life at around 10% per annum for men and 15% for women (Shepherd *et al.* 1966). The evident reluctance to refer the elderly for specialized help (as contrasted with "disposal") reflects the multiple problems of attitude, knowledge, skill and resources which bedevil the care of old people.

The Elderly in Psychiatric Hospitals (DHSS 1971*b*, 1973, 1975*a*)

One hundred years ago people of 65 and over were only 1 in 10 of the inmates of our asylums (Lewis 1946). Now they are half of in-patients in psychiatric hospitals, and since 1954 the proportion of residents aged over 75 has doubled (DHSS 1973). Of the 50 000 old people in mental illness hospitals in England and Wales half are over 75 — and they are the only group of adult psychiatric patients whose residence rates have increased over the recent period of "rundown" whereby mental hospital beds have been reduced by some 30%. On these trends a further eight or nine thousand beds for these over 75s may be needed by the 1980s, and old people may then comprise two-thirds of psychiatric in-patients (DHSS 1971*b*).

Admissions of over 75s to psychiatric units more than trebled between the early 1950s and the end of the 1960s; over half are first admissions, reflecting the inward tide of the dementias. However in the first years of the 1970s there has been a fall in the first admission rates of old people. The significance of this fall in unclear, and its durability uncertain; possible causes may include the availability of more places in communal residential homes (DHSS 1975*b*) and it may be that increased investment in community services is beginning to tell. But it is likely, too, to be becoming more difficult for old people to gain admission to psychiatric hospitals, because of the growing pressure to ease crowding.

But by far the largest group of the elderly in these hospitals are those who were admitted much earlier in life and who have aged there; they are mostly diagnosed as schizophrenics. (In Goodmayes Hospital, for instance, despite vigorous rehabilitation programmes, over half of all our old people have been in hospital for over ten years). Nevertheless, some 12 000 of psychiatric in-patients have been admitted in old age for senile dementia (DHSS 1975*a*) and in 1971 there were some 10 000 such admissions (DHSS 1975*b*). There are grounds for concern in regard to the training of doctors to deal with this common and taxing condition, for in the same year teaching hospital psychiatric units in the whole of England and Wales (DHSS 1973) admitted only 67 demented patients, and at the end of the year there were only 29 such patients in all these teaching units (DHSS 1975*a*).

Despite the fact that dementia should now normally be the only condition which makes it necessary for old people to remain in psychiatric hospitals permanently, both depression and paranoid states still account for a great deal of time spent in hospital through multiple admissions. Dr David Jolley and I have studied our own use of beds over five years (Jolley and Arie 1976). We found that one quarter of patients admitted with paranoid disorders, and 13% of those with affective disorders had cumulative stays of six months or more. Functional disorders in old age, although they carry a generally good outlook for the individual episode, nevertheless have a tendency in old age to recur or to grumble on — which has a bearing on the organization of services, which I shall be discussing later.

It should be noted that in the United States and the United Kingdom the diagnosis of dementia appears often to depend on different criteria. Eighty per cent of old people first admitted to state mental hospitals in the United States in the late 1960s were labelled demented, whilst the corresponding figure for England and Wales was only 43% (Copeland *et al.* 1974). Demented patients are often, in our country, admitted to geriatric rather than to psychiatric hospitals, but nonetheless these figures give cause for disquiet. There was a comparable discrepancy between Queen's County of New York City, and Camberwell in London, but when psychiatrists of the US/UK project examined these patients, one quarter of those who had been labelled as demented in Queen's were reclassified as suffering from functional illness. Misdiagnosis of dementia is fraught with dangers for the patient, for it generates self-fulfilling prophecies by inducing both pessimism in management and the deterioration which occurs almost inevitably when the depressed are treated as if they were demented.

Public Policy and the Organization of Services

Successive British governments have committed themselves to policies of "community care". These seductively reassuring and alliterative words command instant assent — to be in favour of community care is self-evidently to be on the side of the angels. It is indeed no ignoble aim to seek to avoid unnecessary "uprooting" (Roth 1973) and to preserve the dignity of the sick and the frail as private citizens in their own homes. But there are limits to what can be done adequately, economically and even humanely at home, and the often meagre care of institutions may be replaced by no effective care at all (Hawks 1975).

A parallel development of public policy has been towards the desegregation of the mentally ill. By 1971 16% of all psychiatric admissions were to units in *general* hospitals, but this proportion ranged from nearly one half of all admissions in the Manchester Region to less than 5% in the East Anglian Region (DHSS 1973) — an instance of the many regional disparities which still beset our National Health Service. It is envisaged that mental hospitals may ultimately be replaced by a pattern of care based on District General Hospitals, supported by small "Community Hospitals" (DHSS 1975*c*). Leaving aside the effect of our current economic crisis on such developments, many questions are being asked about the capacity of general hospital-based services to provide the range of facilities for the mentally ill which, at their best, can be offered by large psychiatric hospitals.

But life in psychiatric hospitals is becoming difficult, not least because of the climate of scrutiny which has settled over them since the publication in 1969 of the Ely Hospital Inquiry (National Health Service (NHS) 1969), which revealed neglect and demoralization in a hospital for the mentally handicapped. Since then a continuing series of "scandals" have generated opprobrium over the whole of institutional care and the consequences have been many-sided: on the one hand, a long overdue public concern has been accompanied by some redirection of resources into the longstay sector; on the other hand, staff are more reluctant to work in settings in which a "scandal" may be just around the corner, and thereby a further twist is given to the vicious circle by which staff prefer to work in well-staffed settings, causing understaffed units to become still more understaffed, with still more likelihood that things will go wrong in them.

Moreover, with further development of general hospital services there is a danger of a double standard in psychiatry, with accumulations of chronic, mostly elderly patients being looked after by isolated and often demoralized staff in large mental hospitals. And even when general hospital units exist in the locality old people are frequently admitted direct to a mental hospital. Such trends were eloquently documented by yet another Committee of Inquiry at Whittingham, a large mental hospital (NHS 1972) — an Inquiry which, perhaps significantly, took place in that region of the country where general hospital psychiatry has advanced furthest. But in the care of the elderly general hospital units are themselves not immune to having things go wrong (North Western Regional Health Authority 1975). These problems are now documented each year in the reports of the Hospital Advisory Service (NHS Hospital Advisory Service 1970–1975) which was established as part of the government's reaction to the Ely Report, and which has now sent teams to visit every psychiatric and geriatric unit in the country.

The Goodmayes Psychiatric Service for Old People

The pressure of the "psychogeriatric problem", the particular characteristics of old age mental disorders and indeed the predicament of the elderly as such, lead to the conclusion that there may be advantages in the establishment of local psychiatric services specifically for the elderly; moreover those responsible for such services are well placed to act as advocates for the elderly amid competing claims on local resources. It was considerations such as these, that led me to take the opportunity in 1969 of establishing a psychiatric unit for old people at Goodmayes Hospital, a district psychiatric hospital in East London. The origins and development of our service have been described elsewhere (Arie 1970, 1972, 1976) and I will confine myself here only to brief details such as will enable me to draw, in most of the rest of what I have to say, on issues which we have identified in the course of our service and research activities.

Our unit takes responsibility for the entire referred psychiatric morbidity in 52 000 old people in a population of 415 000. We see the whole range of functional and organic disorders and have an excellent epidemiological frame for studying old age psychiatric morbidity in a defined population. The unit's base in the hospital is an acute assessment and treatment ward, and a series of longstay wards. All out patients are seen initially in their homes, and whenever possible are maintained at home by the deployment of extramural services. But we do not hesitate to admit to hospital either for assessment or treatment, or indeed for permanent care where this seems right. Each year we now see some five hundred patients, about half of whom are admitted to hospital, but two-thirds are home within two months, and only some 12% of admitted patients remain for permanent care. We found that we were able rapidly to reduce the number of beds which were needed in the hospital, and so to reduce the crowding which is characteristic of wards for the elderly, and to improve greatly the quality of the hospital environment. Our initial 350 beds eventually were reduced to 198 despite an increase of over 40% in the referral rate over the first five years, despite increased admissions and despite a sharply diminished death rate in admitted patients. These results were achieved by a variety of factors — careful home assessment, willingness to spend a great deal of time and effort on formulating and reviewing solutions for the maintenance of old people in their homes by collaborative programmes with other agencies, and careful pre-assessment to ensure that those patients who needed the services of medical or surgical units were not wrongly admitted to a psychiatric hospital; and perhaps above all, by the quality of our staff.

It is to my mind of great significance that we have been able to attract to our team able young doctors of whom we have now had some twenty or more. They have included of late some who have come from abroad, including North America, seeking experience in this field, and several have gone on to establish similar units of their own. The problems of recruitment to services for the elderly are notorious (Green 1975) and so I emphasize this, for we are satisfied that if the work is done well and with something approaching adequate resources it is an eminently satisfying field of professional work for able people from all the health disciplines.

In recent years posts for psychiatrists "with a special interest in the elderly" have come to be increasingly established in our health service, and the Royal College of Psychiatrists has a very active Group for the Psychiatry of Old Age which has over one hundred members. It seems likely that psychiatric services for the elderly will come to be established in many districts and several are already flourishing, with a fruitful diversity of approach (e.g. Baker 1974, Bergmann 1972, Donovan *et al.* 1971, Godber 1975, Pitt 1975, Robinson 1972, White 1975, Whitehead and Mankikar 1974).

In such work much depends on effective collaboration with other related services, expecially the social services and the geriatric service. The Joint Patient Unit which we have established together with the geriatrician, Dr Tom Dunn, is an instance of such collaboration (Arie and Dunn 1973). This unit of five beds (initially four) is in one of Dr Dunn's wards in nearby Chadwell Heath Hospital, and serves the population of some 170 000 which is common to our two services. It arose out of our wish to enable any patient who made contact with one of the two services to get the benefit of the resources of either or of both. In this way "misplacement" of old people in psychiatric or geriatric hospitals respectively, the subject of much debate in recent years (Kidd 1962, Mezey *et al.* 1968, Langley and Simpson 1970), has been eliminated in our District. The government in 1972 published guidance on the division of responsibility between psychiatrists and geriatricians (DHSS 1972), a division which rests essentially on the sensible basis that those patients whose care needs are primarily behavioural are the responsibility of the psychiatrists, while those with primarily physical dependency belong in geriatric units. Nonetheless there are many patients whose disability is either mixed or needs joint assessment or treatment, and it is for these that we established our short-stay joint unit.

We admit three main types of patient to this unit: those who on home assessment appear to have both physical and behavioural problems which need further evaluation in hospital; those who have both physical and behavioural problems of such significance that they need joint medical and psychiatric care; and finally patients with frankly psychiatric disturbance who develop serious physical illness — of whom a large group are the deeply depressed patients who become dangerously dehydrated — and who need specifically medical treatment before their psychiatric treatment can proceed.

During the first twenty months, 85 patients passed through the unit, half of them admitted by each of us. The mean length of stay was 20 days; one-third were discharged home direct from the unit, whilst 14% died there. Of the patients whom I admitted 44% were either ultimately transferred to the geriatrician's care, or died soon after admission, indicating the high incidence of serious physical disorder in old people referred to a psychiatric service. Three months after admission 54% of the patients had been discharged and 25% had died in hospital.

Such a joint enterprise can be mounted with no extra resources beyond goodwill and willingness to co-operate (commodities admittedly often in shorter supply than money). We now regard it as an indispensable part of our resources, though we remain equally willing to admit patients direct to each other's wards when they appear simply to have been misreferred to one or other of us. In 1970 the government recommended the establishment of larger and more ambitious "Psycho-Geriatric Assessment Units" (DHSS 1970) but we feel that simpler and less costly units such as ours are likely to become much more widely established.

The Staff Factor

I should like now to consider one or two particular issues which arise in this work. Measurement of need and evaluation of the effectiveness with which services meet need are now accepted bases for health service planning. But in this model an essential factor is often overlooked — the needs of staff. The appalling problems of recruitment to geriatric services (Arie 1973, Green 1975) and the issues of "morale" which arise in work with the elderly (Arie 1971) to which I have already referred, emphasize the importance of what I call the "staff factor". Quite apart from the problems of staffing which derive from the very nature of the disabilities of the elderly and of their low status in our society, there are particular problems which derive from the way in which we organize our services. I have already referred to the polarity which may arise when work is divided between relatively prestigious general hospital units on the one hand and large mental hospitals on the other; similarly, in our own unit the very success of the acute sector of care and the strenuous efforts made to avoid unnecessary chronicity within the hospital, mean that those patients who must remain for longstay care are more deteriorated than they used to be and may generate a similar polarity by inducing a sense of distance and deprivation in the staff of the longstay sector.

It seemed of high priority that we should study the work of the nurses in our longstay wards, the sources of their job satisfaction and the relationship between this and the quality of care of their patients. Albert Kushlick has vividly distinguished between "hit-and-run" personnel such as doctors, social workers and psychologists, and people like nurses and relatives who may be in contact with patients around-the-clock (Kushlick 1975). The social and professional distance between doctors and the intimate work of longstay care is such that doctors' views concerning the sources of satisfaction and dissatisfaction of the staff who do this work are unlikely to be very accurate. It seemed important therefore to look more closely at this work, and to consider also the pros and cons of transposing this work — in effect the care of severely demented people who are ambulant — into a setting of residential rather than hospital care; the latter has quite different goals from the traditional medical ones of investigation, treatment and cure which is so little consonant with the realities of longstay care. Analogies for such a redefinition of traditionally medical problems are in the transposition of some services for the mentally subnormal in our country from the medical to the education service. These are large issues, and it might be noted in passing that one constraint on such a redistribution is the fact that in our country only 4% of residential care staff have any training in this field, and such a transposition would at present be from a relatively well-trained professional group in one discipline to an almost wholly untrained group in another.

We have no firm answers yet to these questions, but with such considerations in mind May Clarke, a sociologist working with Margot Jefferys and ourselves and supported by the Department of Health, has been studying the work of nurses in longstay wards (Clarke 1974). There is time merely to indicate the sort of issues which arose. Thus, for example, established caring ideologies which emphasize maximization of independence, personal relationships and talking, often conflicted with the inclination of the longstay ward nurses to "do things for" their patients, and they could not always quite emancipate themselves from the view that "work" is necessarily *physical* work, and felt that they were idling if they were not engaged in some physical task.

May Clarke looked also at strategies for dealing with incontinence (Arie *et al.* 1976). The very effective routine for dealing with incontinence in a humane, clean and cheerful ward was such that it became almost impossible for a patient to remain continent — for independence would have disrupted that routine. By contrast another ward with similar patients was less concerned with the effects of incontinence and patients were less methodically changed and cleaned; yet on that ward the variety and quality of life was in some ways better. For the nurses incontinence was not the most burdensome nor the most disagreeable disability — it was the morose, uncommunicative patients that they least enjoyed nursing and if a patient was outgoing and cheerful — what was often called "a character" — almost no disability was too burdensome to the staff, and with these outgoing patients the nurses spent a disproportionate amount of their time. Questions arise at many levels — questions of values and objectives in this work; practical questions of the organization and style of the work as these relate to the problems of recruiting the staff to do it; and fundamental questions of identifying those aspects of the development of personality which might be influenced to enable us to be more attractive to those upon whom we can expect to depend for care in old age and chronic disability.

Last I want to consider some aspects of the care of the elderly at home. Dementia sets limitations to the feasibility of community care which are not always realistically identified. The global nature of the disability deriving from dementia means that often the mildly demented, and certainly the severely demented, need someone to be around all the time — not necessarily to give skilled care or continuous care, but to be available if needed: this is what is offered by families, or could be offered by a quite unskilled person such as a sensible teenager. It follows that the *episodic* interventions which are all that domiciliary services can normally offer, may be both too much (in the sense that skilled personnel are not necessarily required) and too little (in the sense that such visits fall short of the continuing presence that is called for by the loss of the capacity for self-care and avoidance of common dangers). Such around-the-clock care in the home is one thing that can never be provided by statutory services; institutions exist precisely because they are the only economic way of providing this care for large numbers of people.

There may indeed be scope for tapping much further the resources of the neighbourhood and community in support of its old people, but there is a world of difference between the care needs of the demented and those with more circumscribed, even though possibly much more dramatic disabilities, the support of whom is often feasible on an episodic basis. Such considerations set limitations to the scope also of programmes of day care (Arie 1975*a*) for those demented old people who either live at home, or with a spouse who is almost equally dependent — and it should be noted that one of the Newcastle studies reported that of old ladies with dementia no less than 53% were living entirely alone (Kay *et al.* 1964*b*).

There are limits to the extent to which the pool of resources can be expanded by more flexible and innovatory approaches, such as the use of volunteers (e.g. Griffiths 1975) (including of course the fit "young-olds"), or of married women working part-time (Arie 1975*b*), or the transposition of tasks from highly trained to less expensive personnel (Arie 1972); and translocations of staff into one sector of care are almost always at the cost of denuding another. Certainly early detection and intervention will minimize the frequency of crises in dementia, and may indeed impede the rate of deterioration; but hope that dementia may be prevented by more energetic community intervention has little evidence to support it, and in particular the belief that dementia is largely socially induced seems to conflict with the evidence (Kay *et al.* 1964*b*). What we do know is that the cost to families (Sainsbury and Grad de Alarcon 1973, Hamilton and Hoenig 1966), to say nothing of the old people themselves, of maintaining them at home may be high in terms of family breakdown, marital strife, and other damage to the caring individuals (including, as a recent study has shown (Sanford 1975) chronic misery through sheer loss of sleep) — a cost which is not always adequately counted.

There is a final danger which faces the demented, and it behoves us as professional workers to strive to protect them against it, not least because it comes from ourselves. I refer to the belief that it is necessary only to treat the demented differently, and their dementia will disappear. One version of this belief is the "environmental fallacy", which holds that if only one manipulates the environment sufficiently the demented will be enabled to function as if they were not demented; its counterpart among doctors in particular, is the "diagnostic fallacy", which holds that if only one investigates demented people with sufficient skill one will find them instead to be depressed, anaemic or myxoedematous. Both fallacies are the more dangerous for having *some* basis in truth; but both have in common that they make it easier to turn our backs on the mountain of a problem that faces us and to confine ourselves to displacement activities in its less formidable foothills.

References

Arie, T. (1970). *Lancet* **ii**, 1175–1182

Arie, T. (1971). *British Medical Journal* **iii**, 166–170

Arie, T. (1972). *In* "Approaches to Action: Services for the Mentally Ill and Handicapped". Ed. G. McLachlan. Nuffield Provincial Hospitals Trust. Oxford University Press, London: pp 17–26

Arie, T. (1973). *Modern Geriatrics* **6**, 308–311

Arie, T. (1975*a*). *Gerontologica clinica* **17**, 31–39

Arie, T. (1975*b*). *British Medical Journal* **iii**, 641–643

Arie, T. (1976). *Gerontologist* **3**, 280–281

Arie, T., Clarke, M. and Slattery, Z. (1976). *In* "Incontinence in the Elderly". Ed. F. L. Willington. Academic Press, London and New York; pp 70–81

Arie, T. and Dunn, T. (1973). *Lancet* **ii**, 1313–1316

Atkinson, A. B. (1973). *In* "Needs of the Elderly". Eds. R. W. Canvin and N. G. Pearson. Exeter University Press, Exeter

Baker, A. A. (1974). *Lancet* **i**, 795

Barraclough, B. M. (1971). *In* "Recent Developments in Psychogeriatrics". Eds. D. W. K. Kay and A. Walk. Royal Medico-Psychological Association. Headley, Ashford: pp 87–97

Bergmann, K. (1972). *In* "Gerontopsychiatrie". Janssen Pharmaceutical, Düsseldorf: No. 2, pp 339–354

Carstairs, V. and Morrison, M. (1971). "The Elderly in Residential Care." Scottish Health Service Studies No. 19. Scottish Home and Health Department, Edinburgh

Central Statistical Office (CSO) (1974). Social Trends No. 5. HMSO, London: pp 16–17

Clarke, May (1974). "The Care of Patients on a Long Stay Psychogeriatric Ward and Working with Elderly Patients: Nurses Expectations and Experiences." Research Reports to the DHSS

Copeland, J. R. M. *et al* (1974). *Canadian Psychiatric Association Journal* **19**, 267–271

Department of Health and Social Security (DHSS) (1970). "Psycho-Geriatric Assessment Units." Memorandum accompanying Circular HM(70) 11. (1971*a*). "Psychiatric Hospitals and Units in England and Wales, 1969." Statistical Report Series No. 12. HMSO, London. (1971*b*). "Services for Mental Illness Related to Old Age." Memorandum accompanying Circular HM(72) 71. (1973). "Psychiatric Hospitals in England and Wales, 1971." Statistical and Research Report Series No. 6. HMSO, London. (1974). "Report of the Hospital In-Patient Enquiry, 1972." Part 1. HMSO, London. (1975*a*). "Censuses of Patients in Mental Illness Hospitals, 1971 and Mental Illness Day Patients, 1972." Statistical and Research Report Series No. 10. HMSO, London. (1975*b*). "Health and Personal Social Services Statistics for England, 1974." HMSO, London. (1975*c*). "National Health Service — Development of Service." Community Hospitals. HSC(15) 75. (1976). "The Census of Residential Accommodation, 1970." 1. Residential Accommodation for the Elderly and for the Younger Physically Handicapped. HMSO, London

Donovan, J. F., Williams, I. E. I. and Wilson, T. S. (1971). *In* "Recent Developments in Psychogeriatrics". Eds. D. W. K. Kay and A. Walk. Royal Medico-Psychological Association. Headley, Ashford

Godber, C. (1975). *Journal of the Royal College of Physicians of London* **10**, 101–112

Green, M. (1975). *In* "Specialized Futures (Essays in Honour of Sir George Godber)". Ed. G. McLachlan. Nuffield Provincial Hospitals Trust. Oxford University Press, London: pp 95–153

Griffiths, V. E. (1975). *British Medical Journal* **iii**, 641–643

Hamilton, M. W. and Hoenig, J. (1966). *The Medical Officer* **15**, 193–196

Hart, J. Tudor (1971). *Lancet* **i**, 405–412

Harwin, B. (1973). *In* "Wing and Hafner" (1973)

Hawks, D. (1975). *British Journal of Psychiatry* **127**, 276–285

Jolley, D. J. and Arie, T. (1976). *British Journal of Psychiatry* **129**, 418–423

Kay, D. W. K., Beamish, P. and Roth, M. (1962). Sociological Review, Monograph No. 5. Ed. P. Halmos, Keele: pp 173–193

Kay, D. W. K., Beamish, P. and Roth, M. (1964*a*). *British Journal of Psychiatry* **110**, 146–158

Kay, D. W. K., Beamish, P. and Roth, M. (1964*b*). *British Journal of Psychiatry* **110**, 668–682

Kay, D. W. K., Bergmann, K., Foster, E. M., McKechnie, A. A. and Roth, M. (1970). *Comprehensive Psychiatry* **1**, 26–35

Kidd, C. B. (1962). *British Medical Journal* **ii**, 1491–1495

Kushlick, A. (1975). Some Ways of Setting, Monitoring and Attaining Objectives for Services for Disabled People. Health Care Evaluation Research Team, Highcroft, Romsey Road, Winchester, Hampshire; Research Report No. 116

Langley, G. E. and Simpson, J. H. (1970). *Gerontologica clinica* **12**, 149–163

Lewis, A. J. (1946). *Journal of Mental Science* **92**, 150–170

Mezey, A. G., Hodkinson, H. M. and Evans, G. J. (1968). *British Medical Journal,* **iii**, 16–18

National Health Service (NHS) (1969). Report of the Inquiry on Allegation of Ill-Treatment of Patients and other Irregular Activities at the Ely Hospital, Cardiff. Cmd. 3975. HMSO, London. (1972). Report of the Committee of Inquiry into Whittingham Hospital. Cmd. 4861. HMSO, London

National Health Service Hospital Advisory Service (1970–1975). Annual Reports. HMSO, London

North Western Regional Health Authority (NWRHA) (1975). Committee of Inquiry on the Transfer of Patients from Fairfield Hospital to Rossendale Hospital. NWRHA, Manchester

Office of Population Censuses and Surveys (OPCS) (1973). The General Household Survey. Introductory Report. HMSO, London

Pitt, B. (1975). "Psychogeriatrics". Churchill Livingstone, Edinburgh and London

Post, F. (1972). *British Journal of Psychiatry* **121**, 393–404

Robinson, R. A. (1972). *In* "The Elderly Mind". British Hospital Journal/Hospital International, London; pp 22–24

Roth, M. (1973). *In* "Wing and Hafner" (1973): pp 215–238

Sainsbury, P. and Grad de Alarcon, J. (1973). *In* "Wing and Hafner" (1973): pp 239–255

Sanford, J. R. A. (1975). *British Medical Journal* **iii**, 471–473

Shanas, E., Townsend, P., Wedderburn, D., Friis, H. Milhoj, P. and Stenhouwer, J. (1968). "Old People in Three Industrial Societies." Routledge and Kegan Paul, London; Atherton Press, New York

Shepherd, M., Cooper, B., Brown, A. C. and Kalton, G. W. (1966). "Psychiatric Illness in General Practice." Oxford University Press, London

White, D. M. D. (1975). *Lancet* **i**, 27–29

Whitehead, T. and Mankikar, G. (1974). *Lancet* **i**, 1213–1215

Williamson, J., Stokoe, I. H., Gray, S., Fisher, M., Smith, A., McGhee, A. and Stephenson, E. (1964). *Lancet* **i**, 1117–1120

Wing, J. K. and Hafner, H. (Eds.) (1973). "Roots of Evaluation." Nuffield Provincial Hospitals Trust, Oxford University Press, London

World Health Organization (WHO) (1972). "Psychogeriatrics." Report of a WHO Scientific Group, Geneva

Environmental Factors in Dependency

Elaine M Brody
Philadelphia Geriatric Center,
Philadelphia, Pennsylvania

Sorting out dependencies due to advancing age — that is, those intrinsic to the very processes of aging — from those due to the psychological, social, and physical environment, is a task that has been a focus of research and practice since the inception of scientific and professional interest in aging. Though knowledge is far from complete, there is abundant evidence that a significant amount of the dependencies of older people is environmentally induced.

At the same time, the general direction in old age is decline in level of functioning. Previous speakers have delineated the physiological and disease-related changes that are a part of aging and that lead to dependency. Even if scientific breakthroughs should eliminate the major diseases of old age, it is unlikely that the foreseeable future will witness "cures" of the "normal" dependencies. The arc of decline (which varies widely among individuals) would not change to a horizontal line of continuing maximal functioning that drops suddenly when programmed life runs out (Hayflick 1974).

Recognition that some decline is inevitable compels re-examination of the value judgment often implicit in attitudes toward dependency — specifically, the notion that dependency *per se* is "bad" and independence is "good." Though the number and nature of supports required vary over time, normal healthy inter-dependence is a constant throughout the life-span. Beginning with total dependency in infancy, as the individual moves through childhood and adolescence and gains competence, he assumes more and more responsibility for himself; with maturity, he assumes a care-giving role towards others. In the aging phase of life he again may become more dependent. This time, the goals of care are different. The dependencies of old age are chronic rather than transitional; they may foreshadow continuing or increasing dependency. Chronicity dictates that supports provided on any level aimed at maximizing independence must be sustained.

While environmental influences are important to all human beings, the special vulnerability of older people has been expressed by Lawton and Simon (1968) as the "environmental docility" hypothesis: "As the competence of the individual decreases, the proportion of behavior attributable to environmental, as contrasted with personal, characteristics increases". Examples in the sphere of physical function are the sensory, perceptual, and physiological changes that impede the use by older people of physical spaces such as buildings and neighborhoods. (Pastalan 1973).

An analogy can be drawn with respect to reliance on the social and psychological environment. To quote Rosow (1967) "... the crucial people in the aging problem are not the old, but the younger age groups, for it is the rest of us who determine the status and position of the old person in the social order." Attitudes towards old people and aging are the basic determinants on every level of what is done (or is not done) to find solutions to the dependencies of older people. The new word that has been added to our vocabularies — "age-ism" (Butler 1969) — on the macro-level determines such matters as priorities in the allocation of resources for income, the provision of health and social services, and attention to housing and neighborhood environments. On the micro-level, attitudes creep insidiously into incorrect psycho-dynamic clichés such as "parent–child role reversal" and "second childhood" (Brody 1974*a*). One is reminded of the injunction of Grey Panther Maggie Kuhn not to turn older people into "wrinkled babies." Weinberg (1976) has written eloquently about psychological vulnerabilities unique to the elderly that are exacerbated by the injuries inflicted.

The vulnerabilities of children and their dependence on the physical, social, and psychological environment are *expected*, *accepted*, and *provided for* by the family and society. In the main, the dependencies of old age have not yet been similarly legitimized. Within certain parameters, children are "programmed" developmentally for a somewhat orderly progression in the reduction of dependence. Society distinguishes between their normal, healthy dependence and that which is extreme or pathological. The dependencies of old age appear with great variability and irregularity, over much wider time spans, and in different sequential patterns. There are no normative standards for evaluating the appropriateness of dependency in old people. Among unsettled issues, therefore, is determining precisely when and how (quantitatively and qualitatively) to provide environmental supports to meet dependency needs and to avoid fostering unnecessary dependency.

In attempting to distinguish "normal" from environmentally induced dependencies, it cannot be assumed that the slope of decline is so inevitable that we become therapeutically nihilistic. The goals are (1) to identify and reduce the "excess disabilities" that are environmentally induced and do not reflect actual impairment (Kahn 1965) — that is, to close the gap between actual function and potential function, taking nothing for granted, and (2) to meet residual dependencies in such a way as to maximize independence and well-being. The word "potential" is key, for realistic goals with the frail elderly include improvement as well as maintenance of function and retardation of decline.

An apparent paradox should be made explicit: "meeting dependency needs," rather than fostering dependence, can foster independence. Misunderstanding of this concept led to polarized attitudes about whether the aged should be urged towards independence and activity or whether concerted efforts should be made to meet their dependency needs. The balanced view now generally held is that appropriate service- and physical-environments, selectively provided, maximize independence. The road to maximum independence is often paved with supports of various types.

The series of stresses that have been called the "insults" of aging contribute to dependency. Unique to this phase of life is the clustering of intrinsic and socially induced stresses occurring at a time when the individual's coping capacities are diminished: the loss of physical and/or mental capacities; loss of income, employment, and status; interpersonal losses of spouse, other relatives, peers, and the special poignancy of loss of adult children.

A theme reiterated in the literature on stress is that its negative impact is due to the existence of the stress perceived as such, coupled with an inability on the part of the individual to cope with it (Selye 1970, Holmes and Masuda 1974, Rahe 1974, Colligan 1975). The helplessness and hopelessness engendered are powerful contributants to breakdown which manifests itself as illness or even death. Some sense of mastery, then, is critical not only to the integrity of the human personality, but to physical integrity as well. The contribution of lack of control to the downward spiral of stress leading to illness (mental or physical) leading to dependency has obvious implications. It is not for ethical reasons alone that gerontologists emphasize the need for options and choices.

The role of cumulative stresses in the etiology of illness has been dramatized by the Social Readjustment Rating Scale developed by Holmes and Masuda (1974) and Rahe (1974). The clustering of events that required changes in the life pattern of the relatively young people used in their research is a prominent feature of the lives of old people. Though the scale was not designed specifically for the population in which we are interested, many of the events to which dependent old people have been exposed are those it weights most heavily in ranking stresses. Death of a spouse and of a close family member are numbers 1 and 2 respectively; personal illness or injury and retirement are in the top 10 of 43 items. One can only speculate as to the number of "points" that would be assigned to death of a care-giving adult child;

to permanently disabling illness; to the onset of chronic brain syndrome; to the trauma of institutionalization (for which their phrase "change in residence" is scarcely adequate); or to the assaults so common on frail old people in high crime areas.

The stream of research focusing on one type of stress, that of environmental change of older people, illuminates the role of environment in producing dependency (Lawton and Nahemow 1973, Brody 1974*b*, Liebowitz 1974). Early in the 1960s, a handful of studies documented the existence of a phenomenon called the "relocation effect" — i.e. the apparent negative impact, including excess morbidity and mortality, of moving institutionalized older people from one environment to another. Subsequently, the moves studied were expanded from the focus on institutionalized populations. Attention was turned to the identification of qualifying factors such as the characteristics of the most vulnerable and of the facilities from which and to which they were moved, the reasons for the move and its meaning to the mover, and the ways in which the moves were managed.

It became apparent that relocation effect cannot be attributed globally to a change in environment *per se*. The most vulnerable were found to be the physically ill, the depressed, confused, and disoriented, and those who were moved involuntarily. Disorganization during and immediately after a move increases mortality. In seeking a solution to their problems, and in contrast to the low mobility of older people in general, many older people move several times in rapid succession prior to institutionalization (Townsend 1965, Friedsam and Dick 1963, Brody 1969). The stress of such multiple changes in environment has not been calculated. Improvements in movers have been noted for those who were physically well and those who chose to move. For example, moves into Senior Citizens' housing resulted in positive effects and the lack of negative effects has been attributed to their voluntary nature. Other factors that reduce or avoid negative effects are the provision of opportunities for choice, careful individualized preparation through counselling and pre-move orientation to the receiving facility, and participation of the older person in the decision-making process.

The dependency-fostering implications of such findings are self-evident in a context in which moves of the frailest old people most often are frenetic and chaotic; in which it is rare that they are involved in decision-making or their preferences considered; in which orderly assessment seldom takes place and when it does, focuses on physical functioning to the exclusion of psycho-social needs; in which options are conspicuously scant and there is generally a lack of careful consideration of the few that do exist; and in which placement decisions are determined not by suitability for the individual, but in response to fiscal supports provided by the controlling system which in turn governs bed-availability (Brody 1975*a*).

Even more striking are unequivocal findings about the role of the environment itself. Lieberman's study of the effects of entry into institutions (Lieberman 1969) attributed negative effects to institution-like environments, vastly different from previous more natural living styles, that over-loaded the old person's adaptive capacities. In his report (Lieberman *et al.* 1971) on the relocation of elderly mental patients, the strongest association with outcome status was the psycho-social milieu of the receiving environment. "Patients placed in cold, dehumanized, dependency-fostering environments show declines. The psychological characteristics of the relocation environments were considerably more influential on outcome than any combination of the characteristics of the discharged patients themselves."

A similar study by Marlowe also assessed environmental dimensions (Marlowe 1973). Two groups of highly comparable individuals experienced diametrically opposed outcomes: one group did very well and the other "fell apart." "The answer to this anomalous situation," she wrote, "is to be found in a consideration of the environments." The improvers went to environments that: encouraged autonomy (the resident's control over his own life); fostered personalization (privacy and respect); offered less succorance (did not foster dependency by doing things for an individual that he could with encouragement do for himself); fostered community integration (access to the outside world); had a lower tolerance for deviance; encouraged social interaction and did not expect docility or passivity; and treated residents with warmth and positive attitudes. Under opposite conditions, the same type of people withdrew and deteriorated.

Marlowe's finding that the characteristics of the improver environments cross-cut different types of facilities comments on the heterogeneity of institutional environments and their positive potential. It supports the steady procession of reports on successful experimental treatments of institutionalized older people that involve modification of the social and physical environments (Gottesman and Brody 1975).

Interest in the effects of relocation has not been matched by the same degree of concern with the opposite condition: the negative impact of failure to change the environment when a move is needed or wished for by the older person. That phenomenon might be characterized as the "immobilization effect." It can be produced by a lack of options, by psychological resistance to moving despite acute need, or by subtle declines that hamper the individual's capacity to mobilize the necessary psychic or physical energy and lead to "giving-up". For example, the negative effects generally attributed to institutional environments were produced by waiting on a list for admission

(Lieberman *et al.* 1968). In the Philadelphia Geriatric Center's (PGC) Intermediate Housing study, those who wished to move but did not do so experienced a precipitous drop in psycho-social adjustment between baseline and 6 month follow-up (Brody and Kleban 1976).

The most dramatic illustration of immobilization is the failure of older people to move from harsh environments. Concentrations of elderly poor are isolated in changing neighborhoods, locked in by low-cost housing often in deplorable condition; subject to ills such as malnutrition; lacking appropriate transportation to medical and other services; and often imprisoned in their own homes by acute fear of robbery and attack. In several studies, they resisted moving even when offered help in relocating (Pollack 1969, Thurman 1970). Threats to life and safety in high-crime neighborhoods have become so well known that a telecast of Monty Python's Flying Circus reversed the situation. A gang of elderly women called "Hell's Grannies," hung around on street corners, tripped passing girls, beat up adolescent boys, and rode their motorcycles destructively in and out of stores (Public Broadcasting System, February 17, 1975).

Many elderly in the PGC project resided in such areas. Our data show that the experimental housing environment was extremely significant in the sharp rise in its tenants' (in contrast to the controls') satisfaction with housing, enjoyment of life, and happiness. While many variables undoubtedly are at work, the case records tell us that escape from the active persecution, states of acute anxiety and fear, and even murder that were the fate of the non-movers has played a role in improving our tenants' well-being.

It is hypothesized that the immobilization effect can be caused not only by the older person's failure to move when indicated, but by the environment changing while the old person remains in place, or by failure to change the existing environment by application of services, physical modifications, or protection. Whether the change is in the individual or in the environment, the net effect is that the environment is not congruent with the capacity of the older person to function in it.

A major lesson to be learned from the clinical and research data is that *the process* by which environmental change is effected is as important as the fact of change itself. Stress that leads to dependency, even stress that is potentially lethal, can be mitigated by appropriate psycho-social services and environments. Similarly, when the individual himself is experiencing changing capacities, services can facilitate adaptation and therefore promote function.

In turning to consideration of community and housing environments, their importance is reinforced by the fact that poor health, low income and enforced disengagement increase the dependence of the elderly for services, amenities, and social relationships (Lawton *et al.* 1976). A significant amount of research (Lawton and Nahemow 1973, Schooler 1970, Lawton 1969*a*, 1975; Rosow 1967, Carp 1966, Lawton and Kleban 1971) has identified some aspects of well-being that relate to living arrangements: morale; satisfaction with housing; participation in activities; mobility; socialization and interaction with family, friends, and neighbors. Environmental factors that foster well-being and enhance the older person's capacity to function are proximity to and accessibility of relatives and friends; necessary health, recreational, shopping, religious and occupational resources; availability of appropriate transportation; safety and convenience; spatial opportunities for socialization; availability of adequate funds for rent and repair; and varying degrees of age-integration. Environmental inadequacies result in isolation, poor health, or robberies and attacks.

Studying thousands of older people across the country in housing environments, Lawton affirmed the usefulness of design and planning solutions for some problems of old people. "Environmentally based interventions in the form of community development, planned housing, favorable neighborhood location and crime control may significantly enhance well-being" (Lawton *et al.* 1975). Site location, for example, affects satisfaction and motility which in turn is highly related to functional health. The investigator postulates a transactional model designed to relate the aging individual to his environment that includes the degree of individual competence, environmental press, adaptive behavior, affective responses, and adaptation level. Environments should be planned so as to encourage the exercise of skills without over-taxing the tolerance for stress (Lawton and Nahemow 1973).

Though the role of services requires additional exploration, it is known that the amount and nature of the services actually provided in various housing environments are major determinants of the characteristics of people who move in. Data on the effects of moves to specialized housing are "unanimously positive", with service-rich housing attracting older, less healthy, less socially active people and those with lower morale than housing without supportive services (Lawton 1975). Simply stated, older people self-select to go where their level of service-needs can be met.

When tenants who moved to a service-rich high-rise were compared with those who moved to a building with fewer services, it was found (though the effect was small), that the service-rich building produced higher morale and housing satisfaction, and reduction in solitary status in its tenants. The low-service group improved (or had less decrement) in participation in activities and social interaction (Lawton 1976). The investigator suggested that maximum choice be provided for potential applicants along the continuum between no-service housing and service-rich housing; that sensitized management of congregate housing attempt to compensate for tenants' reduction in interaction with the community by stimuli such as proximity to resources, access to transportation, and programming for outside involvement; and that both inner satisfaction and behavior maintenance be used as criteria in evaluating the impact of environments.

Though the issue as to whether over-service has potential for increasing dependency has not been settled, it is suggested that the critical factors are the selection of appropriate services and the manner in which they are offered to particular groups. At this time the preponderance of evidence makes it safe to conclude that there is no imminent danger of saturating old people with services or of creating a surfeit of supportive environments. It is self-evident that services that enable older people to improve their functioning are not "over-service". On the other hand, dependency is fostered by the over-provision of services in the interest of the provider, as when the institutionalized elderly are fed and dressed routinely because it is less demanding of staff than encouragement of self-care. When total care facilities such as hospitals and institutions are over-used because lesser levels of care are not available, that too is "over-service".

In general, it seems safe to trust older people to exercise self-determination in the selection of the services and facilities they need. When options are real, they do not seek over-nurturing environments. Most, for example, do not apply to institutions until they cannot function in their current environments and unless suitable options are not available.

It has been argued that in some situations, freedom to be dependent actually fosters independence. Goldfarb has written extensively about his therapeutic techniques resting on the psycho-dynamic formulation that "patients can be helped toward self-sufficiency if they are permitted to be emotionally dependent" (Goldfarb 1969). Confirmation from a different setting is provided by a report of a special clinic for demanding, "thick-chart" patients in which any number of appointments are made upon request. The utilization of services dropped off because the flow of dependency satisfaction was not shut off but was gratified in a way "that does not divest the patient of his autonomy, self-control, and therefore self-esteem" (Lipsitt 1969).

The simple existence of services and resources has no effect unless they are both known and accessible through linkages such as counseling, communication, and transportation. Lack of such linkages impedes older people's capacity to obtain services and entitlements that maximize independence. Transportation emerged as a topic at the 1971 White House Conference on aging and continues to be a major concern of older people and professionals. Its absence can foster dependency through isolation and the inability to obtain food supplies, health care, or enrichment services. The reduced sense of mastery and control creates barriers to independence both psychologically and functionally.

Aspects of the tangible environment such as the design, construction, and furnishing of buildings for older people have been receiving increasing attention (Byerts 1973). Architects, planners, and gerontologists agree that architectural features can increase functional independence. Barriers and hazards should be identified and eliminated (e.g. steps, slippery surfaces, poor lighting) and prostheses be provided through such devices such as color-coding, ramps, grab-bars, clearly demarcated spaces, special lighting, orientation supports such as clocks and calendars, reachable light switches, counters and storage spaces. Two recent buildings — Highland Heights for the physically handicapped (Sherwood *et al.* 1972) and the PGC's Weiss Institute for the mentally impaired aged (Lawton 1969*b*, Kleban 1969) attended to incorporating design and architectural features to enhance the functioning of their respective target populations.

Review of findings regarding the impact of specific environments on older people should not obscure the direct link between social policy and the functioning of the individual. Reference must be made to policies that created and perpetuate a system in which flagrant abuses abound in nursing homes and in bootleg nursing homes called "boarding homes". Unscrupulous profiteering, dangerous conditions, downright neglect and cruelty, lack of health and psycho-social care, over-drugging and the like in the "litany of nursing home abuses" (United States Senate Special Committee on Aging 1974) do not foster independence.

Apart from such abuses, social policy and professional influences that are more subtle because the intent is benign, also increase dependency. Long-term care of older people is being shaped into a medical rather than a social health model both in institutions and in the community. The long-term facilities in which people reside for the rest of their lives are entered for social as well as medical reasons. Yet increasingly they are assuming the physical and social attributes of the short-term general hospital with its crisis-and-cure orientation, supremacy of medical routines, shrinkage of roles open to the older person so that the patient role is often the only one left open, and lack of attention to psychological, social, and recreational needs. Procrustean approaches that try to tailor the people to the institution rather than the reverse, engender institutional neuroses (Brody 1973). The resultant passivity, depression, less competent behavior, infantilization, desexualization, low self-esteem, submissiveness, anxiety, and other indicators of poor adjustment and dependency are among the best documented findings in gerontology.

One of the broadest areas of neglect in the US has been in the development of social/health community services that enable community dwellers to maintain independence. They, too, are being linked to the medical prescription as the point of entry into the systems. S. J. Brody points out that the focus "is on short-term relief rather than long-term functioning and on medical rather than on psycho-social needs. Environmental or stress-causing factors may be overlooked or considered of secondary importance" (Brody S. J. 1976*a*). The medical emphasis on "patient compliance" — that is, the "doing for" and "doing to" approach—encourages passivity and diminishes the opportunity for patients to comprehend their treatment and participate in it.

Clearly, there is now an inadequate range and number of facilities and services. The unanimous call of those who are knowledgeable is for a continuum of environments ranging from totally independent living in one's own home on the one hand to institutions providing total care on the other, and with many intermediate points between (Beattie 1970). The intermediate arrangements may be the delivery of services to the home, bringing the individual to the service, or living arrangements offering varying kinds and amounts of service. A critical ingredient is the capacity to move the older person along the continuum as his changing needs dictate. The heterogeneity of the elderly population requires a wide variety of options. There is a false dichotomy in the current emphasis on community care services as "alternatives" to institutionalization rather than on the primary need for them in their own right. When an impaired older person requires round-the-clock care or supervision, unless economics permits the creation of a nursing home in his own home, there is no "alternative." Institutional care should be improved, and community care services developed.

Approaches that determine the nature of these options and the identification of those for whom they are appropriate require examination. Assessment techniques designed to facilitate matching of individual to environment in the main are focusing on physical function, neglecting assessment of the individual's social, psychological, and recreational functioning and social support system (Brody 1976). No matter how sophisticated the assessment system, people, not instruments, make decisions. The wishes of individual and family must be considered. The service worker is often confronted with a dilemma in advising acceptance of a more environmentally dependent situation or in recommending any move from one environment to another.

Also fostering dependence is the separate treatment of either medical or psychiatric illness, each without taking note of the other (Schuckit 1974). Further, older people and their families often regard complaints as to be expected, with the result that many illnesses are un-reported, un-diagnosed, and therefore un-treated. Shanas' survey revealed that in the US a substantial number of the bedfast elderly are not visited regularly or occasionally by a doctor (Shanas *et al.* 1968). Another study reported a disconcerting ill-preparedness and lack of sophistication about illness on the part of elderly people, a reliance on "folk-fatalism" rather than on scientific medicine, and an "appalling" lack of knowledge about health care (Litman 1971). Older people and their families, then, do not have the information required to strengthen their own capacity to prevent dependency (Brody 1975*b*).

Discussion of environmentally-induced dependency must acknowledge attributes of the elderly individual's personality and the family personality as determinants of the need for environmental supports. It would be simplistic to assume that the same environmental prescription affects the dependence or independence of all older people in the same way, given similar health and social status. The heterogeneity of older people in personality, life-style, resources, culture, and perceptions of their environments elicit widely varying responses. The richness or poverty of the individual's social support system is often the critical determinant of a living arrangement plan, and the family is a most significant component of that system.

The literature on personality in old age emphasizes individuality, diversity and heterogeneity; it tells us that personality is continuous over time as are the widely varied capacities to cope with and adapt to stress (Neugarten 1973). There are many patterns of aging and no one path to "successful" aging. Some individuals, such as the developmentally disabled and the emotionally fragile have been dependent all their lives; for others the dependencies are age-related. In a similar vein, the same event may be perceived and experienced by different individuals to produce differing degrees of stress (Lowenthal and Chiriboga 1973). Stereotyped expectations and prescriptions are therefore inappropriate. The indomitably independent elderly person will be able to maintain herself in her own home long after her equally disabled but fearful, timid, "dependent" neighbor must move to a more protected setting. To deprive the dependent old person of the support the more independent does not require may constitute an additional stress leading to more, not less, dependency.

The family environment is of primary importance. Overall, the responsible behavior of families towards older people has been so thoroughly documented that it is no longer at issue in gerontological research. The cultural rejection of the aged has not been acted out on the individual or family level, despite the vastly increased pressures created by larger numbers of old people for whom the younger generations are responsible. However, the "family personality" differs, depending on the historical pattern and quality of its relationship (Brody 1974*a*). Environmental interventions to reduce dependency must take that fact into account.

The family's reality circumstances as well as the family personality determines the extent to which it can meet the dependency needs of its old. Where they have families, applicants to the PGC's institutional facilities illustrate constraints on family capacities. (Only about half of institutional residents nationwide have at least one adult child.) The middle-aged adult child of the applicant, with responsibility for more than one old person and for members of generation 3 as well, has long been a familiar figure. The very old who are the bulk of institutional applicants, and who most require environmental supports, are likely to have "children" who themselves are old or aging. In a study at the PGC, the ages of adult children were as high as 74, and 40% of the applicants had at least one adult child over the age of 60 (Brody 1966). Expectations of "old" children must be qualified by recognition of their own beginning or existing dependency needs.

Examples of other emerging family patterns are:

The 84-year-old woman, disabled after a stroke, who has outlived her husband and 3 children and now lives uncomfortably in the home of her grandson and granddaughter-in-law, sharing the bedroom of 2 young children in generation four. The granddaughter-in-law also gives care to her own elderly parents and a schizophrenic brother.

The devoted couple facing separation after 55 years of marriage because the intact but frail wife can no longer give care to the incapacitated confused husband.

The 90-year-old mother and her 65-year-old mentally retarded son.

The stress of caring for impaired elderly relatives often produces negative effects on family members. It points to the need for services to the family to supplement its efforts to meet the older person's need for care (Grad and Sainsbury 1966). Since the well-being of the generations is interlocked, solutions to the dependencies of old people must focus on the family. Parenthetically, it is ironic that at a time when new roles for older people are being sought, the role of care giver to the very old has emerged. A distinction must be drawn between the role of providing emotional support (visiting, availability in emergencies, affectional bonds) and that of providing instrumental services (shopping, cooking, cleaning, personal care). It is the former that older people want from their families, and the latter that the community must supplement to prevent family breakdown.

What does the future hold?

Data on the proportion of old people who are particularly vulnerable and the nature and number of their needs are in the early stages of development. Shanas estimates that one-fourth of all elderly dwelling in the community require home care services including those who are bedfast or housebound (8%) or able to go out but with difficulty (6 or 7%) (Shanas 1974). Depending on the nature of services included, others estimate one-third (Brody, S. J. 1973), 41% (Pfeiffer 1973), and 27% (Gottesman *et al.* 1975). To these must be added the 5% who are in institutions at any one time. At present 38% of the 65 plus group in the US are 75 or over. By the year 2000, the proportion of very old will increase to 44% of the 30.6 million elderly individuals (Brotman 1975). Since dependencies increase with advancing age, the target population by then may well be 10 million individuals.

The dependencies of older people already have moved beyond what Blenkner (1969) characterized as the "self-solution" and the "kinship solution"; they require societal solutions. This trend will continue. At present families, primarily the women in the next generation, provide 80% of the health services given to old people (Department of Health, Education and Welfare 1972). The projected increase in old people proportionate to the supportive generations undoubtedly will diminish the latter's capacities for giving care. Further, the career-orientation of today's young women will in future make them less available to provide such services (Brody, S. J. 1976*b*). A question unanswered for the present is whether changing life-styles that increase the participation of men in the tasks traditionally carried by women will extend to giving care to the elderly.

Finally, Brotman alerts us to the constant turnover in the elderly population (one-third every 5 years) and therefore to changing characteristics, needs, preferences, and expectations (Brotman 1968). Changes also occur constantly within each aging individual, in the environmental context, and in available resources. There can be no permanent solution to individual or group dependencies. Effective solutions are those that can be flexible in responding to change.

References

Beattie, W. M., Jr. (1970). *Gerontologist* **10** (1), 190–193

Blenkner, M. (1969). *In* "Kalish (1969)," pp 27–37

Brody, E. M. (1966). *Gerontologist* **6**, 201–206

Brody, E. M. (1969). *Gerontologist* **9**, 187–196

Brody, E. M. (1973). *Gerontologist* **13**, 430–435

Brody, E. M. (1974*a*). *Family Process* **13**, 23–37

Brody, E. M. (1974*b*). "Social Work Guidebook for Long-Term Care Facilities." National Institute of Mental Health. US GPO, Washington

Brody, E. M. (1975*a*). *In* Symposium on "Human Factors in Long-Term Health Care". Sponsored by the National Conference on Social Welfare and the Division of Long-Term Care, Bureau of Health Services Research, US PHS, San Francisco

Brody, E. M. (1975*b*). "Mental and Physical Health Practices of Older People."

Research Proposal to the National Institute of Mental Health. Philadelphia Geriatric Center; mimeo
Brody, E. M. (1976). *Medical Care* **14**, No. 5, Supplement; pp 72–82
Brody, E. M. and Kleban, M. H. (1976). "The Fate of Those who do not Move." (In preparation)
Brody, S. J. (1973). *Gerontologist* **13**, 412–418
Brody, S. J. (1976*a*). *Health and Social Work* **1**, 14–31
Brody, S. J. (1976*b*). *Gerontologist* **16**, 181–183
Brotman, H. B. (1968). *In* "State Conference", Iowa Commission on the Aging. De Moines, Iowa; mimeo
Brotman, H. B. (1975). *In* "Staff College", National Institute of Mental Health; mimeo
Butler, R. N. (1969). *Gerontologist* **9** (1), 243–246
Byerts, T. O. (Ed.) (1973). "Housing and Environment for the Elderly." Gerontological Society, Washington
Carp, F. M. (1966). "A Future for the Aged." University of Texas Press, Austin
Colligan, D. (1975). *New York* July 14, pp 28–32
Department of Health, Education and Welfare (DHEW) (1972). "Home Care for Persons 55 and Over in the US, July 1966–June 1969." Vital Health Statistics Series 10, No. 73. Public Health Services, US GPO, Washington
Eisdorfer, C. and Lawton, M. P. (Eds.) (1973). "The Psychology of Adult Development and Aging." American Psychological Association, Washington
Friedsam, H. J. and Dick, H. R. (1963). "Decisions Leading to Institutionalization of the Aged". Unpublished Final Report. Social Security Administration Cooperative Research and Demonstration Grant Program, Project 037 (C1) 20–031
Goldfarb, A. I. (1969). *In* "The Dependencies of Old People", pp 1–14 Ed. R. A. Kalish. Occasional Papers in Gerontology No. 6. Institute of Gerontology, Michigan-Wayne State University, Michigan
Gottesman, L. and Brody, E. M. (1975). *In* "Long-Term Care: A Handbook for Researchers, Planners and Providers". Ed. S. Sherwood. Spectrum. New York: pp 405–510
Gottesman, L., Moss, M. and Worts, F. (1975). *In* "10th International Congress of Gerontology", Jerusalem
Grad, J. and Sainsbury, P. (1966). *Milbank Memorial Fund Quarterly* **44**, Part 2, 246–278
Hayflick, L. (1974). *Gerontologist* **14**, 37–54
Holmes, T. H. and Masuda, M. (1974). *In* "Stressful Life Events: Their Nature and Effects". B. S. Dohrenwend and B. P. Dohrenwend. John Wiley, New York: pp 45–72
Kahn, R. L. (1965). *In* "The York House Institute on Mentally Impaired Aged." Eds. M. P. Lawton and F. Lawton. Philadelphia Geriatric Center, Philadelphia
Kalish, R. A. (Ed.) (1969). The Dependencies of Old People: Occasional Papers in Gerontology No. 6. Institute of Gerontology, Michigan-Wayne State University, Michigan
Kleban, M. H. (1969). Architecture and Behavior: The Mentally Impaired Aged. National Institute of Mental Health Grant, MH 16139. Philadelphia Geriatric Center; mimeo
Lawton, M. P. (1969*a*). *Gerontologist* **9**, 15–19
Lawton, M. P. (1969*b*). "Prosthetic Architecture for Mentally Impaired Aged." DHEW. HSMHA, HS 00100-HSR. Philadelphia Geriatric Center; mimeo
Lawton, M. P. (1975). Final Report; Social and Medical Services in Housing for the Aged. Philadelphia Geriatric Center: mimeo
Lawton, M. P. (1976). *Gerontologist* **16**, 237–242
Lawton, M. P. and Kleban, M. H. (1971). *Gerontologist* **11**, 277–283
Lawton, M. P. and Nahemow, L. (1973). *In* "The Psychology of Adult Development

and Aging". American Psychological Association, Washington. Eds. C. Eisdorfer and M. P. Lawton (1973). pp 619–674

Lawton, M. P., Nahemow, L. and Grimes, M. (1976). "Services in Housing for the Elderly: a Cross-Sectional View." Philadelphia Geriatric Center: mimeo

Lawton, M. P., Nahemow, L. and Teaff, J. (1975). *Journal of Gerontology* **30**, 601–607

Lawton, M. P. and Simon, B. B. (1968). *Gerontologist* **8**, 108–115

Lieberman, M. A. (1969). *Journal of Gerontology* **24**, 330–340

Lieberman, M. A., Prock, V. N. and Tobin, S. S. (1968). *Journal of Gerontology* **23**, 343–353

Lieberman, M. A., Tobin, S. S. and Slover, D. (1971). "The Effects of Relocation on Long-Term Geriatric Patients." Final Report to Department of Mental Health, State of Illinois. Project 17–328: mimeo

Liebowitz, B. (1974). *Gerontologist* **14**, 293–295

Lipsitt, D. R. (1969). *In* "The Dependencies of Old People", pp. 17–26. Ed. R. A. Kalish. Occasional Papers in Gerontology No. 6. Institute of Gerontology, Michigan-Wayne State University, Michigan

Litman, T. J. (1971). *Medical Care* **9**, 67–81

Lowenthal, M. F. and Chiriboga, D. (1973). *In* Eisdorfer and Lawton (1973) pp 281–310

Marlowe, R. A. (1973). Effects of environment on elderly state hospital relocatees. *In* "44th Annual Meeting of the Pacific Sociological Association". Scottsdale, Arizona; mimeo

Neugarten, B. L. (1973). *In* "The Psychology of Adult Development and Aging". Eds. C. Eisdorfer and M. P. Lawton, American Psychological Association, Washington: pp 311–335

Pastalan, L. A. (1973). *Proceedings, Environment Design Research* **1**, 383–392

Pfeiffer, E. (1973). Multidimensional quantitative assessment of three populations of elderly. *In* 26th Annual Meeting of the Gerontological Society, Miami Beach

Pollack, J. (1969). "Aged People Caught in the Decay of the Inner City." Central Bureau for the Jewish Aged, New York; mimeo

Rahe, R. H. (1974). *In* "Stressful Life Events: Their Nature and Effects". Eds. B. S. Dohrenwend and B. P. Dohrenwend. John Wiley, New York: pp 73–86

Rosow, I. (1962). *Gerontologist* **2**, 182–191

Rosow, I. (1967). "Social Integration of the Aged". Free Press, New York

Schooler, K. (1970). *Gerontologist* **10** (1), 194–197

Schuckit, M. A. (1974). Unrecognized psychiatric illness in elderly medical-surgical patients, *In* 27th Annual Meeting of the Gerontological Society, Portland, Ore

Selye, H. (1970). *Journal of the American Geriatric Society* **18**, 669–680

Shanas, E. (1974). *American Journal of Public Health* **64**, 261–264

Shanas, E., Townsend, P., Wedderburn, D., Friis, H., Milhoj, P. and Stenhouwer, J. (1968). "Old People in Three Industrial Societies." Atherton Press, New York; Routledge and Kegan Paul, London

Sherwood, S., Greer, D. S., Morris, J. N. and Sherwood, C. (1972). Final Report on the Highland Heights Experiment: mimeo

Thurman, D. (1970). Coordinated services to the aged: The Dorchester–Mattapan Experience. *In* National Association of Jewish Center Worker's Conference, Sheraton Boston

Townsend, P. (1965). *In* "Social Structure and the Family: General Relations". Ed. E. Shanas and G. Streib. Prentice-Hall, Englewood Cliffs: pp 163–187

United States Senate Special Committee on Aging, Sub-committee on Long-Term Care (1974) Nursing Home Care in the United States: Failure in Public Policy: Introductory Report. US GPO, Washington

Weinberg, J. (1976). *Gerontologist* **16**(1), 4–10

Commentary

Nelson H Cruikshank

National Council of Senior Citizens,
Washington, DC

When I read the papers by Dr Busse and Professor Exton-Smith I found myself, as a man entering his seventy-fifth year, becoming somewhat alarmed. These papers were thoughtful documentations of the biological and psychological problems of the aging process and they were very necessary to a proper approach to the problems to which this conference addresses itself. I cannot, in the time available, make any detailed discussion of these thought-provoking papers, and at the risk of appearing to be nitpicking because there is so much in them that I agree with, I have to search for the questions that arose that did not seem to me to be adequately handled or properly addressed.

I noticed one difference in the approach of the British and the American commentators. The Americans seem to be much happier about the British experience than the British are themselves, and I don't know whether this is just the customary British reticence, but I think it is more than that. It possibly arises from the fact that at least the British have a national policy with respect to the problems of the aging, and we in America have to confess that we don't. So, I think possibly our British colleagues are measuring their achievements against a set of goals and a determined policy, while we are still floundering around without a policy, and therefore they think that they are not doing as well as we think that they are.

There was another element that emerged in the papers and that was an indication of a lack of confidence in the elderly to meet their own problems. Dr Jefferys calls on the providers to correct the problems which she so beautifully documented, and Bob Ball cites the problems of the increasing numbers of aged in our society and the demographic changes that will bring about crises in our Social Security system. But it seemed to me that both of them ignored the possibility of a militant minority with a growing self-consciousness bringing solutions to the problem themselves. We see the growing number of elderly in this country organizing into groups that are taking their problems into their own hands, and doing something about them. In the problem of housing, for example, the National Council of Senior Citizen for 5 hours picketed the office of Housing and Urban Development. We think this was a watershed in changing the attitude of that department.

One-third of the voters in America who will cast their vote this fall will be people aged 55 and over, and although still a minority, this group representing those retired and those who are facing retirement can have considerable political clout in this country, and this is beginning to have some effect. So the increasing number in proportion to the total population may not be the problem. It could possibly be the solution. I would like to see further exploration of this aspect of the situation.

Then there was the problem of the proprietary nursing homes. A couple of the papers referred to it, but they seem to back off from facing up to the issue. It seems to me that there is really here a fundamental question. Is the nursing home, as the institution we know it in America, an appropriate field for private investment? Can good quality care ever successfully compete with the profit motive? Now, we know that there are instances where it does, but they seem to be so much in the minority that it does raise this question. I got the impression, that because they are here, because they are 95% of the beds in this country, the speakers regarded the problem as too enormous for us to do anything but accept the situation. Well, I don't agree that because a problem is big and because it seems unmanageable and because it seems to be deeply rooted in the profit motivations of our society that we shouldn't face up to it and ask fundamental questions.

Another question that seemed to me not quite being fully dealt with, although Mrs Brody touched on it to some extent, was the proper relationship of the young and the elderly and the various supporting and intersupporting roles they can have, particularly as translated into policy issues. What kind of housing and community housing for the elderly is appropriate? I know that among my own group there are conflicting ideas about this, and I would like to see further study on this question. To what extent is living in a community of mixed ages supportive of old people and to what extent is it destructive and non-supportive?

Another point that was not dealt with in my view is the role of maintaining active interest in later years of life. What part does that play in the extension of life and in the improvement of the quality of life? I have recently looked at the 56 men who signed the Declaration of Independence, and the remarkable thing about them is the fact that so many of them lived long and useful lives, particularly in the light of the normal life expectancy of the 18th century. Of these 56 men, five lived into their 90s, and nine more into their 80s. The average age at death was just above 67 years, and if you take out the one from South

Carolina who died in an accident at sea at the age of 30, the average age at death was about 68. These men, having achieved the independence of their country and having started a new nation, could well have retired and relaxed, but they didn't.

John Adams, who died at the age of 91, was active in the drafting of the Treaty of Paris after the Revolution. He represented our government to the Netherlands in seeking a loan (which incidentally he didn't get). He served as Vice-President under Washington, then was President for two terms and maintained an active correspondence right up to the day of his death. Samuel Adams lived to 81. After the successful work of the Revolution he served as Governor of Massachussets at the age of 72 to 76. Ben Franklin, who was 70 at the signing of the Declaration, lived to be 84 and he served on the Constitutional Convention at the age of 83, the year before he died. Thomas Jefferson, who lived to be 83, was Minister to France, Secretary of State under Washington, served as President for two terms and also maintained an active correspondence.

Now to me, the question about this remarkable galaxy of men is did they live to this long life because they retained activity and interest when they might well have rested on their laurels and retired, or were they just remarkable men that they would have been active anyhow? Which was the cause? Which was the effect? We like to think, and some of our own experience indicates, that retaining an active role, continuing a meaningful activity, both prolongs life and adds to the quality of life. But which is cause and which is effect, we don't know and it seems to me important that we try to find out. We can't go back in history and unearth these men and ask them, but we could make inquiries and studies on what I think is an important question and which has not as yet been touched on in this conference.

Bernice L Neugarten

Behavioral Sciences,
University of Chicago

The papers prepared for this Conference, when considered as a group, have stressed the problem aspects of caring for the elderly. The focus is, understandably enough, upon the group we may call the "old-old", the group whose health problems are most concentrated, for whom the costs of health services are highest, and for whom the problems of administering services are perhaps the most difficult when compared with younger age groups.

Some of the papers have painted not only a bleak picture of the present, but also a bleak picture of the future, for the numbers of the very old are growing rapidly and economic stringencies are pressing, not only for the British but increasingly also for the Americans. It is an unhappy fact that, very generally speaking, the well-being of the aged depends more upon the level of affluence of a society than upon any other single factor — or so, at least, it appears to many of us who have studied the status of older people in various societies at various times in history. Political ideologies and value systems are important, but they seem less significant than the level of economic productivity.

It is worth a reminder, however, that the overall picture is not all bleak. As Dr Eisdorfer put it, there is good news as well as bad news. From the perspective of the society at large, the changing age distribution brings with it the appearance of large numbers of the very aged, and therefore large numbers of the chronically ill, the frail, the mentally and physically deteriorated. But it also brings with it the newly emerging group we can call the "young-old." For the first time in history, industrialized societies are seeing increasing numbers of retirees, relatively healthy and vigorous, increasingly well-educated, increasingly well-off economically *vis-à-vis* younger people, increasingly active politically, a group who seek new ways of self-fulfillment and new ways of community participation. In at least some segments of modern society, the young-old constitute a new leisure class. They are a growing proportion of the population who may be said to be truly reaping the benefits of a longer life-span, and as a group they may become the major agents of social change.

From this very broad perspective, the added longevity that has become the striking feature of the twentieth century is to be regarded as one of man's great achievements. Like other achievements resulting from the growth of science and technology, it has its price. In today's conference we are facing up to one part of that social price — to one, and only one, of the sets of the problems that arise because the numbers of old people have grown so suddenly that modern societies are unprepared to accommodate to their needs. Our difficulties in meeting the health needs of the old is only one of the components of the social price we pay for our added longevity. Presumably it is the goal of gerontologists and geriatricians to reduce that social price — to make life better for the old themselves, and to find ways of hastening social change in ways that will accommodate the old at the same time that we accommodate the young.

It almost goes without saying that it is easier to ask than to answer the question how to maximize the benefits of our extended life span? I want only to remind us that for most societies, as for most aging individuals, the benefits are perceived to outweigh the costs.

With regard to the health status of older people, the costs may be rising. Generally speaking, increased longevity is a reflection of better, not poorer health. This is almost a matter of definition. But as this audience knows full well, the relations of various forms of morbidity to mortality are not well understood; nor the relations of mortality rates at younger ages to mortality rates at later ages. We have various definitions of health, and various indices for measuring it. Better levels of health for older persons are the results, not only of advances in medicine, but of improved public health measures, of rising levels of education in the population at large, and particularly of diminishing rates of poverty over the life-cycles of successive cohorts of persons.

All this says little, however, regarding the period of disability that can be expected to occur for most people in the very last phase of life. For the moment we have little basis for predicting that this period of disability will become shorter. Presumably another long-term goal of both gerontology and geriatric medicine is that people should remain physically and psychologically intact through the eighth or ninth decade, then die quickly without a long period of terminal illness. But the prospect may well be the opposite: that with increasing age, people will have a drawn-out period of physical and psychological disability, with medical and social services that can keep them alive, but keep them neither healthy nor happy. This is, of course, the spectre that haunts medical and social planners when they think about the aging society, just as it is the spectre that haunts each of us when we think of our own old age.

In this connection, I have recently been informed by Dr Ernest Gruenberg of Johns Hopkins University of a set of data gathered in a Swedish community that indicate that the course of senile brain disease has been lengthened over the past few decades from about 3 years to about 12 years. Evidently the conquest of pneumonia has had its effects, for one thing, one of them the prolongation of certain slowly progressive diseases which in earlier decades were shortened by fatal complications. If broader sets of data become available, it may turn out that added longevity in the years beyond 65 is accounted for more by the extension of the lives of the seriously deteriorated aged than by the extension of the lives of the less seriously ill — in short, we may be experiencing a *differential gain* in longevity that is far from desirable. This is one possible example of the added price we may be paying for added life expectancy for those aged over 65.

Turning now to problems of health care itself, I hesitate to add still another factor to the already complicated picture that faces us at this conference. Yet I wish to comment briefly on the role of the family in the care of the aged. There has been attention given in these papers to the role of public agencies; to problems of housing; to the hospital, the nursing home, and the long-term care institution; to the problems of manpower; and to the use of volunteers. Surprisingly, with the exception of Mrs Brody's mention of "family personalities" as they affect the relationships of older people, no one has addressed directly the place of the family — surely, from many points of view, the most important social institution of all in caring for the aged. What *is* the role of the family, and what will it be in the next two or three decades?

Keeping in mind that "family" is not synonymous with "household," we know that the four- and five-generation family is becoming more frequent, and will be the norm by the year 2000. In United States, because of changing birth rates in the past — especially the post-war "baby boom" of the 1950s — the person who will be old in 1990 and 2000 will have more, rather than fewer children and other relatives. (For example, it has been calculated that a 65-year-old woman in 1970 had, on the average, 2.1 surviving children; but a 65-year-old woman in 2000 will have 2.99 surviving children.) These rates will change, of course, in the decades beyond 2000 as the lower birth rates of the 1970s show their effects, but persons who are presently middle-aged will have larger kin networks than their predecessors.

Numbers of surviving children do not tell us about the interactions or patterns of assistance between parent and child. Yet the data from a wide variety of studies show that the family has remained a strong and supportive institution for older people. Most old people today want to be independent of their families as long as possible, but when they can no longer manage for themselves, they expect their children to come to their aid. Not only do such expectations exist, but they are usually fulfilled. A complex pattern of exchange of services exists across generations, and both ties of affection and obligation remain strong.

In the United States, there has been a marked trend toward separate households for older persons, due, so it is usually interpreted, to rising levels of income (the generations move apart when they can afford it), to the greater availability of housing, and to the fact that the telephone and automobile make it possible to maintain family ties without living under the same roof. Yet in 1970, the latest year for which we have good data, it was clear that the older the individual, and the sicker, the more likely he or she would be living with a child. Of all persons aged 75+ in United States, one of five women — and one of ten men — was living with a child. It often goes unnoticed that at present, in United States, for every older person living in an institution, there are some 2.5 others living with a child.

For the larger numbers who live in their own households, the overwhelming majority live very near to at least one child, and see children and grandchildren regularly and frequently. The latest national survey in United States shows that of all older people who have children, some 80 to 90% reported seeing a child or a grandchild within the last day or last week.

But it is not the number of contacts alone which are indicative of the "caring" attitudes. There are other indices. Dr Maddox's paper will point out that of older persons receiving home care, 80% are receiving that care from family members.

We need much more data regarding the important topic of *parent-caring*, but there are growing indications that the parent-caring role is becoming a major life task for middle-aged people, especially, of course, for middle-aged women, many of whom tell us, in our own studies, that they feel they move almost immediately from preoccupations with child-caring to preoccupations with parent-caring. "Care" and "responsibility" do not necessarily mean daily physical management, or sharing one's household with an older relative, but they do mean social and emotional responsibility, feelings of diminished self-worth or guilt if the aged relative is not perceived to be content or comfortable, the frequent visits and phone calls, the arranging of services and help. Indeed, it is a noteworthy gap in our researches and in our expressed concerns over the care of the aged that the attention given to the family as the support system has been so much focused upon the inter-generational household, to the neglect of the much wider pattern of family support that undoubtedly exists.

In this connection, it is often lamented that the family is a "vanishing" institution; that the changing roles of women are making it increasingly impossible to provide the tender, loving care for old people that was presumably more characteristic in earlier times in history — in short, that the care needed by the sick old cannot be provided by the modern family, just as it cannot be purchased on the labor market; that the changing value pattern, at least in United States, is one in which the virtues of "duty" and "service" and "sacrifice" are no longer rewarded, and where personal service is regarded as demeaning — and that there is no other solution than the warehousing of old sick people in nursing homes and old-age homes. It is true, with regard to the "vanishing" family, that divorce is on the rise, and that increasing numbers of children are being raised in one-parent households (in United States it is now one of every 16 children), and there are other signs of the fragmentation of the family with regard to marital and child-rearing roles. But it remains to be seen if the same fragmentation will become true of the parent-caring role. Middle-aged children may continue to come to the aid of their aged parents in the future just as they are doing in 1976. It is even possible that inter-generational ties may become more rather than less important in the future; for as other social institutions take over the financial support and the health care of the aged, the ties between generations may become more important with regard to human values and the expressive side of life — that is, in providing lasting emotional ties and a sense of identity and self-worth.

We do not know what will occur to aging men who, divorced and remarried, have produced two sets of children rather than one; or to the increasing numbers of women who may remain single or divorced — but who, if they have borne children, seem to remain closely attached to those children whether or not a husband is present in the home. Indeed some persons are predicting that the stable family of the future will increasingly take the form of child, mother, grandmother, great-grandmother — rather than the form of child, mother, father. Whatever these future trends may be, changes in horizontal family relationships (marital and sibling relationships) are not necessarily generalizable to vertical or inter-generational relationships.

Thus it would be premature, to say the least, to discount the role of the family in the care of the aged. There is little evidence that adult children do not "care about" their parents. Caring *about* one's parent is not the same as caring *for* one's parent, but how the two will be related in the future remains to be seen.

Perhaps it is relevant in this connection that a group of women graduate students took pains to point out to me recently that, first, they feel very closely tied to their mothers, especially in those cases where their mothers are divorced or widowed; second, that one result of the women's liberation movement has been to make them more sensitive to the needs of their mothers; third, that they themselves, will not automatically give priority to their husband's rather than to their mother's needs as they perceive to have been the case with less liberated women. All this may be unrealistic — to say nothing of the implication that men may become more emotionally detached from the family in the future than they are today, itself a bleak prospect — but it provides food for thought. At least we should not take it for granted that changing family patterns will mean increasing neglect of the aged.

I am suggesting therefore that we count the family in, not out, when we talk about policy issues; and that we think about the family as the focal point when we think about community and home care of the aged. Important policy questions relate to the underlying question, how do we strengthen the family as the care-giving institution, whether or not the family lives in one household? How do we help the middle-aged meet their sense of obligation to their parents? How do we alter our housing policies and our social security policies accordingly? How do we educate family members to the alterable and unalterable changes of aging and to the support functions of the family? How can we Americans build upon the experience of our British colleagues in this respect?

Further still, can we begin to think of the family as the unit, rather than the aged individual as the unit? Can our health services and our social services be aimed at the multi-person and multi-generational family unit? Is this the direction we should take for improving the care of the present aged and the future aged?

D J Newell

Department of Medical Statistics,
University of Newcastle upon Tyne

The proper allocation of the available resources for the care of the elderly, and the plea for the increase in those resources, are both at risk of being dominated by the emotive rather than the factual. Since individuals differ one from another, medical statistics are required, as the facts must be based on figures. One sentence from Dr Eisdorfer's contribution sums this up: "The data base is often characterized by the substitution of idiom for ideas, and demagoguery for data." Nevertheless, the first two papers show the extent of the routinely collected and special survey data which are available in the two countries, particularly when the authors work as assiduously as Professor Jefferys and Dr Ball at collating them.

Many British readers will be surprised at the very great strides which the United States has taken in recent years to assure the income of the elderly. They will also note that the proportion of pre-retirement income to be guaranteed in the USA is higher than that in the UK, on the basically higher financial standards of living in the USA. The USA would appear to have had resources available for solving most of these income problems, and has now demonstrated the will to do so.

Turning now to the provision of care for the elderly, each country has much to learn from the other. In the gross figures, giving national averages, there are certain to be some errors of data collection and interpretation on both sides of the Atlantic. More important than this, the national figures also obscure important differences between different areas in each country. Nevertheless, taking the two national sets of data as they stand, it appears that British care is polarized between the high-intensity, high-cost hospital, and the low-cost domestic care, with relatively little in the middle ground where supportive care with less intensive medical presence could be given. It is likely that the reorganization of care on an area basis will lead to some redistribution of whatever resources are available proportionately away from hospitals. Some of the redeployed resources might profitably go towards experimental schemes providing "intermediate" care of the type available in some American (and British) nursing homes.

This polarity may also be noted in that the hospital service in particular, and the health service in general, aspires to be a total service, whereas the social services are a partial service, supplementing the existing domestic, financial, kinship and friendship resources of the elderly individual.

The first two papers of the conference make it clear that the elderly are going to form an increasing proportion of the total populations on both side of the Atlantic, unless the definition of "elderly" is changed. A time of high unemployment is not a good time to propose a change, but we do well to remember that retirement ages, though traditional, are entirely arbitrary. In this context, as in others, the role of the employment of women should not be overlooked.

What are the *needs* of the elderly? Two papers (Gedling and Newell 1972, Gilholme and Newell 1972) admirably summarized by Somers (1976) were more concerned with the *demands* of the elderly for admission and retention in non-psychiatric beds; demand as interpreted jointly and successively by the patient, the general practitioner and the hospital physician. In non-surgical cases, where unsatisfied demand did not obscure the picture, it emerged that demand is higher for urban than rural patients, because of the diseases of urban dwelling, including pollution. And it depends on the expectations of the patient and the attitude of the physician. Further, low social class patients, independently from these other variables, require more hospital care than do others. Despite my earlier differentiation of hospital care being total, where social service care is "topping-up" care, it now becomes clear that the increased morbidity of the poor is not the sole determinant of their hospital demands, but so is the unsuitability of their homes.

Two anecdotes will serve to illustrate very important points made by the speakers. Although I report them anecdotally, they were to the best of my knowledge based on very sound numerical studies. My apologies to the unnamed authors.

Elderly people rehoused in an excellent modern European housing scheme with central heating, elevators and all modern conveniences were compared in health status with a control group of their contemporaries. These controls remained in their old housing, where heating was by coal fire, and the old people had to carry the coal up the stairs from the back yard. In fact, they spent a lot of time on the stairs, because the privy, which they shared with neighbours, was also across the yard. The outcome of the ten-year study was that the rehoused people had much worse health status than the others, not only from isolation, but from decreased physical activity, which had led to immobility for some of them.

A second study, in Britain, has compared aspects of different Residential Homes. A group of Homes under one administration had far more fractures, particularly of the femur, amongst its residents than did other homes. An obvious and immediate conclusion might be that these were the types of institution, mentioned in the conference papers of Margot Jefferys and Tom Arie, which had been found guilty of cruelty or neglect. In fact, these were the sort of institution which would have earned the praise of Elaine Brody, as they encouraged independence and activity by the elderly, which of course, as pointed out by Professor Exton-Smith, carry with them the possibility of falls and fractures. If the alternative is to keep the patients immobile and often bedfast, very serious questions arise about the quality of their lives.

Of course, these two studies should not be interpreted to mean that the elderly should not be rehoused nor that they should be restrained in bed to avoid fractures. I merely use them to illustrate that the secondary effects of beneficial programs must be taken into account. These two anecdotes illustrate studies where there was a specific measure of *output*, health status after some form of intervention. Too many of our studies of care try to assess results in terms of numbers of patients treated, or number of hostel places provided or nurses employed or dollars expended, for example. These are really only measures of input. We need to clear up the meanings of some of the words we have been using.

One of the first real attempts to clarify this concept in Britain came from a medical administrator in the Ministry of Health. Matthew (1971) insisted that "*need* for medical care must be distinguished from the *demand* for care, and from the use of services, *utilization*. A *need* for medical care exists when an individual has an illness or disability *for which there is an effective and acceptable treatment or cure* . . . need is not necessarily followed by utilization . . . there can be demand and utilization without real underlying need."

An American commentator (Boulding 1966) insisted that these concepts of a treatment being effective and acceptable should not be left to the physician and the experts, but should rest largely with the patient himself. His reasons were partly financial, and partly from the American citizen's characteristic attitude of independence (and we join with you this year in celebrating our mutual Independence).

Mathew (1971) made a valuable advance in insisting that "need" has no real meaning if there is no effective treatment. Cochrane (1972) in an important monograph, "Effectiveness and Efficiency in Health Services" shows that a number of commonly accepted treatments have not passed the test of effectiveness. But while we must do nothing to inhibit the great task of testing all the widely used or recommended treatments for common diseases and disabilities, it is now time to go further. We must now admit that it is unrealistic to say that there is a need for an effective treatment, however expensive it may prove to be. To take a ridiculous example, injections of moon dust may cure rheumatoid arthritis, but we could not now say that all arthritics need it.

All of our proposals for improving health care would merit examination by what statisticians called a decision–theoretic approach, which is similar to some forms of operations research, and which economists call cost-benefit analysis. It is tempting to quote from an economist's view of health and medical care (Fuchs 1972): "When an economist enters an area such as health, he runs a high risk of being either irrelevant or wrong." But the same applies to all of us, including health professionals themselves, statisticians, sociologists, administrators or whatever. We can learn by interdisciplinary discussion and working together. An economist who insists that the only sensible economics are those of the free market, and that therefore medical care should be organized entirely subject to market forces, when he will be able to analyze it, has little to offer us. But a number of economists, particularly in the USA, but including the group at York under Professor Alan Williams (1974*a*, 1974*b*), are making valuable progress in the relevant welfare economics. The details are not appropriate here, but one important aspect on the cost side is that we should sometimes concern ourselves more with "opportunity costs" (what would these personnel, these resources be doing if they were not used in the specified way) than with average costs, which are often misleading. On the health benefits side, many of the variables cannot be measured in financial terms, and we fool ourselves if we try to do so. Ultimately, the trade-off decisions of one kind of care for another, with their associated costs and benefits, are often political. The role of research workers, and conferences such as this, should be to inform the decision makers, and then encourage them to make informed decisions.

References

Boulding, K. E. (1966). *Milbank Memorial Fund Quarterly* **44**, 202–218

Cochrane, A. L. (1972). "Effectiveness and Efficiency in Health Services". Nuffield Provincial Hospitals Trust. Oxford University Press, London

Fuchs, V. R. (1972). "Essays in the Economics of Health and Medical Care". Columbia University Press, New York

Gelding, P. and Newell, D. J. (1972). *In* "Problems and Progress in Medical Care", 7th series. Ed. G. McLachlan. Oxford University Press, London: pp 131–145

Gilholme, K. R. and Newell, D. J. (1972). *In* "Problems and Progress in Medical Care", 7th series. Ed. G. McLachlan. Oxford University Press, London: pp 146–161

Matthew, G. K. (1971). *In* "Portfolio for Health". Ed. G. McLachlan. Oxford University Press, London: pp 27–46
Somers, A. R. (1976). *Annals of Internal Medicine* **84**, 466–476
Williams A. H. (1974*a*). *British Journal of Preventive and Social Medicine* **28**, 196–202
Williams, A. H. (1974*b*). *Proceedings of the Royal Society of Medicine* **67**, 1293–1296

Discussion

Sir George Godber (*Late Chief Medical Officer, Department of Health and Social Security, London*) I find myself identifying very closely with Mr Cruikshank, probably because I am another statutory old person. He spoke about the British having a national policy. We do, but from some of the things that have been said recently I wonder if many of us have short memories and think we have only had it for the last 3 or 4 years. In fact, it is implicit in the 1948 recognization of our legislation. So far as old people are concerned, a report was published about 1956, and a detailed programme was set out by ministers in 1963; that we are far short of attaining the targets as defined I entirely agree.

It has been suggested that in Britain we are short of nursing homes. I think that is a deficiency I welcome. I don't think we want nursing homes. I think we want geriatric departments and other similar departments in general hospitals with suitable longer stay establishments associated with them. We want a comprehensive service, although it has been rightly emphasized that most of all it is families who are looking after old people.

I don't think the figures that we have been given today have been always accurate. Mr Ball said that the proportion of old people over 65 being looked after outside institutions was the same in both countries but my sums don't lead to that conclusion. My sums lead me to the conclusion that 4.1% of the over 65s in Britain are in institutional care, and my calculations based on Mr Ball's own figures lead me to the conclusion that about 6% of over 65s in the United States are in some kind of care of that kind.

I don't think that statistics can tell the whole story. It is far more important that we should have some more subjective idea of what improvements have been made and in considering the way our old people were looked after in institutions 40 years ago there has been a far greater improvement than people recognize. One of the reasons why we have scandals now is that people look for them; if you look for scandalous conditions you will find them.

I don't think British conditions are vastly better than American, but even by the year 2000 the USA won't face anything like the proportion of over 65s with which the British now have to deal. I hope we will all be doing it a great deal better by then, because we certainly don't do it well enough now.

Mr Elliot Stern (*US House Select Committee on Aging*) I would like to encourage either the principal speakers or others to comment on Professor Newell's suggestion of helping some of the policy-makers come to informed decisions. From any of the panelists' or speakers' perspectives, which items of national policy, either in the United States or in Great Britain, need the most attention now; and if one has to make that leap of faith from data and statistics to concrete policy issues, which area or specific point should one choose for first attention by the appropriate administrative bodies?

Mr Cruikshank If I were to name a priority, I would like to see the Congress in this country move from a concept of health insurance to a concept of health provision and planning on a structured basis. Then as a part of that process we would need to separate the medical problems from the custodial problems and devise appropriate plans for both. My view, not universally accepted among my colleagues, is that long-term care is not a proper part of a basic health security program, and if it were separated, I think we could do it better by far than we are now doing. There are many lessons that we have learned from 10 years of Medicare. The two primary ones are: (1) a mechanism for payment is inadequate to the total job, even for the elderly; and (2) closely related to that, you can't have a good health plan for the elderly by setting up a system just for the elderly. The cures for the shortcomings in Medicare will be found not just in patching up Medicare, though we may have to do that on an interim basis, but will be found as a part of a comprehensive plan for the total population. I don't think you can properly do this for any one segment of the population, particularly a high risk segment.

Mr Stern Dr Neugarten, you mentioned that you had some scientific and other data showing that there is a shift in family structure, in effect a redefinition of the family. That should have some implications for national policy, but you stopped short of saying what those implications might be. Could you explicate a little further and maybe go beyond the data and speculate. What program is going to be the first, or the most directly affected, and how might we begin to plan now for the year 2000?

Dr Neugarten Unhappily, I am going to have to evade the issue from one perspective, because I did not come prepared for a response to that question. First, I do not think our data clearly establish that four and five generations of women is the stable family but as I said some people are predicting that this will be the stable family by the year 2000. I think if one presumes that some priority attention ought to be given to social change that is not just ameliorative but is more long-range, then I think it is time maybe to think about some of the kinds of legislation that would have long-term effects. How do you support a middle-aged woman with a mother of 65 and a grandmother of 85? How do you come to her assistance when in most cases you can count on the fact that she wants to continue meeting her responsibilities? I don't know how you spell that out in legislation right now but I would give that pretty high priority. For one thing, I would look at housing policies that establish age-segregated communities in which a family is cut apart because there is an age restriction on people who can have subsidized housing, where younger people cannot move in with their old people because they don't meet the eligibility requirement.

Dr Eisdorfer I would like to respond from two points of view. Nelson Cruikshank and I, as well as several others in the audience, are members of the Federal Council on Aging, a group which presumably helps to make federal policy. This year we have embarked on a very interesting excursion, looking specifically at the approximately 15% of the elderly population who are defined as the frail elderly, very much overlapping with Bernice Neugarten's description of the "old-old". One of the issues that we have come to look at very hard is related to the presence or absence of social policy. I think Bob Ball mentioned that we have an economic policy; we also have an acute medical care policy in aging. What we don't have, oddly enough, is a policy of social services, and what has happened in consequence is that certain kinds of social services have been appended as part of health care, and this has confounded both health care, on the one hand, and the social service delivery system on the other. I think that the kind of input that is being generated here, with much more accurate knowledge of statistics of health and social service needs could go a long way toward explicating this policy.

I would like Elaine Brody to comment on an issue that Bernice Neugarten has raised. The role of the family in caring for the frail elderly, in contrast to the role of professionals, has to be a significant point of social policy. Current social policy in manpower is for the Federal Government to withdraw support or categorical support at a time when most of us feel very strongly that one of the crucial variables is the absence of trained person-power. A conviction that the family is really the primary source of support would justify such a social policy strategy, but I would challenge that.

My own feeling, on the basis of some work by Elaine Brody, is that families tend to over-extend themselves, and may so prevent good psychological, psychiatric, and in some cases medical care from being distributed to the elderly; and that family guilt and the necessity of taking care of an aged grandparent or parent lead to as much harm as good. I would question a social policy which facilitates this process in place of providing professional services to support the elderly in maintaining an independent existence.

Dr Neugarten I agree, of course, that those problems exist, but I would put the question differently. How do we educate the family for good care of the elderly; not how do we by-pass the family and educate the professional. What we know about older people and about ourselves, is that an older person looks to the family and feels supported by the family. but maybe the family is uneducated or unable, and that is where I would like to see some of our effort go.

Mrs Elaine Brody I think education for the family certainly is a necessity, because there is so much documentation of the fact that older people and families themselves lack health information. But it is very satisfactory in gerontology when a stream of research occurs in different parts of the country in relation to different kinds of institutions and comes up with the same findings. The area of the road to institutional care is one of those areas of research that has been consistent, whether it is the road to mental hospitalization (Marjorie Lowenthal's (1964) work), or decisions leading to institutions (Friedsam and Dick (1963) in Texas), or work we have done at our institution.

The unanimous findings is that families over-extend themselves. By the time they get the older person to the door of an institution, they have exhausted themselves personally, financially, physically, emotionally in their attempt to avoid institutionalization. I think in terms of policy we tend to confuse two different kinds of support that families give to their older relatives. One kind of support is the emotional bond and the caring, and one hopes this will continue. There is no evidence that affectional ties are diminishing among members of the family. The other kind of support that families can provide are the instrumental activities, the specific things like shopping, cooking, bathing, and so on. Those are two quite different kinds of things.

I think in the future older people will continue to want, expect, and get from their families emotional support in times of crisis, the presence of the child, the caring, the visiting, and so on. I think the things that the community must supply are the instrumental kinds of support — transportation, shopping, cooking, housecleaning, personal care, and the like. The middle generations are being stretched beyond the endurance point in their effort to give that kind of care to the many more older people who are now in those families. The community care services have got to focus on the needs of the family rather than specifically and exclusively on the needs of the older person.

I would like to comment on Professor Newell's examples of good environment having a bad effect on older people. There are several examples of that sort in the United States, as well. In relation to the affair of the hip fractures, one has to remember that this involves a value judgement. In institutional settings we are constantly faced with the issue of whether we should tie old people into geriatric chairs to avoid the danger of hip fracture, or let them roam and take the risk. Essentially this is a value judgment. With respect to the housing environment that continued to keep people active, I think again we should not accept a false dichotomy saying either we have a housing environment poor in services or we have poor health. What we have to look at is the possibility of having a good housing environment and yet providing in that environment opportunities for the older person to exercise his or her physical and mental capacities fully to offset whatever potential negative effects there might be from having services.

Dr Wadie Kamel (*Professor and Director of International Health, University of Illinois Medical Center in Chicago*) I would like to identify with Mr Cruikshank in his aim of developing contributions by the elderly. I think Sir George Godber has done well in saying that we need less nursing homes, not more nursing homes. This brought to my mind immediately our arguments in the medical school about positive epidemiology. Instead of talking about epidemiology of disease, we should talk about epidemiology of health, and instead of concentrating all the time on caring for the elderly we should think hard about it and have a thorough discussion of contributions by the elderly.

The question certainly relates to preventive geriatrics. There is a tremendous need for collection of statistics and especially in places where longevity has been noticed and quantified, such as Georgia in the USSR, Ecuador and the Himalayas, and certainly this would open study and discussion of the positive aspects of old age. In this context I would like to bring to your attention some of our recent studies on the prevalence of heart disease where the ambulatory status of the elderly has been decreased by foot diseases (Jerath *et al.* 1976). There is the thought that people who have had a very successful aging life may contribute to our knowledge on the benefits of exercise and other aspects of their way of life including being kept on their feet.

Dr Dolores Davis (*Executive Director, National Center on the Black Aged*) I would like to reinforce Dr Neugarten's concepts about the family as it relates to the black family. The Senate Committee on Aging Report on the failure of nursing home policies in the United States points out that less than 2% of the 1.6 million black elderly receive any kind of institutional care. It is also well known that black elderly do not rely primarily on doctors and nurses because the care is so poor, discrimination is great, and also because they cannot afford it. So therefore, I think everyone in the audience should look to the black family as a rich model of how community networks and the inter-generational family provide care for the black elderly in their homes and in their communities. I would also like to relate this to the manpower problems. I agree with Dr Brody that we should not use an "either-or" approach. The call is for teamwork, professionals helping elderly people, showing them how, and then working together, because you cannot rely on professionals to provide all the services that the elderly need.

Ms Mary Marshall (*Virginia State Legislature*) I am Chairman of a special committee on the needs of the elderly, and I am, I hope, the target of some of this educational effort of which we have been speaking. I would like to just lay out some of the problems with which I am coping quite unsuccessfully. How do we provide for preventive care? We have been talking mostly today about crisis care. How can we provide the elderly with something like the well baby clinic, which keeps children from getting sick instead of treating them when they are sick? We heard a little bit earlier about dark adaptation problems, and that is almost all I have heard on what we do to teach people to keep well and to perceive disability before it becomes serious and when it can still be met.

How do we cope with the multiple problems? Most of the elderly that I know of have more than one problem, and so a Stroke Center or a Heart Disease Center do not begin to meet all of their problems. If we are going to look for non-institutional care, which is a field in which this country, and particularly my State, is very weak indeed, how do we provide the mix of health, cure, homemaker services or home aides, which enable people to stay in their own homes? (At this point I would like to emit a cry of despair as a state legislator trying to design a program that will combine Medicare, Medicaid, Title XX and the Older Americans Act!)

If we do succeed in producing that battery of home aides that will enable someone to stay at home, are we then going to encourage too much dependence, contributing to the further debility of the older person — and of the taxpayer? When those questions are answered, I would like some help on the issue of compulsory retirement, because I have been trying to get legislation seriously considered on this subject. I have not been able to draft anything that satisfies me or will even interest anybody else.

Mr Peter Meek (*Ridgewood, New Jersey*) I am a retired individual very much interested in trying as a volunteer to solve some of these questions. I would like to ask some of the British representatives a question. At the risk of oversimplifying the situation, I gather that there are far fewer nursing homes in Great Britain than in the United States and that, relatively speaking, there are more domestics, what we call home care or homemaker services. We have in this country commercial interests in the nursing home field, and we are at a critical point in the development of our home services in that, as Mr Cruikshank indicated in relation to the nursing homes, we are about, I think, to decide if commercial interests shall enter the home-care field in a big way. Now, has it been the British experience that the reason they do not have many commercial nursing homes and have a well-developed domestics service is because this was set up under government auspices? It is critical for us now, because a number of us in the non-profit field are concerned about the entry of the for-profit group, having seen what happened in the commercial nursing home field where uncontrolled profit-making is rampant. Our business people contend that the non-profit sector cannot meet the need, ever, and that therefore it takes business with capitalization, subsidy, and so forth, to move into the field.

Professor John Brocklehurst (*University of Manchester*) I hesitate a little to come into this question, but I think that really it is one of history. In Britain there has been no tradition of commercial care which has been in any way significant and I think that we have a tradition of what is in effect State care, going back probably three-and-a-half centuries. As you heard from Margot Jefferys this morning, a good deal of this has been bad, and a good deal of our long-term care is still in inadequate buildings and is inadequate in many other ways.

I would like to make one other point, about the family, because this is what our discussion has mainly been about. Clearly for large numbers of elderly people their families have to cope, and therefore we ought to identify the problems. The papers today have indicated that the great problem is dementia; in the UK six out of seven demented people are living in the community, and dementia is the factor that produces the greatest stress on families. So I think this is what we should concentrate on. Of course, there is the essential need for research to discover what is the cause and how to treat and prevent senile dementia, and governments should give more resources for this. But apart from that, community care is essentially episodic, and we must look for the best ways of relieving family strains in an episodic fashion.

Mr Marcus Walker (*Johns Hopkins University*) I want to react against certain attitudes which seem to underlie some of what has been said. For example, it seems that the Women's Liberation Movement has largely ignored the plight of older women in terms of re-marriage. If women outlive men our continued social prejudice against women marrying men younger than themselves may be maladaptive. It is perhaps through modification of fundamental social attitudes of this nature that we could make a radical attack on the problems faced by the non-institutionalized elderly.

Mr Stern I have a point of clarification on the home health care requirements and the possibility of profit-making organizations entering the field. There were some regulations proposed by the Administration last year on the entry of for-profit entities into home health care programs under Medicaid. There was a joint hearing by the Senate and House Committees on Aging, which took testimony from all sides. One of the results was that HEW then reconsidered the regulations for more study, and it stands now that Secretary Mathews intends to hold hearings himself.

It is far from certain whether for-profits will be put into the mainstream of Medicaid reimbursement. But it is more complex than that since proprietary organizations can and do act as homemaker services under other titles of the Federal Government. So it is a very mixed picture. We do have for-profits now providing chore services and homemaking services, but whether they will provide home health services is still an open question.

Mrs Edith Robins (*Division of Longterm Care Public Health Service*) I might just point out that at the Federal level, there is great interest in prevention but in terms of the elderly this is too often interpreted as referring only to primary prevention. I would suggest that we should all make a deliberate effort, if we really feel that prevention should include prevention of disability and dependency to speak loud and clear about it.

Mr Martin Loeb (*Institution on Aging, University of Wisconsin*) My comments and questions are rather specific. Today we have heard the problem of the care of the elderly in largely statistical terms. Indeed, the problem is vast. But whether it is large or small, it seems to me that the actual treatment of the elderly would be the same whether there were a great many or a few. I would be interested in whether there are new treatment approaches to the elderly. What do the psychiatrists do for those who have dementia and depression these days that is different from what it was when I came into this field 35 years ago? What research is there going on in either of our countries to improve the treatment modalities for dementia and depression and, if any, how do they get known by the practitioners.?

I have one other comment related to the fact that the United Kingdom doesn't have nursing homes. I have in my time studied some of the mental hospitals in the United Kingdom, and found them so much better than anything we had here. We have an experience in this country that the United Kingdom can learn from: don't close those mental hospitals, because all you will do is to get something infinitely worse, as we have in the United States now, the use of nursing homes without resources to treat or care for the mentally ill. The notion that Great Britain ought to build nursing homes frightens me a little because it might mean that some of those very good mental hospitals would close as has happened in this country.

Dr Evan Calkins (*Suny-Buffalo, New York*) I am out of my depth here a bit because I am a professor of medicine, not specifically involved in geriatrics as a circumscribed speciality, but heavily involved in trying to care for older patients, and in the educational aspects of the medical field. If we are going to try to solve this kind of problem, intuitively I and many others would turn to our young people and to the educational system. We must obviously put a lot more emphasis on education in the field of geriatrics if we are to be able to resolve these problems. I am interested that several centers seem to have sent a number of people who have contributed to our discussions here today, and other centers are less actively involved. I was wondering if I could ask a question, perhaps of Professor Newell and Dr Neugarten. Professor Newell, I note that Newcastle on Tyne has several people interested in this field. Do you have a whole interdisciplinary team interested in geriatrics or gerontology, or does this just happen to be a hobby of a few of you, and what suggestions would you have on the development of the educational mix, the interdisciplinary mix, that will help us educate our young people in this field? Similarly, Dr Neugarten, I wonder whether in your interest in behavioral sciences, you have got cross-fertilization with the Department of Medicine, or others in the medical field? Have you got an interdisciplinary program that crosses departmental barriers as you try to develop educational programs related to this field? What suggestions would either of you have on ways in which we can foster that? I would like to ask the folks from Duke the same question, because I see they have several people that have contributed to this discussion.

Professor Newell You have raised a very interesting tactical point. How does one go about initiating developments in a new and not universally acceptable field? In Newcastle there are research and teaching activities in the broad fields of gerontology, geriatric and psychogeriatric medicine taking place in several different University and clinical departments. These activities are becoming increasingly coordinated but in a largely informal way based on personal contacts and cooperation between the people involved. There are precedents in Newcastle for this type of development, social medicine being one. The alternative approach, setting up a monolithic department of gerontology and geriatrics, might well be an appropriate development in other centres but would, I suspect, be resisted in Newcastle not merely because of the inevitable conflict of interests it might involve but because it might to some degree go against the Newcastle philosophy in its approach to the old. My colleague, Professor Grimley Evans, has persuaded us that the tendency to separate the elderly from the rest of the human race as a problem group requiring different doctors, special hospitals, extra privileges, and so on, while overcoming some difficulties may in the long term create or consolidate others. We therefore aim to integrate teaching about the elderly into broader programmes. The social problems of old age are taught in a context covering a survey of modern social structures as a whole, showing how disability, poverty and cultural alienation will have predictable effects. We are about to initiate some formal teaching of biological gerontology in the medical undergraduate curriculum but this is deliberately integrated into a course including development and behaviour. Similarly, the plan is to expand the teaching of geriatric medicine firmly within clinical medicine as a whole so as to avoid giving it the image of a branch of knowledge which only a few doctors need to know about. Time will reveal whether this approach proves too subtle to be effective.

Dr Neugarten These abstract problems in education work out in individual ways in different institutions. At Chicago we began in the behavioral sciences and that is where we have worked most extensively. The program now does extend into the professional school, although we do not happen to have on our campus many professional schools. The medical school is now beginning to see that there might be some advantages if the walls that have existed on our particular campus for a particularly long time between the medical school and the rest of the university were to fall. This new attitude did not shape up around aging but aging may be the way to bring it about. The study of aging is having all kinds of social implications.

Ms Cleonice Tavani (*Federal Council on the Aging*) In searching for some of the differences between the care of the elderly in this country and the United Kingdom, and in particular in terms of the social care and the social support we provide, I wonder if we don't have to look at the financing arrangements and arrangements for the provision of health and social services. If I understand the British system correctly, there are to a greater or lesser extent universal social services for the whole population. We have nothing like that. We have the voluntary agencies but the government intervention for social services is related to those in poverty. Implicit is that the need for social services is connected to poverty.

The funding of our health and social services, again, with my limited knowledge of the British system, is very different. Our health care system is primarily a reimbursement of fees for service. The desire of many of us to separate the health care needs and the social service needs of the elderly is to take advantage of the values and benefits that already exist in some of the provisions of our social services.

I am no expert in the nursing home field but if I understand correctly, up until the passage of our Medicare and Medicaid financing provisions, the nursing home field in this country was primarily non-profit; what we have now is a consequence of financing arrangements that we are beginning to question. These questions about financing hopefully will enter into any kind of new social policy in this country for the care of the elderly, especially the oldest of the old.

Ms Vera Riddick (*Institute of Gerontology, Federal City College*) Not all nursing homes are as bad as we are inclined to think, and one way that we could deal with the problem is to set standards so that all staff members of nursing homes should be educated in the concepts of aging and the needs and interests of the aged. How can they adequately deliver services to the aged if they are not aware of the relevant needs and interests?

Dr Michael Green (*Royal Free Hospital, London*) Although in Britain we have few nursing homes, there are more than 100 000 places in local authority homes, many of which overlap in function with what you call nursing homes. I think we should question what these are for. They may be well-designed, but people sit there waiting for the next meal or the next departure rather like an airport lounge.

Dr Eisdorfer In response to Martin Loeb's question about getting improved treatment modalities out to the practitioners, there are a number of examples, including the one at King County, Seattle, of community-based geriatric screening programs. In our case we have a program which has over 2 years screened — 85% of them in their own homes — more than 1000 older persons referred to us for psychiatric reasons, virtually all of whom were sent to us because they were "senile". We have a team of psychiatrists, nurses and social workers, and we discovered that 56% of the referred patients had untreated, typically undiagnosed, medical conditions which we could help with, and 36% had pseudo-dementia: about 10% were clinically depressed. About 26% had some acute medical illness, primarily due to the misuse or the side effect of drugs. So by approaching the problem as a diagnostic one, we have already reversed a considerable number of the difficulties.

The point Elaine Brody made is well worth taking. We know precious little about the natural history of the dementing diseases. We are only now beginning to separate out the vascular from the non-vascular types, and in fact much of what we see clinically is not dementia per se but a combination of dementia and poor treatment. We can certainly reverse the effects of poor treatment and so restore people to an optimal level of functioning.

Let me name one other thing. At one time I didn't believe there was such a thing as paraphrenia; I thought it was something the British made up to confuse American psychiatrists. I was wrong. We now have a group of about 20 persons in the community, all over age 65, all exhibiting significant paranoid symptomatology. We entered into each case at the point at which they were about to be evicted and would have wound up literally on the streets of a major city, some of them becoming institutionalized, some of them dying a premature death. We are treating almost all of them at home with medication.

One comment on education; I have long labored against the absurdity of putting all or most of our community's educational resource into the first couple of decades of life. This is at best ill advised, and at worst, creates an unplanned obsolescence which is roughly analogous to putting one tankful of gas into a new car and discarding it after the gas runs out. I think we create significant social problems by failing to recognize that lack of the exercise of learning is significant in aging in addition to changes in the information base as knowledge advances. I think we must include education in an integrated lifelong program of care.

References

Friedsam, H. J. and Dick, H. R. (1963). "Decisions leading to institutionalisation of the aged". Unpublished Final Report, Social Security Administration Co-operative Research and Demonstration Grant Program, Project 037 (CI) 20-031

Jerath, B. K., Moses, V. K. and Kamel, W. W. (1976). Prevalence rates of foot disorders and co-existing heart disease. Illinois College of Podiatric Medicine Publication Series 3, No. 2

Lowenthal, M. (1964). "Lives in Distress". New York. Basis Books

Institutional Care: United States and United Kingdom

New Approaches in the United States

Herbert Shore
Dallas Home for the Jewish Aged

It is a great privilege to be a participant in this historic meeting, which comes at a time when long-term institutional care in the United States is in the throes of a series of crises of confidence in the health delivery system. Institutional care has been the concern of a Presidential Initiative Program, has seen the creation of an Office of Nursing Home Affairs (ONHA) in the Department of Health, Education and Welfare and the prestigious Senate Special Committee on Aging has been issuing a series of reports on Nursing Homes and the Failure of Public Policy. Hopefully we can explore important approaches and issues which can improve the lot of the dependent aged.

The Director of the ONHA stated recently (Abdellah 1976):

> Long-Term Care (including home health, day care, and special institutions, in addition to approximately 23 000 nursing homes) is a $5 billion industry in the United States. Approximately 96 percent of the nursing home beds in this country are in proprietary homes. Of the total of 23 000 nursing homes, about 16 000 are certified to receive Federal funds under Titles XVIII (Medicare) and XIX (Medicaid) of the Social Security Act. Only about 2000 of this group are certified to serve both Medicare and Medicaid patients.
>
> During Fiscal Year 1975, a total of $302 million was spent on Medicare (Title XVIII). An additional two and one half billion dollars were spent on Medicaid (Title XIX). In toto, over three billion dollars are spent by the Department for long-term care services including Medicare and Medicaid for such services as provider certification, surveyor improvement, provider training, long-term care training and nursing home data collection.

The number of people served and the cost; human, social and financial, make this more than a matter of academic interest.

This presentation will concern itself with the need to develop a rethinking of the role and function of long term care; the changes taking place in evolving from single service in-patient facilities to geriatric agencies and centers, the problems of homogenization of the patient population and the problems of financing long-term care.

It is my essential premise that one of the reasons why we are having so many problems with long-term institutional care is that the context chosen as the criterion for modeling and for measurement is not only inappropriate, grossly inefficient and costly, but harmful to all as well. The medical model which has been used to describe the disease-oriented, acute, short-term hospital care system (emphasizing illness and cure) doesn't fit long-term care. Yet it is the absence of other models of care which contributes to our problems. I believe a different model is necessary — a psycho-social health model.

For instance, much has been said and written about the "medical model" which generally implies the perception of the consumer of a human service as a "sick patient" who, after "diagnosis" is given "treatment" or "therapy" for his "disease" in a "clinic" or "hospital" by "doctors" who carry primary administrative and human management responsibility, assisted by a hierarchy of "paramedical" personnel, and "therapists" — all this hopefully leading to a "cure" (Wolfensberger 1972). This objective of curing must not be overlooked or understated — it is central to much of the issue. Medical care has been keeping people alive longer, but cure, not long-term care, is medicine's stock in trade. This fact begins to establish the conflict of the medical model on one hand, with chronicity on the other.

Another illustration of the fact that Homes are considered mini hospitals, comes from a recent communiqué from the Assistant Surgeon General, Dr Faye Abdellah (ONHA Policy Memorandum No. 14 (mimeo not dated), Implementation of Conditions of Participation, Medical Direction. US Department of Health, Education and Welfare) which, in question and answer form, says:

> 3. What are the types of agreements that a physician may enter into with a Nursing Home that would satisfy the condition of medical direction?
>
> First, he may be a member of the medical staff of the nursing home. This is comparable to the Hospital Model, in which there is an organized medical staff from which a member is chosen. . . . . Thus, we can see the Nursing Home conceptualized as a Hospital by those setting government policy.

The medical, the disease, the hospital model maintains the centrality of the physician, and benefits follow the supposition that such care is provided in the hospital or in the post hospital extended care facility when ordered or directed by an MD. It is essentially and fundamentally conceived of as acute care followed by short-term or convalescent stay. Thus, long-term care, the major characteristic of which is chronicity, is inappropriately modeled on short-term care, whose major characteristic is acuteness. Attention has been directed (unfortunately without apparent success!) to this difference between the hospital (medical) model and the nursing home. Those responsible for the provision of long-term care have attempted to point out the significant difference between the acute vs. the chronic, short stay vs. long term, disease orientation vs. disabled impairment orientation.

While the hospital has been characterized as the physicians' domain (we have a few known as "doctors' hospitals") — the nursing home borrowing its name from a proud profession has unfortunately not attracted the professional nurse in significant numbers.

We need to make the distinction between the medical model, medical care and medical capability. Certainly there is a significant role for medical care in the psycho-social model just as there is medical capability, but these must not be dominated by the medical model.

Among the factors which have further impeded clarification have been ownership (commercial, proprietary, usually recognized for profit) vs. sponsorship (non-profit, charitable and philanthropic, usually identified for service), as well as lack of standard nomenclature, identification of service by facility design (residential, custodial, congregate institutional), etc. Confusion abounds also because of lack of public policy, because of chronic shortages of funds, fear of the open-endedness of chronic illness, artificial payment mechanisms locked into law, etc.

What has often been overlooked in this state of affairs is that the differences between the hospital and nursing home are not the only differences. Differences exist also between the nursing home as it is generally conceived and the home for aging as a long-term care facility and geriatric health center, which is not understood. The differences exist in philosophy, in thrust, in organization, and they are just as real and compelling.

Constance Beaumont (1975) ably points out that the very terms "skilled nursing facility" and "intermediate care facility" are so awkward, so unfamiliar to most people and so deficient with respect to conjuring up any kind of image, that the public, the press and even members of Congress avoid these terms, and simply label everything a nursing home. The traditional nursing home generally attempts to follow the medical-hospital model, while the long-term care facility (geriatric health center) generally follows the psycho-social health, total person care model.

Other differences between nursing homes and homes for the aging exist. The patients in nursing homes tend to remain there, sometimes on a temporary basis, and even when they do reside permanently in these homes, their length of stay is about half of the length of the stay of the average resident in a home for the aging. Moreover, as the headlines have repeatedly indicated, some for-profit homes tend to warehouse older people, while it is more generally true that homes for the aged tend more fully to meet the psycho-social needs and may do a more adequate rehabilitation job. Nursing homes may be age integrated, while homes for the aging are age segregated. It might be a subjective judgment, but I think that many observers would agree with me that the nursing homes' atmosphere is usually more sterile than the more home-like atmosphere of the non-profit facilities. In addition, nursing homes seem to foster dependency in their patients, since dependency will provide the nursing home with a more substantial profit. Homes for the aged, on the contrary, tend to foster the highest degree of individual independence.

Long-term care is total care emphasizing an appropriate balance between social and health services. While it includes essential medical and nursing care, it must be recognized as separate from the hospital and medical model.

Several points emerge from this analysis. First, the geriatric total (psycho-social) health facility as it exists is substantially different from the nursing home (and unfortunately it follows that if we have no public policy for nursing homes we certainly do not have it for long-term care), and secondly, the characteristic of long-term care is chronic illness, be it physical or mental, or both.

A recent article on "Problems in Chronic Illness Care" points out:

> In the mid-1970's three major problems in the health field are beginning to merge into a larger and more complex series of problems for public policy. These are: (1) the increasingly chronic character of the illness load suffered by the total population; (2) the increasing emphasis, both within the medical profession and in general public discussion, on problems of quality of life; and (3) the increasing attention being given to the organization of health care focusing both on reducing costs and on improving the quality of care, and that
>
> 1) Chronic illnesses are long term.
> 2) Chronic illnesses are uncertain in a variety of ways.
> 3) Chronic diseases require proportionately large efforts at palliation.
> 4) Chronic diseases are multiple diseases.
> 5) Chronic diseases are disproportionately intrusive upon the lives of patients.
> 6) Chronic diseases require a wide variety of ancillary services if they are to be properly cared for.
> 7) Chronic diseases imply conflicts of authority among patients, medical workers and funding agencies.
> 8) Chronic illnesses are expensive.
> 9) Chronic-disease care is primary care.

Among the reasons long-term care was patterned on the acute hospital medical model appears to be the economics of long-term care. We are immobilized by the lack of a public policy which defines what an older person is worth in our society. With our utilitarian bent, we invest in things with a productive future. Sick old people are consumers, no longer producers. What are they worth? How long do we support them? How open-ended is their care? The dilemma exists that as we extend life and conquer disease, as we invent pacemakers and pressure breathing machines, we increase the cost of support. If we use the hospital model, we can arbitrarily limit benefit days and thus theoretically dispense with our obligations.

One of the interesting illustrations of the fiscal bankruptcy of present policy is the recognition that Medicare essentially ends when long-term helplessness and surveillance begins. The purpose of this legislation was to provide assistance with the cost of acute care episodes. To that end Medicare has been most helpful to older people, but it has misled them in their understanding and in their needs for long-term financing of chronic care.

Once an inappropriate and costly model was selected, a series of consequences follow which have continued to prove expensive and confusing to the nation. However, we have a circular problem of ever increasing enforcement of rules and regulations which won't and can't work because the model won't and can't work. Jerome Kaplan (1974) summed it up when he pointed out, "The aged-serving institution is to become a national mold of an imperfect model."

If the hospital/medical/acute disease model changes, a host of other inappropriate and costly consequences of the model must change. These include the use of the patient's medical chart (endless documentation) as the regulatory document, the use of medical directors (when paraprofessionals, health assistants, geriatric nurse practitioners, etc. would do as well at far less cost) and certainly the regulatory, inspection and enforcement process. All must be rethought.

Our problems are compounded because government and institutions visualize a delivery system from different vantage points. Institutional care providers see the government's approaches as rigid, arbitrary, and indifferent to the needs of the individual, while the government sees the institution as inefficient, wasteful and inappropriate. The government believes that it is acceptable to pay for medical care but questionable to support social care. The government doesn't understand long-term care, yet it controls the regulatory and payment mechanisms. We must redirect and redefine long-term care to the psycho-social model.

The medical model implies that all patients in nursing homes are alike, that all have the same needs, and that nursing care is the way to care for all! But patients come for different reasons, although a health crisis usually precipitates the need for care. The average nursing time given to patients in homes is 2½ hours per 24-hour day. Patients need psycho-social services, such as sensory awareness, educational, creative, and religious activities. These strengthen the patients' self-image so that they will believe they are a vital significant part of society, not an unwanted burden. These programs often determine whether a long-term care patient will recover, or will regress into a hopeless, inevitable slide toward death. Psycho-social services are provided by social workers, activity directors, chaplaincy personnel, community volunteer workers, and so forth. Paradoxically, these are the services that are most important to the well-being of the patient, yet least recognized by the medical model. The result is that these vital services are not paid for by government programs. As long as the medical model, with its emphasis on acute hospital care, dominates the evaluation of, and the rate setting process in the delivery of health services, the overemphasis on medical care and the unwarranted denigration of health-social and psycho-social services will continue.

Patients Differ

There are several different types of patients in homes. The so-called "well aged" function because they are in a protective environment. For this group of patients, with their chronic impairments, the medical model does not fit. A different social support system of care is necessary. Another group is patients with chronic physically disabling illnesses. This group of patients requires nursing care and rehabilitative services. They need nursing care as well as nurturing.

Perhaps the most underserved and neglected but the most challenging are the patients with mental disabilities. In the medical model, if complex nursing procedures are not used, the patient is not deemed in need of skilled care. Thus the ambulatory, confused, impaired resident is not linked to the payment mechanism, though he requires additional therapeutic, skilled care.

Because the rationale imposed by government for nursing homes is to reimburse for physical illness and disability, another self-defeating cycle is assured. The negative incentive pays to keep the patient on his back and dependent, instead of stimulating functional improvement.

Although many federal studies report an alarming overtranquilization of patients, it was the psychopharmaceutical revolution that made possible the wholesale dumping of confused, elderly patients from state hospitals to nursing homes. These patients require a vast array of treatment modalities, including resocialization and remotivation. Because those who seek the specialized care of a home do so because they need treatment, the home should be an organization of treatment centers where specialized care will be provided according to the patient's needs.

I have attempted to call attention to the issues of the medical model vs. the psycho-social health model, the problems of homogenization of the population, and the changing nature of homes from single service institutions to geriatric serving agencies. Limitations of time make it impossible to deal with all the issues, but some discussion of economics is essential.

Present American health care is an intricate "non-system" (it has been characterized as an "illness system") of various disconnected categorical health delivery programs. The faulty functioning of any one program affects the actual workings of all the other partial health delivery efforts. Obviously the goals of health care are related to the courses of financing for health care. The *Wall Street Journal* (Robbins 1975) in an article on health costs says:

> . . . The administration and the costs of hospitals are determined by physicians and especially by surgeons. Somehow this condition must be changed and hospitals forced to operate with reasonable efficiency for the convenience of the community and in ways that will reduce the enormous drain on national resources and personal income now being devoted to health care — without a sacrifice of quality. Can it be done? We must start with a NEW PUBLIC POLICY OBJECTIVE: TO PROVIDE HIGHER QUALITY HEALTH CARE AT SIGNIFICANTLY LOWER COST

We have often heard these perpetual demands for unlimited services, high quality and low cost.

But Rashi Fein (1975), the noted economist of the Harvard Medical School, further debunks the myths about Health Care:

> The basis of the myths about health care, is the fallacy that the health industry is like other industries and that the health care market is governed by the same economic principles of supply and demand.
>
> It is that view — that we are really dealing with a market that we have met before in other areas of economic life — that leads to explanations of behavior that are incorrect, insufficient and inappropriate — that, in a word, are myths.

We have unfortunately had some political and simplistic solutions that the problems of long-term care would be solved by phasing out the for-profit homes. This is impossible: if the commercial proprietary homes were outlawed, they would become non-profit, but what happens to the massive infusion of capital that this sector has "invested" in the creation of physical plant? The real problems lie in our creating a public policy that recognizes long-term care and that is willing to infuse funds for care not only for enforcement and inspection! We cannot continue to use laws designed primarily for illness care to meet the psycho-social health care needs. We must take long-term care out of the means test. Our States face bankruptcy and the programs strain under financial stresses. We can reduce dependency or foster it — which we do will depend on our choices and fiscal policy.

In summary: I have selected those statements of importance: Hobart Jackson (1961) thoughtfully said:

> The modern institution is becoming aware of its significant potential for reversing and correcting undesirable societal trends that promote the deterioration of older people. In many ways the institution is expected to undo the ills of social practices by furnishing a corrective atmosphere for older residents. Instead of perpetuating the inhumane attitude of a dispassionate society, the institution must become the ideal society, giving the older client within the confines of the facility what is lacking in the outside world.

Lucille Nahemow (1975) said, "We must conclude that under the conditions of modern population trends and our ability to deliver health services, institutions for the elderly are here to stay."

Jerome Hammerman (quoted by Sack *et al.* 1975) said, "The question is not, will institutional care be needed in the future; rather, what form will the institution take and what functions will it serve within a continuum of optimally developed, linked and supported services for long-term care."

Indeed we believe they need to take on a new form and to be viewed as a network of service system of care. I am hopeful that this meeting will be a beginning in the creation of new approaches to public policy.

References

Abdellah, F. G. (1976). Conference on Public Policy, National Association of Jewish Homes for the Aged, Washington, DC: mimeo p 3

Beaumont, C. (1975). *Congressional Record* July 24, p 7482

Fein, R. (1975). *Group Health and Welfare News* December, p 7

Jackson, H. (1961). Proceedings of Arden House Conference (November) American Association of Homes for Aging; p 8

Kaplan, J. (1974). *Gerontologist* **14**, 275

Nahemow, L. (1975). *Gerontologist* **15**, 58–65

Robbins, I. D. (1975). *Wall Street Journal* May

Sack, A., Friedman, R. and Sheldon, T. (1975). *Journal of the American Association of Homes for Aging* **1**, No. 3, p 25

Wolfesberger, W. (1972). "Normalization: The Principles of Normalization in Human Services." National Institute on Mental Retardation; p 8

Current Issues in the United Kingdom

J Grimley Evans
Department of Medicine (Geriatrics),
University of Newcastle upon Tyne

My brief is restricted to institutional care for the elderly although this is only one of the modalities of care offered by a comprehensive geriatric service and separate consideration necessarily distorts the total picture. At any one time about 5% of persons aged 65 and over (here referred to as "the elderly") are in some kind of institution, if only temporarily. Table 1 sets out the organization of institutional care for the elderly in the United Kingdom and makes some estimate of separate numerical contributions as estimated from various data available for 1970 to 1971. You will note the very small contribution made by private and voluntary agencies. The administrative arrangements within the statutory organizations are complex: in theory the various institutions in the public sector provide for the necessary continuous spectrum from minimal to total dependency (McKeown and Cross,

Table 1

Institutional care for the elderly — England and Wales 1970–71
Prevalence Rates per 1000

	Local Authority		*Private Sector*	
COMMUNITY	(Sheltered housing)		(Sheltered housing)	
	Residential homes	16.2	Hotels	2.2
	Homes for elderly mentally infirm	0.4	Voluntary homes	4.9
			Nursing homes	0.2
HOSPITAL	*Non-Psychiatric*		*Psychiatric*	
	Geriatric service	8.2	Psychogeriatric service	8.7
	Other	10.0	Other	

1969) but because of discontinuous administration (Local Authority and Hospital Services being run by separate agencies) problems may arise if a patient is misplaced or if her state changes while under care. Implementation of the Seebohm Report (1968) on the organization of Local Authority Social Services has made an integrated geriatric service impossible and a co-ordinated one difficult unless the links between the different agencies involved are much closer than legislation requires. Basically the problem is one of possible incommensurability of priorities between the different agencies. There is, for example, no statutory provision for medical assessment or even involvement in application for residential care even though an old person's failure to cope in her own home might be due to unrecognized but treatable disease. The increasing development of joint geriatric and social service assessment facilities, often based in a Day Hospital is one way in which local initiative overcomes deficiencies in statutory communications between the two services. Analogous difficulties may arise between

Physician and Psychiatrist; where there is good co-operation placement of a patient is arranged on a mutually agreed basis of functional status and nursing needs rather than diagnostic categories, which form the major basis of statutory guidance. A further problem arises in the psychological disturbance for an elderly patient of transition between one type of care and another, particularly in the change from Residential Care to Hospital in the event of illness requiring more nursing care than is normally provided in Residential Homes. It is a tribute to the devotion of residential home staff that they will usually try to continue caring for an old person who has deteriorated to the point at which officially she should be placed in hospital, in order to save her the trauma of removal from what has become her home. The burden this may place on the staff can be immense and explorations have been made of ways to provide some type of care intermediate between Residential Homes and Hospitals. Joint establishments set up by Hospital and Local Authority have been mooted but raise problems because of the separate administration and funding of the two services. In Newcastle we are exploring the possibility of special Local Authority Residential Homes for the more physically handicapped with high staffing ratios and regular visits from Hospital medical staff similar to the Local Authority Specialist Homes for the elderly mentally infirm in our City. One idea which recurs is that of comprehensive settlements for the elderly with all grades of care from retirement bungalow to sick ward sharing the same site and staff. Such complexes are to be found in Britain particularly in the voluntary sector but they have the theoretical disadvantage of increasing the social distance between the elderly — even the fit elderly — and the rest of the community, which is one thing that in the long term we are trying to prevent.

The conventional image of service development for the elderly in the United Kingdom over the last two decades has been that of a progressive shift from an institution-intensive to a community-intensive strategy but it is difficult to assess the success of this re-orientation. Census data can be used to compute institutionalization rates among the elderly for the Census years. Figure 1 shows that, in fact, there has been an increase in the institutionalization of persons aged over 80 particularly among women. Using Census data again Fig. 2 shows that this increase is predominantly in Residential Care. To some extent this may reflect an increase in social need since owing to a fall in birth rate between the Wars the average number of potentially dutiful middle-aged children available to give support to elderly parents fell by 19% during this period calculated from fertility data and corresponding life tables, as Table 2, shows. This Table also demonstrates that this process is going to continue through the twentieth century. Widowhood rates and outward migration of younger families

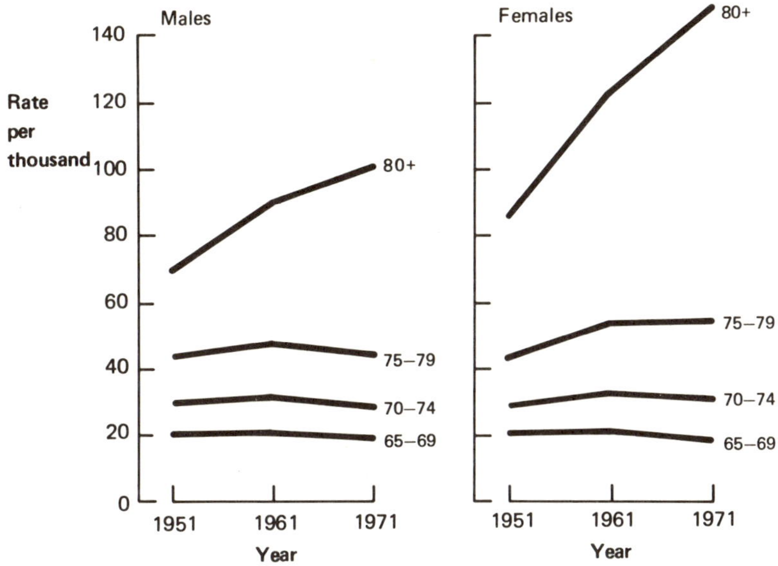

Fig. 1 *England and Wales census: persons in institutions on census day, age – specific rates per thousand*

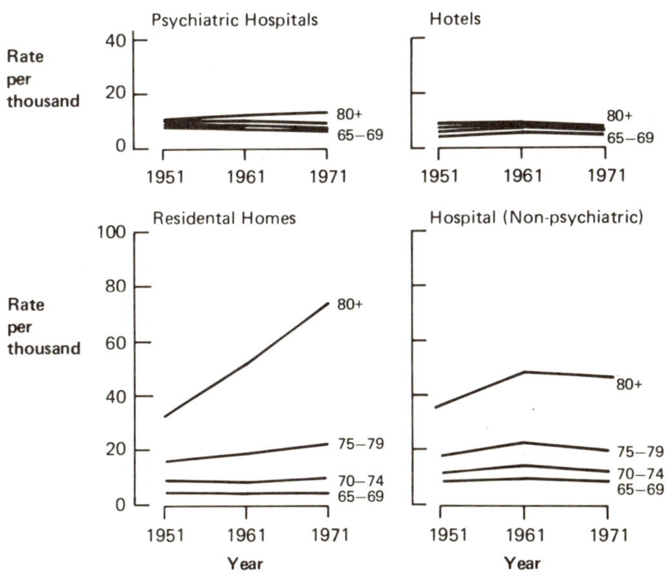

Fig. 2 *England and Wales census: persons in institutions on census day, age – specific rates per thousand*

Table 2

Estimated average number of children to parents born in different years 1811 to 1921

Year of Birth of Parent	*Average Number of Children*	*Average Number of children Surviving to Age 45*
1871	4.8	2.7
1881	4.1	2.5
1891	3.3	2.2
1901	2.6	2.0
1911	2.2	1.7
1921	2.0	1.6

may have also contributed to a decline in family support. It could be that criteria for admission to Residential Care are becoming less stringent. One survey suggests on the contrary that persons currently being admitted to Residential Care are more disabled than their predecessors. The evidence presented is not convincing (DHSS 1975*b*) but this conclusion falls in with the personal impression of staff working in the homes (Brown 1974). Clearly it would be of great interest to know more about these phenomena: are these elderly people who would once have ended their days in hospital or are they new survivors from chronically disabled middle aged? Whatever the explanation the figures show that progressive institutionalization of the old is continuing in the United Kingdom and this is confirmed by the steadily increasing norm set by Government for the provision of Residential Care places, the current figure standing at 25 places per thousand elderly population.

Bosanquet (1975) has pointed out that more money is spent on the running costs of Residential Homes than on all the domiciliary services put together. Many Geriatricians (e.g. Williamson 1971) consider that there is need for greater provision and more flexible and discriminating management of sheltered housing and Bosanquet (1975) shares this view. Clinicians are well aware that some old people are driven into Residential Care not by their disabilities but by their inadequate housing and the impossibility of doing anything about this within a reasonable length of time. Wroe (1973) has summarized the evidence that the elderly are on average in worse housing than younger age groups and their houses may even be discriminated against when money for upgrading is available. Table 3 is derived from data of the General Household Survey (Office of Population Censuses and Surveys 1972). Carstairs and Morrison (1971) estimated that two thirds of

Table 3

General household survey (GB) 1971–72
Household amenities

	Elderly		Others
	Alone	Not alone	
No bath or shower	17.3%	12.3%	5.5%
No indoor WC	15.1%	13.7%	6.7%
No central heating	74.0%	71.0%	57.5%

Scottish people in Residential Care could live in sheltered housing were it available but in England and Wales the proportion is probably much lower. Bosanquet (1975) estimates it is at least a quarter but in Newcastle the figure is no higher than 15% at most (Brown 1974). Townsend (1962) suggested a target of 50 sheltered housing places per thousand elderly population but Bosanquet (1975) estimates present provision of purpose-built accommodation at 50 000 units or less than 8 per thousand. A survey of Local Authority Community Services (Health and Welfare 1967) suggested that in 1965 some 65 000 elderly people were in special housing (not necessarily purpose-built) and planning predictions were of 24.6 places per thousand by 1971. There were gross differences in the scale of provision between different Local Authorities ranging from zero in some urban areas to 70 places per thousand in some County areas. Clearly there may be some uncertainties about definitions.

Sheltered housing provides two main facilities for the elderly, a physically undemanding environment and good communication with outside help usually provided through a resident warden. If this second function could be provided within patients' own homes by a reorganization of community staff and appropriate use of modern communication devices as is currently being proposed (Michael Davis, personal communication 1976) some of the capital cost of sheltered housing might be saved. Not everyone is convinced that more sheltered housing and less residential care is an appropriate strategy. Coleman (1976) has suggested that this view represents "unreal idealism" and he draws attention to evidence that many old people, he suggests the majority, in sheltered housing are so disabled that they should be in residential care. Co-ordinated research and planning in this vital area is made more difficult by another fragmentation of administration, for sheltered housing is provided and administered not by the Department of Health and Social Security and Social Services Departments but by the Department of the Environment and Local Authority Housing Departments.

Although overall hospitalization rates revealed by Census data have shown little consistent trend over the last 20 years there have been changes in the pattern of hospital use. The British National Health Service provides a much simpler base for routine statistics than does a Free Enterprise pattern of care but there are still tantalizing gaps and anomalies in the data available. The two main sources of data relating to non-psychiatric hospitals are the Hospital Annual Returns (SH3 returns) and the Hospital In-Patient Enquiry (HIPE). Published figures from the SH3 data give average number of beds available and occupied by specialty and for the more acute specialties average length of stay. Until recently waiting list figures were also published by specialty. HIPE data are based on approximately 1 in 10 sample of hospital discharges and give estimates of number of beds occupied and length of stay per completed hospital admission by age, sex, specialty and region. HIPE data are unlinked so that length of stay figures can take no proper account of hospital transfer or re-admission. Theoretically the number of beds occupied should be the same in both SH3 returns and HIPE data but there are consistent differences. In particular, according to HIPE approximately 4000 geriatric beds fewer (and a similar number of general medical beds more) are occupied than are claimed by SH3 figures. This discrepancy amounts to about 8% of

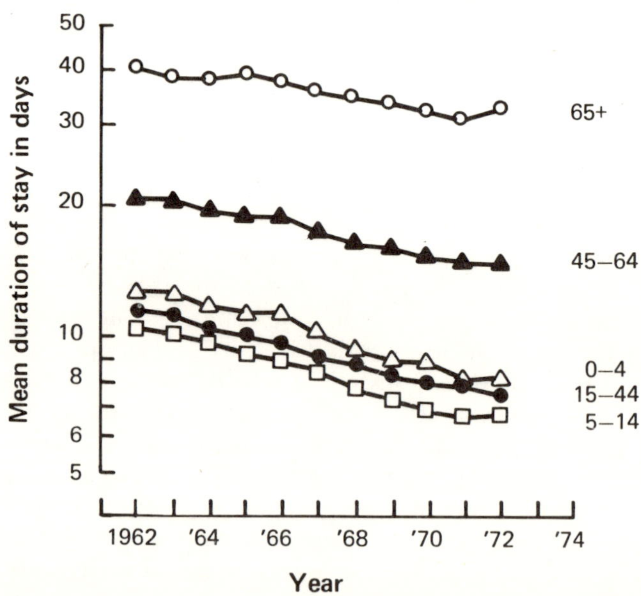

Fig. 3 *HIPE data. Mean duration of stay (all departments) by age group*

Geriatric beds. There are also sampling biases in HIPE data. Ashley (1972) for example, has drawn attention to the deficiency of hospital deaths revealed by HIPE. The reasons for such discrepancies are probably complex and it is to be hoped that Hospital Activity Analysis, a new system of routine statistics based on total coverage, will overcome these difficulties. Meanwhile, some caution is necessary in accepting hospital usage statistics particularly for the elderly.

Figure 3 shows how mean length of stay by different age groups estimated by HIPE have changed over a recent decade. On this semi-logarithmic plot it seems that the proportional reduction in length of stay of the elderly is no greater than that in other age groups. If we distribute the care of the elderly in-patient according to specialty as shown in Fig. 4 we find uniform proportional trends for general medicine, geriatric medicine and even general surgery. At first glance it would seem that Geriatricians have not achieved anything very

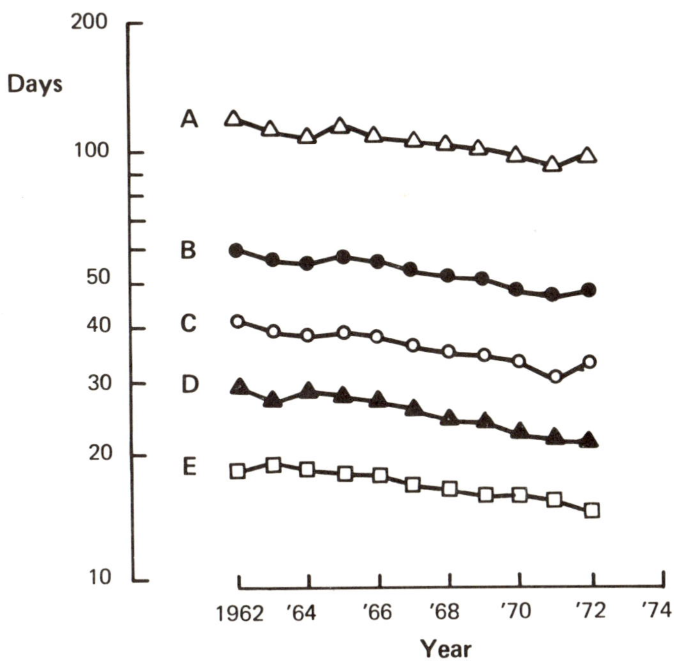

Fig. 4 *HIPE data. Average duration of stay by persons aged over 64. A. Departments of geriatrics and chronic sick. B. All medical specialties. C. All specialties. D. Major medical specialties excluding geriatrics and chronic sick. E. General surgery*

remarkable but two points bear emphasizing. First is the actual magnitude of the reduction of mean length of stay which amounts to 25 days per patient in geriatric units compared with 7 days in general medical and 3 days in general surgical units. Second, Geriatricians have achieved this result despite the fact that they receive patients highly selected for severe and chronic handicap and social disadvantage (Isaacs *et al.* 1972). The achievement is no mean one if it represents improved rehabilitation rather than simply increased hospital transfer or re-admission rates, a distinction the data do not permit us to make. There is also the factor of an increasing proportion of deaths occurring in hospital rather than in private homes: a trend that is affecting the elderly as well as other age-groups. Although age adjusted hospital fatality rates for the elderly changed little from 22% in 1962 to 18% in 1972 the proportion of elderly deaths occurring in hospital rose over the same period from 43% to 53% (calculated from HIPE and Registrar General data). Several different interpretations might be put on these trends and only record linkage (Acheson 1967) could have enabled us to identify the correct one.

Figure 5 sets out the basic modalities of geriatric or psychogeriatric in-patient care and outlines the main lines of patient flow. Depending on local circumstances these modalities may or may not be in the same place. A study in rural England showed that visiting of elderly patients

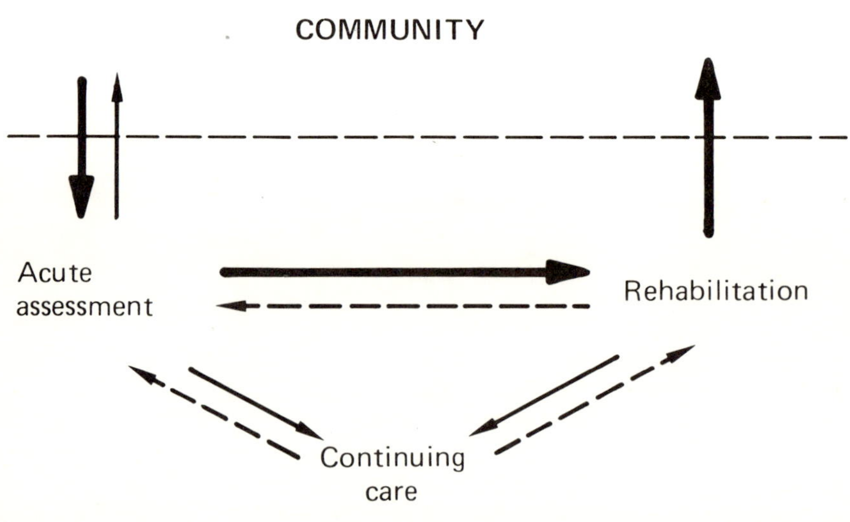

Fig. 5 *Hospital inpatient modalities*

in hospital by relatives or friends falls off with time if travelling distances are too great so that although assessment and short-term rehabilitation facilities can be centralized in a District General Hospital (as they need to be) longer-term facilities should be provided close to a patient's community which may mean placement outside the General Hospital (Cross and Turner 1974). This finding falls in neatly with recent Government guidance on the provision and use of Community Hospitals (DHSS 1975*a*). Geriatricians were called into being 25 years ago to supervise long-stay beds in outlying hospitals and received their cases as therapeutic failures from other hospital sources. The contemporary Geriatrician receives his patients as direct referrals from General Practitioners and spends most of his working time in acute high turnover wards, rehabilitation units, day hospitals, out-patient clinics and home visits. The explicit reasons for this revolution are that it is more humane and less expensive to keep old people out of hospital as much as possible, but neither of these assertions is necessarily true and as with all revolutions one problem is to know when to stop. A major issue in contemporary British hospital geriatrics is the balance to be drawn between the continuing care and the acute and rehabilitation services. Some Geriatricians (e.g. Hodkinson and Jeffery's 1972) consider that there is no need for long-term facilities, that if the acute services are adequate in quantity and quality and run by the right people long-stay patients are no longer generated. Others (Adams 1974, Isaacs 1972) regard this as an extreme view which pays less than appropriate heed to family and individual problems and to local variations in morbidity, demographic factors and development of community and other services for the elderly. The emphasis on the acute and rehabilitation aspects of Geriatric medicine has been intense in the last decade partly because of the deficiencies in facilities for these activities and partly in a determined effort to change the depressing image of Geriatric Medicine in the eyes of the public, the medical profession and health administrators. Voices have recently been raised to protest that in the midst of this commendable activity the special needs of the hospital long-term patient have received less attention than they deserve. Clearly a balance must be defined but this should be determined by the pattern of patient need, and not as is so frequently the case, by the uses to which the obsolescent or poor standard hospital accommodation available to a geriatric service can be put.

Government guidance for the provision of geriatric service beds in England and Wales is that there should be 10 beds per thousand elderly population (Hospital Plan, 1962) and at least half these beds should be in District General (or Teaching) Hospitals (DHSS 1971). Planned provision in Scotland is more generous at 15 beds per thousand but this is associated with a lower provision of other categories of hospital bed

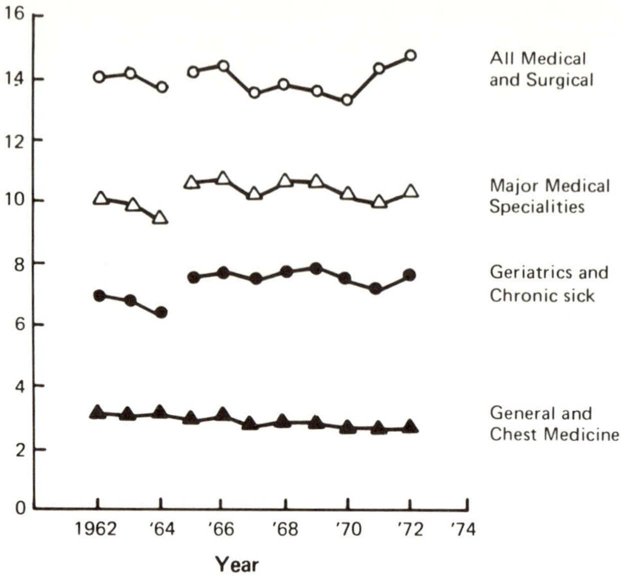

Fig. 6 *HIPE data. Average daily beds occupied per 1000 population persons aged over 64*

(Hospital Plan for Scotland 1962). Figure 6 shows present bed usage by the elderly according to HIPE data for a recent decade. The discontinuity from 1964 to 1965 shown in the curves is due to a change in the method with which HIPE estimates were derived. Geriatric bed usage is running at about 7.5 beds per thousand and a further 2.7 beds in general medical and chest wards are occupied by the elderly and these figures have been fairly stable. We should note, however, that total non-psychiatric hospital occupation by the elderly is estimated by HIPE at 14 to 15 beds per thousand but the Census figures for 1971 suggest 18 to 19 per thousand. Accepting the HIPE data at their face value, approximately 11.2 beds per thousand are therefore needed to maintain present services and yet during the decade shown in Fig. 6 the waiting lists for admission to geriatric units rose slowly to almost 9000 so this provision can scarcely be claimed as adequate. And yet at least two geriatric services in Britain can provide all the medical in-patient care for an elderly population within a provision of 10 beds per thousand (Gedling and Newell 1972, O'Brien *et al.* 1973). There is clearly an anomaly here, and, although it would be dangerous to jump to conclusions without knowing more about the other services available, two factors which distinguish the areas in question are, first that virtually all the geriatric beds are in General Hospitals and second that all the medical beds for the elderly are under the management of Specialist Geriatricians. And here, in my view, are the two nettles to be grasped if a radical attack on the problems of providing adequate geriatric care is to be undertaken. The first is for Health Service administrators: in certain circumstances a comprehensive hospital medical service for the elderly can be provided within 10 beds per thousand but not 10 cheap beds per thousand. There is no reason to expect that adequate treatment of an elderly patient with all the complex multidimensional problems characteristic of the age group will be any cheaper than treatment of a younger patient and only a philosophy left over from the days of the Poor Law and the Workhouse would suppose that it should be. Not only are geriatric beds currently provided on the cheap in that they are outside major hospitals they are cheap because of poor medical staffing ratios. According to SH3 returns the average number of general medical beds per Consultant Physician in 1971 was about 34. The average number of Geriatric beds per Geriatric Consultant was 189 and no-one can look after even half that number of beds adequately. This situation is made worse by poor recruitment to the Specialty so that some Consultant posts lie vacant. The second nettle is for the medical profession. It is widely recognized by Geriatricians, if not by others, that the elderly carry a great burden of iatrogenic disease. This not only comprises illness due to errors of commission — mostly inappropriate or inadequately supervised drug therapy (Shaw and Opit, 1976) — but also unnecessary disability due to errors of omission. Williamson *et al.* (1964) drew attention to the amount of undisclosed physical illness in elderly persons in the community and Bergmann has reported on the high frequency of medically unrecognized mental illness among the elderly both in the community and in hospital (Bergmann *et al.* 1965: Bergmann and Eastham, 1974). Although a proportion of this undetected illness is attributable to the low expectation of health in old age among the British compared with some other peoples (Shanas *et al.* 1968) part must be attributed to lack of appropriate expertise and adaptive organization of medical care. The high rate of failure of family practice follow-up for elderly patients discharged from hospital is well documented (Age Concern 1973). Geriatric Medicine like most other specialties calls for no great intellectual gifts among its practitioners but it does require interest, application, orientation and some management skills, and an elderly patient has a right to expect any doctor under whose care she falls to have these attributes in appropriate measure. There are several ways in which this might be achieved. One is to ensure that the next generation of doctors have acquired more experience in the care of the elderly during their training than did their predecessors: this is the only method of carrying good geriatric care out into the community where it matters most, but calls for a revision of medical school curricula and possibly a reappraisal of methods of selecting students for medical training. Another step which some consider necessary is for Geriatrics to become a strictly age-defined specialty and for all patients over a certain age to receive hospital medical care under the supervision of an accredited Geriatrician. Alternatively, every medical team in a hospital could include a Physician with special interest in and responsibility for the elderly and with appropriate executive powers. This approach has some theoretical advantages but is not yet of proven benefit in practice (Evans 1974). Neither of these aims could be universally achieved on current levels of recruitment of doctors into the specialty of Geriatric Medicine and solution of this problem is fundamental to any advance.

Further contentious issues centre on psychiatric institutional care for the elderly. Guidance on psychiatric bed provision for the elderly is complex since it falls under the shadow of the long cherished ambition of the Ministry of Health to abolish the mental hospitals. Currently, guidance implies that care for the elderly mentally disturbed requiring psychiatric in-patient care will be provided within the 0.5 to 1 acute beds per thousand total population to be provided in psychiatric units at General Hospitals (DHSS 1972) together with 2.5 to 3.0 beds per thousand elderly to be provided for physically fit dements in Community Hospitals (DHSS 1975*a*). In addition a 10 to 20 bed psychogeriatric assessment unit is envisaged for each Health District of 200 thousand to 250 thousand total population (DHSS 1970). Reduced to a common denominator and assuming that about one third of the beds in the District General Hospital units will be occupied by elderly patients (DHSS 1975*c*) all this amounts to between 4.2 and 6.4 beds per thousand elderly population. Andrews *et al.* (1972) reported the conclusion of a working party of Geriatric Physicians and Psychiatrists on the planning of psychogeriatric care. The working party started from the assumption that placement should be determined by a patient's behaviour and needs rather than by a diagnostic classification. As we implied above this is an essential basis for fruitful co-operation but it does require adequate provision for immediate and continuous cross-consultation if not joint simultaneous assessment. The need for a special psychogeriatric assessment unit may therefore be determined more by the local geography of hospital buildings than by more universal factors. There are other considerations however: our personal experience in Newcastle, where we are particularly fortunate in our colleagues in the psychogeriatric service, suggests that a psychogeriatric assessment unit provides a stimulating and effective ambience for undergraduate and post-graduate teaching. Perhaps this reflects the particular education needs of the present time when so much medical thinking appears to be dominated by distorted stereotypes of the elderly patient, among which are ideas that all physical disease in old age is nonspecific and degenerative and that all mental disturbance is due to dementia and is not amenable to treatment. The psychogeriatric unit is also a dramatic demonstration to students that the needs of patients may transcend the professional barriers between specialties and this is a useful lesson to be carried forth into wider fields.

The second point brought out by Andrews *et al.* (1972) is that although previous articles in the literature have dealt with the proportion of patients "misplaced" in either geriatric or psychiatric institutions there is, in fact, a sizeable group of patients who can be equally well managed in either. The authors make a plea for planning in terms of total place provision instead of the present system of separate norms for each administrative division of the services for the elderly. This concept requires administrative arrangements to ensure that all beds are equally available and subject to the same measures of admission priority. Andrews and his colleagues go on to suggest that this total provision will have to be greater than that allowed for in the present planning guidelines for England and Wales (Scottish planning is more generous). In contrast to the 14.2 to 16.4 beds per thousand proposed for hospital geriatric and psychogeriatric services (see above) Andrews *et al.* (1972) suggest that 20 to 23 beds per thousand will be needed but that 3 to 5 of these places could be in specialist Residential Hostels rather than hospitals. Actual provision will be responsive in the long term to local need, but if current planning for the 7 million elderly people of England and Wales is as wide of the mark as this, the implications are daunting. In fairness to the Government planners one should add that they have attempted to include in their equation some estimate of future increase in the efficacy of geriatric treatment while Andrews *et al.* (1972) assume that present practice will continue unimproved.

Mention of specialist Residential Homes brings us to a further important current issue. For some years there has been a development of special residential homes for mentally disturbed elderly people commonly known as EMI homes (Elderly Mentally Infirm). Meacher (1972*a*, 1972*b*) on the basis of 151 hours observation in six residential homes has launched a swingeing attack on the whole concept of separate homes for the elderly mentally confused. Meacher's appreciation of the psychiatry and pathology of old age is incomplete and his concept of what constitutes a medical model of a disease is decades out of date, facts which emerge from his book and from an exchange of letters with Dr Klaus Bergmann (Bergmann 1972, 1973, Meacher 1972*c*). Meacher's viewpoint can be exemplified in his own words on the subject of senile dementia, which in this context is what the problem is chiefly about. "Senile dementia should not be regarded as a pathological condition, but rather as an attempted adaptation, executed with varying degrees of ingenuity and meeting with varying degrees of success, to an environment which is inauspicious in terms of the needs of the pre-existing personality pattern, which has already itself been moulded by the steady accretion of earlier experiences which cumulatively tend to strengthen or weaken the reaction on each subsequent occasion to adverse or alien surroundings" (Meacher 1972*a*, p 46). In this one recognizes the authentic voice of the fashionable twentieth century heresy that all biological variation must be environmental in origin which has achieved influential exposition in the work of R D Laing and T D Lysenko among others. And being in a fashionable vein, Meacher's views have had a great deal of influence among the susceptible. No one will deny the importance of environmental factors in the manifestations and behavioural severity of senile dementia; medical workers among the elderly have long emphasized the various forms of institutional neurosis to which the elderly, and particularly the brain-damaged elderly, are prone. But the idea that senile dementia is exclusively a psychogenic disorder without primary organic pathology seems in the present state of knowledge frankly perverse and not in the patients' best interest. But even if we were to accept Meacher's premise, his conclusion that demented old people will be better off among a reasonable cross-section of other elderly people does not necessarily follow. His own work draws attention to what he calls the ostracism with which the mentally confused are treated by their more fortunate fellow residents in non-specialist homes (Meacher 1972*a*, p 161).

A valuable contribution of Meacher's work is to draw attention to the unsatisfactory administration and supervision of some homes for the elderly mentally infirm. Such homes must be specialist, catering for the particular needs of mentally impaired residents, rather than simply separatist, a means of preventing confused residents from offending the susceptibilities of more fortunate companions or the expectations of inadequately trained or selected staff. If this is to be achieved the Homes must be architecturally suitable and close to a defined catchment community, staff ratios should be high and include psychiatric nurses but appropriate training for all grades of staff should be mandatory, and both for patient welfare and staff morale supervision by a Consultant Psychiatrist should be close and continuous, and there should be full integration with hospital and other services for the elderly. It is on the basis of the work of units set up to this specification and on their general feasibility that the principle of specialist EMI homes should be judged. My personal view on the second point at least is that the question is still an open one and my quarrel with Meacher is that he has attempted to close it prematurely.

We have frequently alluded to the use of "norms" by central government for planning purposes. This whole concept has received a great deal of justified criticism. Although it may be officially promulgated as a statement about average level of current provision, in practice a norm may become interpreted as a minimal standard so that potentially the system is spiral, as Bosanquet (1975) pointed out. A further criticism of norms is that they are based on the population aged 65 and over but are not sensitive to local or national variations in the age structure within that group. Figure 7 shows that some institutional care usage mounts steeply through old age and Wroe (1973) summarizes similar evidence for the use of other services. Gedling and Newell (1972) suggested that planning non-psychiatric hospital beds for the elderly on the basis of the population aged over 65 might, in fact, be

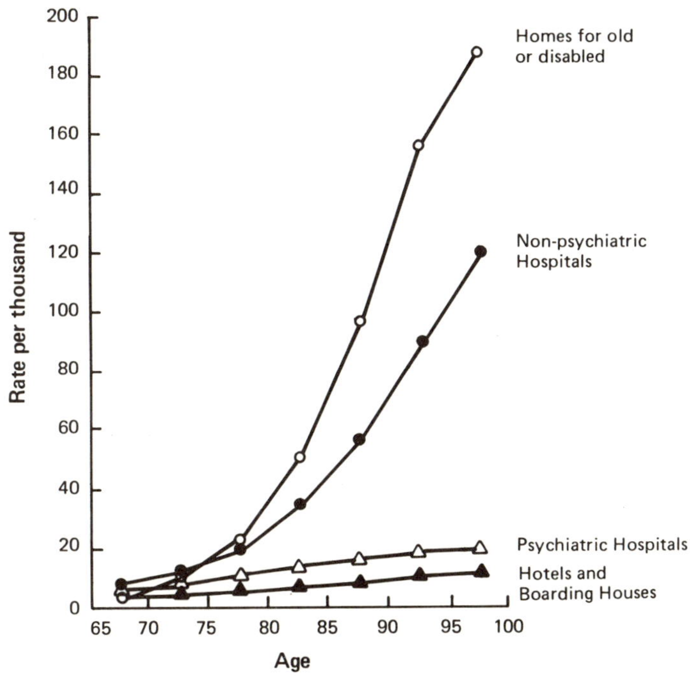

Fig. 7 *1971 census. Persons in institutions on census day per 1000 population*

adequate in the areas they studied to embody the prospective increase in the population of persons aged over 75 in the general population, but presumably there will be areas where this approximation will not suffice. Although most official norms embody a rider to the effect that they should be interpreted and implemented with such modifications as are appropriate to local conditions and needs, there is little conscious effort to do this and no agreed methodology is definable. Several factors affecting the needs of an elderly population are demonstrable (Gedling and Newell 1972), and Bleddyn Davies (1964) has made notable advances in multifactorial analyses of demographic data which might form a basis for what we need for planning at a local level (Davies *et al.* 1971). It is not realistic to plan separately for the different modalities of geriatric care. We have dealt at some length with the point made by Andrews *et al.* (1972) that geriatric and psychogeriatric care should be treated as a continuum: presumably equivalences or equations can be found to link modalities as diverse as home helps and hospital beds. Indeed, if no equation to link community and hospital facilities can be demonstrated then the whole basis of contemporary geriatric practice, namely that we are keeping people out of institutions by means of domiciliary services, will have to be questioned for it will imply that the different facilities are serving predominantly mutually exclusive groups. Maddox (1971) has commented on the preference of the British Civil Service to base planning on the opinions of prestigious advisers rather than on appropriate data. As far as care of the elderly is concerned this is not due to lack of opportunity; there is a wide range of different local mixtures of services in Britain and one would like to see a comprehensive and integrated data base established within sampled communities which could be used to generate an adaptive model for care of the elderly. Such a project might interest a nation facing a decision on shifting from an institution-based to a community-based system of care; for the conflicting and ill-defined data available, together with the service deficiencies endured by the elderly and those whose work with them in Britain make it clear that the British experience has not yet established the parameters of a successful system, but a failed community system can cause more hardship than does over-institutionalization.

References

Acheson, E. D. (1967). "Medical Record Linkage." Oxford University Press, London

Adams, G. F. (1974). *British Medical Journal* **iii**, 789–791

Age Concern (1973). "Care is Rare." Age concern, Mitcham, London

Andrews, J., Barddon, D., Gander, D. R., Gibson, K. B., Mallett, B. L. and Robinson, K. V. (1972). *Gerontologia clinica* **14**, 100–109

Ashley, J. S. A. (1972). *British Journal of Preventive and Social Medicine* **26**, 135–147

Bergmann, K. (1972). *New Society* **21**, 595–596

Bergmann, K. (1973). *New Society* **23**, 201–202

Bergmann, K. and Eastham, E. J. (1974). *Age and Ageing* **3**, 174–188

Bergmann, K., Foster, E. M. and Kay, D. W. (1965). "The Need for an Integrated Geriatric Service in Psychiatric Disorders in the Aged." Geigy, Manchester

Bosanquet, N. (1975). "A New Deal for the Elderly." Fabian Society, London (Tract No. 435)

Brown, D. (1974). "A Survey of the Dependence of Residents of Homes for the Elderly in Newcastle upon Tyne" (unpublished)

Carstairs, V. and Morrison, M. (1971). "The Elderly in Residential Care." Scottish Health Service Studies No. 19. Scottish Home and Health Department, Edinburgh

Coleman, P. (1976). "Balanced Provision of Sheltered Housing and Residential Homes for the Elderly: Contrasts between Britain and the Netherlands." Paper presented to British Society of Social and Behavioural Gerontology.

Cross, K. W. and Turner, R. D. (1974). *British Journal of Preventive and Social Medicine* **28**, 133–139

Davies, B. (1964). *Sociological Review* **12**, 5–38

Davies, B., Barton, A., McMillan, I. and Williamson, B. (1971). "Variations in Services for the Aged." Occasional Papers on Social Administration No. 40. Bell, London

Department of Health and Social Services (DHSS) (1970). Psycho-Geriatric Assessment Units. HM 70(11). (1971). Hospital Geriatric Services DS(329)71. (1972). Services for Mental Illness Related to Old Age. HM 72(71). (1975*a*). National Health Service Development of Health Services Community Hospitals. HSC (1S)75. (1975*b*). The Census of Residential Accommodation: 1970. 1. Residential Accommodation for the Elderly and for the Younger Physically Handicapped. (1975*c*). Census of Patients in Mental Illness Hospitals and Units in England and Wales at the End of 1971. Statistical and Research Report Series No. 10. HMSO, London

Evans, J. G. (1974). *Lancet* **ii**, 282–283

Gedling, P. and Newell, D. J. (1972). *In* "Problems and Progress in Medical Care." Ed. G. McLachlan. Seventh Series No. 10. Oxford University Press, London; pp 133–145

Health and Welfare (1967). "The Development of Community Care." Cmnd. 3022

Hodkinson, H. M. and Jefferys, P. M. (1972). *British Medical Journal* **4**, 536–9

Hospital Plan (1962). "A Hospital Plan for England and Wales." Cmnd. 1604. HMSO, London

"Hospital Plan for Scotland" (1962). Cmnd. 1602. HMSO, London

Isaacs, B. (1972). *British Medical Journal* **4**, 729–730

Isaacs, B., Livingstone, M. and Neville, Y. (1972). "Survival of the Unfittest." Routledge and Kegan Paul, London

Maddox, G. L. (1971). *Medical Care* **9**, 439–488

McKeown, T. and Cross, K. W. (1969). *British Journal of Preventive and Social Medicine* **23**, 34–39

Meacher, M. (1972*a*). "Taken for a Ride." Longmans, London

Meacher, M. (1972*b*). *New Society* **21**, 458–459

Meacher, M. (1972*c*). *New Society* **21**, 708–709

O'Brien, T. D., Joshi, D. M. and Warren, E. W. (1973). *British Medical Journal* **4**, 277–280

Office of Population Censuses and Surveys (1972). General Household Survey. HMSO, London

Seebohm Report (1968). "Report of the Committee on Local Authority and Allied Personal Social Services." Cmnd. 3703, HMSO, London

Shanas, E., Townsend, P., Wedderburn, D., Friis, H., Milhøj, P. and Stenhouwer, J. (1968). "Old People in Three Industrial Societies." Routledge and Kegan Paul, London; Atherton Press, New York

Shaw, S. M. and Opit, L. J. (1976). *British Medical Journal* **i**, 505–507

Townsend, P. (1962). "The Last Refuge: a Survey of Residential Institutions and Houses for the Aged in England and Wales." Routledge and Kegan Paul, London

Williamson, J., Stokoe, I. H., Gray, S., Froher, M., Smith, A., McGhee, A. and Stephenson, E. (1964). *Lancet* **i**, 1117–11120

Williamson, J. (1971). *Health Bulletin* (*Edinburgh*) **29**, 97–103

Wroe, D. C. L. (1973). *The Elderly in Social Trends* **4**, 23–34

Community and Home Care: United States and United Kingdom

The Unrealized Potential of an Old Idea

George L Maddox
Center for the Study of Aging
and Human Development,
Duke University Medical Center,
Durham, North Carolina 27710

The human and economic cost of excessive dependence in late life is very high. In both the United States and the United Kingdom we have become increasingly aware of how high that cost is already, and worse, how high it might become. Modern technology has tended to produce affluence, increased life expectancy at birth and, concomitantly, a high proportion of older persons in our populations. Unfortunately, improved life expectancy has not ensured freedom from disease, impairment, and disability; on the contrary, among adults, the risk of disease, impairment, and disability remains a function of age (National Center for Health Statistics 1971, Harris 1971). Societies that know how to prolong life regrettably do not know how to ensure personal independence for older persons. This is why reduction of excessive dependence in late life demands our attention.

The proportion of older persons in the United States and the United Kingdom has more than doubled in this century. Currently, more than 10% of the population in the United States are 65 years of age or older; in the United Kingdon the proportion is already over 13%. About one third of the older persons in both societies are very old, that is, 75 years of age and over. If a Zero Population Growth rate is achieved and sustained in the two countries, which is a realistic possibility, an additional 6% might be added to those proportions. The implications of this possible outcome for future demands on health and welfare services are staggering. But we should not dwell on the conjectures of demographers about the future. The aging individuals already with us appear to be quite enough to test the ingenuity of the managers of our social institutions in the foreseeable future. Long average life expectancy, a distinct achievement of modern societies, has proved to be an embarrassment and a current threat to existing institutional arrangements not only for health and welfare but also for income maintenance, transportation, housing, and education. Medical education and health delivery systems in both countries were designed for acute, not chronic illness; they are therefore mismatched with the particular needs of older persons for preventive, primary, and long-term care and, one might add, with the general needs of most adults. The mismatch is troublesome in the United Kingdom (Anderson 1974, Andrews *et al.* 1971, Harris 1971, Somers 1976) and dramatic in the United States (Glazier 1973, Garfield *et al.* 1976). The trouble and the drama flow from statistics on how the health and welfare needs of older persons translate into the utilization of health and welfare resources. Among adults in the two countries, utilization of health and welfare services is a function of age; as a rule of thumb, older adults consume health and welfare services at a rate of about two and a half to three times greater than adults generally.

The threat to established ways of doing things has been perceived most acutely by the managers of health and welfare institutions, where the pressure is most immediate. It is small comfort to recognize that those who are responsible for transportation, housing, and education are beginning to share in the general discomfort with institutional arrangements that were not designed with late life in mind. There has been an understandable tendency for all of us who are not yet old to discuss with academic detachment the "problems of the old" or "the old as a social problem". A more accurate assessment is that many, if not most, of the "problems" we associate with older people may lie in our institutional arrangements, not in older people.

Social systems that are ostensibly designed to help solve our problems sometimes have an opposite effect. This is well known to social scientists, as indicated in Robert Merton's phrase "the unintended consequences of purposive action" which he used to describe the latent functions of institutional arrangements. Simone de Beauvoir has made a similar point about modern, technological societies with great force in "The Coming of Age" (1971, p 807):

> . . . Society cares for the individual only insofar as he is productive. The young know this. Their anxiety as they enter in upon social life matches the anguish of the old as they are excluded from it. Between the two ages, the problem lies hidden by routine . . . Between youth and age there turns the machine, the crusher of men — of men who let themselves be crushed because it never occurs to them that they can escape it. Once we have understood what the state of the aged really is, we cannot satisfy ourselves with calling for a more generous "old-age policy," higher pensions, decent housing and organized leisure. It is the whole system that is at issue and our claim cannot be otherwise than radical — change life itself.

Simone de Beauvoir's insight anticipates the basic conclusion of this paper: the substantial potential of community and home care, a type of care which has particular relevance for older persons, will be realized only when such care is an integral part of a comprehensive, coordinated health and welfare delivery system. The necessary integration, I will argue, has in fact been achieved to a substantial degree in the United Kingdom and, for the most part, not at all in the United States. Thereby hangs the tale which will be developed in this paper.

The Argument in Brief

My argument is as follows. In the first place, community and home care for older persons are a common sense response to common problems of dependency in late life. Community and home care are old ideas which reflect such obvious good sense that arguments about evidence to document need, feasibility and merits appear to be gratuitous and dilatory. The great majority of the health needs of older persons in both the United Kingdom and the United States are currently met, more or less adequately, in the community and at home. More of these needs can be adequately and economically met there.

Second, discussions of the economics of community and home care have continued to be inconclusive and controversial. Intuitively, non-institutional care ought to be cost-effective and there are many who assert that it is. However, this imputed cost-effectiveness has been more convincingly asserted than demonstrated. As we will see below, few attempts have been made to demonstrate the cost-effectiveness of community and home care with adequately designed studies in the United States, where there is some compulsion to have research evidence when such matters are under consideration. No such compulsion is in evidence in the United Kingdom, where traditionally there is a preference for reliance on the testimony of experienced practitioners rather more than on the data of social scientists.

Third, in any case, the issue of cost-effectiveness is probably a diversion and not the crucial issue which must be addressed. The fundamental issue appears to be the presence or absence of a comprehensive, integrated system for delivering care to older persons. Whether such a system of care exists determines whether community and health care are cost-effective and, more importantly, whether the substantial potential of community and home care can be realized. Each of these points will now be developed.

More Non-Institutional Care of Older Persons is Needed, Feasible and Desirable

The basic argument for community and home care may be summarized as follows. The social process by which health care is allocated is complex and imprecise. Older persons appear to be particularly vulnerable to binary "all-or-none" responses; they tend to receive too little care or too much care. Consider mental health services, for example. Older persons are under-represented in community mental health clinics and over-represented in mental institutions. Moreover, the probability of a mismatch between clinically established medical needs and receipt of appropriate types and quantities of service is high (Williams *et al.* 1973). An established impairment is clearly not the only consideration in decisions to institutionalize older persons. In a systematic assessment of carefully drawn samples of older persons living in the community and in long-term care institutions, using a reliable valid instrument for evaluating functional status, colleagues at the Duke Center for the Study of Aging and Human Development have found about 12% of the individuals surveyed appear to be interchangeable; that is, at least 12% of the institutionalized older persons in the study had demonstrated personal and social resources which were sufficient to sustain them in the community and about an equal percentage of older persons living in the community were so impaired that experienced clinicians would expect them to be institutionalized (Pfeiffer, 1975).

There are understandable but consequential tendencies to equate health care and medical care and to use hospitals extensively in both the United States and the United Kingdom, particularly the former. The first three-quarters of this century have been a veritable golden age of scientific medicine. Common infectious diseases have been substantially mastered. Hospitals, which played a relatively minor role in health care at the turn of the century, now assume a dominant role in health care. Hospitals, especially teaching hospitals and the medical specialists who control them, now consume more than half of the economic resources allocated to health care in both countries. In the United States the total allocation for health care is currently about 8% of the Gross National Product and in the United Kingdom, about 5%.

Although concern has been expressed in both the United States and the United Kingdom about the total cost of health care, much more concern has been expressed about over-specialization of medical care, maldistribution of services, excessive concentration on in-patient facilities, neglect of preventive care, and provision for long-term care outside of medical facilities (Glazier 1973, *Scientific American* 1973, Maddox 1971, Shanas and Maddox 1976). A review of the epidmiology of health and of related health care needs among older persons illustrates the basis for these concerns.

Risk of chronic disease, impairment and disability is a well documented function of age among adults (National Center for Health Statistics 1971, Harris 1971). In one substantial comparative study which included older persons living in the community in both the United States and the United Kingdom, Ethel Shanas and her colleagues (1968) found very similar patterns of impairment and disability. The

United States National Health Survey (US Vital and Health Statistics 1975*a*) reports that a large majority of older Americans have at least one identifiable chronic condition; 46% of older persons have a chronic condition which limits their normal activity and 36% experience some limitation in a major activity. Amelia Harris (1971) has documented that 70% of the impaired individuals identified in a large national sample in the United Kingdom were 65 years of age or over. She reported impairment rates of 22% for persons aged 65 to 74 and 38% for persons aged 75 and older.

A number of important observations are suggested by this documentation of high levels of impairment and disability among older persons in both countries. On the one hand, we would expect what we in fact observe about the utilization of health care by older persons in both countries; as a rule of thumb, older persons consume most types of health care resources at a rate of about two and one half to three times higher than adults generally. In the United States a health care industry, the nursing home, has been developed in the private sector primarily to serve disabled older persons. This industry has generated almost 16 000 facilities and 1 175 000 beds and produces 369 million resident days of care at an average monthly cost per resident of $479 and an annual total cost of over $8 billion (US Vital and Health Statistics 1975*b*). There is evidence that a substantial minority of individuals in long-term care institutions could be appropriately served in the community or at home (Williams *et al.* 1973, Pfeiffer 1975, Controller General of the United States 1974, Hurtado *et al.* 1971). The economic costs of unnecessary institutionalization and inappropriately high levels of care are consequential.

On the other hand, while the demand for health care is high among older persons, it is well below its theoretical maximum. This is so, in part, because morbidity in a population is never translated perfectly into demand for health care services (Maddox 1972). As cases in point, we should note again that community surveys of impairment and disability in both the United States and the United Kingdom have identified far more older people who are at risk for seeking health care than in fact do so. In the United States, for example, we are impressed — intimidated might be the more accurate word — by the over one million older persons who occupy beds in nursing homes at any point in time. We hear very little, by contrast, about at least an equal number who are receiving care at home, primarily from a household member (Maddox 1975). And among older persons who are receiving whatever care they receive at home, about one third require constant care over a long period of time. In the United States, e.g. among persons 65 years of age and over receiving care at home, 25% have received care for over five years; 63% of those aged 65 to 74 and 73% of those aged 75 and over receiving care at home have received that care for over one year (US Vital and Health Statistics 1971). It is reasonable to assume that a comparable situation exists in the United Kingdom. Amelia Harris (1971) documented, for example, that older persons in the United Kingdom were less likely to be registered with a local authority than younger persons with the same level of handicap. Among persons with severe handicaps, 47% of those aged 16 to 49 were registered with a service agency in contrast to 39% of those aged 50 to 64 and 9% of those 65 years of age or older. Further, a report on social work service in the United Kingdom (DHSS 1973) has noted that, while 80% of home health services are provided to older persons, the unmet need for such services is probably two to three times greater than the amount actually provided.

These facts underlie increasing interest in community and home care in the United States and United Kingdom. Some older individuals currently in health care institutions do not need the level of care they receive, or could leave those institutions sooner if community and home care were available, or do not need to be institutionalized at all. Some individuals living in the community or at home demonstrably can be maintained there adequately with proper support services.

Experience suggests that there are two key support services in the community which are first lines of defense against triage procedures which, once begun, tend to result in inappropriate types and levels of care. These are home health (usually nursing) and home help (a variety of domestic services). Although home health and home help services both have distinct tradition and foci, current practice stresses the importance of coordinating the two (Somers and Moore, 1976, International Federation on Aging 1975). By way of emphasizing the importance attached to this coordination, current discussions of community and home care typically refer to "home health–home help" programs as elementary, basic and complementary components of health care which should receive high priority. For this reason it is useful in this discussion to concentrate on "home health–home help" programs for older persons. We specifically recognize that the designation *community and home care* encompasses a broad array of services which we might but cannot discuss in this brief presentation. These services are as varied as home visits by physicians, meals on wheels, health centers, community mental health centers, day care, day hospitals, special housing and transportation. Concentration on one type of service which is rather well documented will serve our purposes here.

A review of the relevant literature (e.g. Somers and Moore 1976, International Federation on Aging 1975, Calendar and LaVor 1975, Hurtado *et al.* 1971) suggests the following generalizations about "home health–home help" services:

1. Western European countries, particularly the Nordic countries and the Netherlands, have extensive and successful experience with both home health and home help services. The visiting nurse is typically an integral part of the health care delivery system in these countries and formal home help services have built upon established patterns of friendly neighboring and voluntary services.

2. Experience has confirmed that such programs have special relevance for older persons. Older persons typically constitute about 75% of the clients of home health–home help programs; best estimates are that the need for such services exceed available service by at least a factor of two.

3. The ease with which such programs can be established and maintained is well established. Appropriate personnel are available. Training procedures, curricula, and materials are adequately documented.

4. A substantial amount of experience exists regarding adequate personnel/population ratios, expected levels of demand, and approximate cost of home health–home help services. As a rule of thumb, experience suggests that one home health–home help full-time-equivalent is needed for every 100 persons 65 years of age and older. A few Nordic countries are currently near this ratio but most countries are quite distant from it. The ratio in the United States, for example, is about 1:5000 and in the United Kingdom, about 1:750. Although data on average use of services and cost are very ephemeral and difficult to compare from one country to the next, two important conclusions emerge from current evidence which tend to allay concerns about unlimited demands for service and related high cost of programs: first, the length of time the average older person receives home care services and the amount of services received are modest; and second, the average cost of these services per case is well below comparable figures for long-term care in a nursing home or other setting.

Conclusions such as these have apparently been convincing in the United Kingdom. Home health–home help services in particular and more generally community and home care delivery organizations are clearly an intentional and integral part of national policy in that country. The intention is especially clear in the reorganization of the National Health Service in 1974. In contrast, consensus has not emerged in the United States regarding the role of community and home-care services. To my knowledge, no one in this country argues that the need for such services has not been demonstrated or that such services are not feasible. Rather, the stumbling blocks appear to be the continuing commitment in the United States to a medical model of services delivery featuring long-term care institutions and uncoordinated arrays of supportive services which are permitted, but not facilitated, by complex legislation and related administrative rules. When community and home care are authorized at all in the United States, an emphasis on medical certification and on the use of skilled professionals to provide permitted services, presumably in the interest of controlling the cost rather more than the quality of service, is typical. This extreme cautiousness in the United States has resulted in minimal development of community and home-care service. The most frequently stated reason for this cautiousness in the United States is concern about cost. What is the evidence?

The Cost-Effectiveness of Non-Institutional Care of Older Persons

Americans and Britons, it has been perceptively observed, are a people separated by a common language. One might add that they are also a people with very different interests in assessing the cost of health and welfare services. In the United Kingdom, where it would be feasible to design and implement research on the cost-effectiveness of various components of an integrated care delivery system, there appears to be little interest in doing so. In the United States, where it is for all practical purposes impossible to implement adequate research on cost-effectiveness of a fragmented non-system of services, there is a preoccupation with assessing cost.

The most compelling argument from the United Kingdom for increasing emphasis on community and home care in the interest of producing economical, quality services for older people remains largely implicit. This argument can be constructed as follows: the total national health bill in Britain is very favorable in comparison with other industrial countries. Costs have been contained in part by stressing primary health care and care outside specialized medical facilities; there has been some inconvenience but no demonstrable detriment to the health and welfare of the British people. Their health, for example, compares very favourably with the health of persons in the United States whose health bill is considerably higher. The availability of community and home-care services has not resulted in excessive new costs traceable to those services. This is the case in part because, even in the absence of restraints such as medical certification of services, average levels of utilization have been moderate; under-utilization is more likely the problem than over-utilization. Analysis of program costs and total system costs attributable to these needed and apparently useful non-institutional services appear, therefore, to be tolerable. Continued development of such services does not depend on further demonstrations that they serve useful purposes, will be used appropriately in the absence of strict rules of certification, or are more economical than institutional care.

In the United States the comparable argument, both implicit and explicit, may be summarized as follows: Some older persons are hospitalized or are located in long-term care institutions unnecessarily and at a very high cost. Alternatives to institutionalization surely can be found which probably provide more adequate care at lower cost. But commitment of more than a small fraction of our resources to these alternatives is not prudent because total system cost is already too high; new services will add to and not replace existing services, and thus there is no effective way to control utilization and related cost. Consequently, we must repeatedly convince ourselves that alternative types of care are cost-effective or, more specifically, that they are more economical than institutionalization.

There is more to this concern about cost than meets the eye. Lay persons suspect what research investigators have demonstrated in the United States: older persons receive the care they do, where they do, and when they do for a variety of reasons, only one of which is medical necessity. Hence, sympathy can easily be generated for movements to de-institutionalize older persons even in the face of evidence that, for some older persons, the de-institutionalization means less care or no care rather than better care (e.g. Arnhoff 1975, Becker and Schulberg 1976). The alternatives we want to believe, surely are cheaper. The General Accounting Office of the United States has taken this position in a report to the Congress, observing "several studies have pointed out that home health care *can be* (emphasis supplied) considerably less expensive than care in a hospital or a skilled nursing facility." (Controller General of the United States 1974). What explains this cautious endorsement? The answer is supplied in part in a policy statement on Home Health Care by the Board of Governors of the Blue Cross Association (April, 1974):

> ... (home health care) does not appear to create a cost saving to the community except as it may reduce the need for care in a nursing home facility. In fact, it appears to increase total cost of care because it represents an additional level of services which are necessary and appropriate in specific instances but do not, as a rule, reduce the need for other institutional types of health care services.

This statement makes a crucial point. Impact on total system cost of a particular type of program cannot be determined by concentrating on the cost of that program alone. Consider the research findings of Hurtado and his colleagues (1971) at the Kaiser-Permanente facility in Portland. This research was designed to assess the impact on hospital utilization and the economic effects of introducing an extended care service and a home-care service into a comprehensive prepayment health plan with a history of low hospital utilization by subscribers. The effect of alternative service arrangements on hospitalization of Medicare patients was of special interest. The authors concluded that, with an extended care facility and a home care service which were spatially and administratively an integral part of a comprehensive system of care, hospital utilization by Medicare patients could be reduced by 27%. They noted, however, that the reduced hospitalization was attributed principally to the availability of the extended care facility, not the home-care services. Patients reported liking the alternative service; physicians were equally divided in their opinion. Nevertheless, and this is very important, the cost of total days in the extended care facility was greater than the saving attributable to reduced hospital days. Significantly, the report also stressed that the outcome of this demonstration of economy of using alternative care facilities was affected substantially by spatial and administrative arrangements. At the beginning of the demonstration, when the extended care facility used was not spatially and administratively integrated with the hospital, the expected savings were not realized. Reduction in hospital days for Medicare patients was not achieved until the extended care facility was literally integrated into the hospital.

The conclusion suggested by the Kaiser-Permanente demonstration is that an integrated, comprehensive health service can utilize a variety of services, including home services, in the effective management of older patients. This can be done at a cost equal to or not much greater than the cost incurred by using a conventional hospital service. The potential savings attributable to community and home care for older persons are not the only considerations, however. If one could demonstrate that the physical, psychological, or social outcomes for patients managed in the community or at home were in fact superior to outcomes for patients who are managed in a conventional hospital service — and the report does not address this issue — the Kaiser-Permanente (Portland) demonstration would nevertheless be important evidence in favor of an expanded range of non-institutional services even in the absence of reduced cost. The expanded services would be justified not because they save money but because they provide more value for money.

As a sobering reminder that, in the absence of an integrated system of care, costs can be quite variable and unpredictable, we should note a recent report to the Health Resources Administration (Transcentury 1975) regarding the cost of ten day-care centers serving older persons. Day care in the United States, the report indicates, encompasses some programs which provide primarily social support services and other programs which stress rehabilitation. The average daily cost per client in these varied community programs reflected very different services and thus had a range from about $11 to over $60 with an average of about $25 per day per participant. This average figure is much higher than the daily average cost for nursing homes, which was about $16 in 1973–4 (US Vital and Health Statistics 1975*b*). The report concludes hopefully that day care is cost-effective because day care patients are typically served only a few days each week in contrast to the longer stays of nursing home patients. This is why the average monthly cost of day care per older person is said to to be economical. The report does not address several significant questions: Was the level of care given in the day-care programs necessary and appropriate? Were the outcomes comparable to the expected outcomes for alternative modes of care? Did the provision of the services described change the total health care costs in the community attributable to these patients? Conclusions about the efficiency and effectiveness of day care require answers to these questions.

One need not quarrel with the good intentions of the proponents and providers of alternative community and home services and their hope that favorable outcomes can be achieved economically. At the same time, it is incorrect and misleading to argue that community and home care have been demonstrated to be economical and effective; this has not been demonstrated.

My own best estimate is that, in the absence of a comprehensive, integrated system of health care, community and home care do not reduce total community costs. Whether stabilization or reduction of total cost is achievable through coordination remains an open question, although the evidence from the United Kingdom appears to be favorable. An equally important question which has not satisfactorily been answered in the United States is the following: Can more effective, as well as more economical, care be provided to older persons in non-institutional settings as compared with institutional setting? Preoccupation with the cost factor may divert us from the central issue — the systematic coordination of services for older persons.

The Central Issue: Organization of Services

We have argued up to this point that community and home care for older persons are needed, feasible, and possible, though not demonstrably cost-effective in the absence of a comprehensive, coordinated system of care. The unresolved issue of cost-effectiveness in the United States, we have argued, is symptomatic of a more and persistent basic issue of how we organize health care services for older persons. This observation is hardly novel. The United States and the United Kingdom present an instructive contrast in approaches and outcomes.

In 1971 the Department of Health, Education, and Welfare of the United States published a "white paper" which presented a detailed critique of health care in this country. The diagnosis was bleak and the recommended therapy was demanding. Health care in the United states, the "white paper" argued, suffered not from lack of resources so much as from inadequate organization and distribution of resources. The health care delivery system was described as "a cottage industry of small entrepreneurs," "push-cart vending in an age of supermarkets," or, in summary, a non-system. What was to be done? The prescription was complex and included potentially contradictory items. More primary and preventive care was stressed and Health Maintenance Organizations received very favorable notice (see also Klarman 1971). The intriguing suggestion was also made that, if one took the economics of a free market seriously, the most effective way to affect health care was to redistribute personal income rather than to increase investment in medical institutions and personnnel directly. Moreover, public dollars could probably do more for the public health if they were devoted to improving housing and nutrition rather than to increasing medical research and hospital care. The report did not mention community and home care as such and only an incidental reference was made to the health care of older persons. Lest you think the authors of this document were totally out of touch with political reality in the United States, the report announced a preference for keeping health predominantly in the private sector and for a *national* but not *nationalized* system of health care.

Five years after this "white paper," the United States has not enacted national health insurance; has had to tamper incessantly with its basic Medicare regulations; has apparently immobilized Health Maintenance Organizations with very restrictive legislation; has developed a policy of de-institutionalization without insuring provisions for alternative sources of care; and has not developed an effective program for developing personnel and mechanisms to insure adequate care of older people. In the light of such conspicuous non-performance, we would be surprised if community and home care for older persons were established as part of national policy in the United States. But there are no surprises here; community and home care continue to be discussed as though their merits and outcomes still had to be established. The future of geriatric health-care services both in and outside institutions in the United States remains very much in doubt. Lack of resources is not the problem. Our non-system of health care *is* the problem.

The situation in the United Kingdom provides a sharp and instructive contrast. The British National Health Service has its problems; but it represents a considerable organizational achievement as a comprehensive, integrated system of services which has been particularly responsive to the health care needs of older persons. Reorganization of health care in Britain, we should note, did not come easily. Impetus for the creation of the National Health Service was provided to a substantial degree by the imminent collapse of medical care delivery prior to the First World War (Eckstein 1958). The organization which emerged in 1948 — an organization committed to free access to care, salaried practitioners, and a team approach to care — proved to be remarkably stable, effective, and economical over the next two decades.

It was my good fortune to study in Britain in 1968 as a US Public Health Service Research Fellow at a time when various Royal Commissions were assessing the work of the first twenty years. The major points of criticism of the National Health Service were evident in widely circulated reports on every aspect of health and welfare services: control of further medical specialization and renewed emphasis on primary care were needed; geographic redistribution of care was required; the ratio of hospital beds to population needed to be reduced and alternative care settings provided; and most of all, the separation of medical, health, and welfare services was intolerably ineffective and required a new integration. In 1968, the United Kingdom was well on its way to the reorganization of 1974. This American, who was in London to study how a socialistic Labour government made and implemented health policy, admits having been disconcerted by the heavy reliance of National Health Services planners and managers on what might be called the testimony of experienced men in contrast to information based on social scientific research. Health planning in the United Kingdom was indeed captured in phrases like "muddling through" and "disjointed incrementalism." Yet, the observed scientifically inelegant planning procedures had generated, or so it appeared, a sound and effective health-care organization which was delivering value for money (Maddox, 1971). It was my impression then, as it is now, that the United Kingdom has very few health problems that adequate financing could not resolve satisfactorily. A similar conclusion is reached in a recent analysis by Anne R Somers (1976). In providing "an American perspective" on the National Health Service, she documents the major characteristics which insure that geriatric care is an integral part of the total health service. General practice has continued to be emphasized and provides access to primary and preventive care. Geriatric medicine is a recognized specialty. "Alternatives to institutionalization" is not a slogan but a policy which is actively implemented by programs of visiting nurses, home help, health centers, day care and day hospitals, special transportation, and special purpose housing. Mrs Somers also makes a thoughtful comment about the philosophy of care in the United Kingdom, which she describes as an amalgam of public preference and traditional ways of practicing medicine. This philosophy continues to stress free access to care, primary and preventive care, and non-institutional care. In such an environment we would be surprised if community and home care for older persons were not observed.

In summary, barring total financial disaster in the United Kingdom, community and home care for older persons will thrive as an integral part of the National Health Service. In the city of Glasgow under the leadership of Sir Ferguson Anderson and his colleagues, one can observe today a very complete array of geriatric services operated at a bearable cost. Glasgow provides an excellent example when one is conceptualizing a system of comprehensive care which is designed to meet the health care needs of an aging population (Anderson 1974: Andrews *et al.* 1971).

In contrast, in the United States repeated documentation of the unmet needs of older persons and of the probable cost-effectiveness of community and home services are unlikely to produce the needed services until an integrated system of health care and health care financing is achieved. And when that system is achieved, it is my prediction that it will look remarkably like the British National Health Service.

References

Anderson, W. F. (1974). *Alternsforschung* **68**, 341–350

Andrews, G. R., Cowan, N. and Anderson, W. F. (1971). *In* "Problems and Progress in Medical Care", 5th Series. Oxford University Press, London: pp 57–86

Arnhoff, F. (1975). *Science* **188**, 1277–1281

Becker, A. and Schulberg, (1976). *The New England Journal of Medicine* **294**, 255–261

Calendar, M. and LaVor, J. (1975). "Home Health Care: Development, Problems and Potential." Department of Health, Education and Welfare Working Paper

Controller General of the United States (1974). "Report to the Congress on Home Health Care Benefits Under Medicare and Medicaid." United States Department of Health, Education and Welfare, Washington

de Beauvoir, S. (1972). "The Coming of Age." Putnam, New York

Department of Health, Education and Welfare (1971). "Towards a Comprehensive Health Policy for the 1970s": A White Paper. Government Printing Office, Washington

Department of Health and Social Security (1973). "Review of the Home Health Service in England," February–July 1972

Eckstein, H. (1958). "The English Health Service." Harvard University Press, Cambridge, Mass.

Garfield, S., Collen, M., Feldman, R., Soghikian, K., Richart, R. and Duncan, J. (1976). *The New England Journal of Medicine* **294**, 426–431

Glazer, W. H. (1973). *Scientific Medicine* **228**, 13–17

Harris, A. (1971). "Handicapped and Impaired in Great Britain," Part 1. HMSO, London

Hurtado, A. V., Greenlick, M. and Saward, E. (1971). "Home Care and Extended Care in a Comprehensive Prepayment Plan." Hospital and Research Educational Trust, Chicago

International Federation on Aging (1975). "Home Help Services for the Aging Around the World." International Federation on Aging, Washington

Klarman, H. E. (1971). "Health Maintenance Organizations: A Reconfiguration of the Health Services System." Thirteenth Annual Symposium on Hospital Affairs, Graduate School of Business, University of Chicago

Maddox, G. L. (1971). *Medical Care* **9**, 439–448

Maddox, G. L. (1972). *In* "Behavioral Science: A Selective View". Eds. F. Hine, E. Pfeiffer, G. Maddox, P. Hein and R. Friedel. Little, Brown & Co., Boston

Maddox, G. L. (1975). *In* "Long Term Care". Ed. S. Sherwood. Spectrum, New York

National Center for Health Statistics (1971). "Health in the Later Years of Life." Government Printing Office, Washington

Pfeiffer, E. (Ed.) (1975). "Multidimensional Functional Assessment." Duke Center for the Study of Aging and Human Development, Durham, NC.

Scientific American (1973). "Life and Death in Medicine" (articles from *Scientific American* September 1973). Freeman, San Francisco

Shanas, E., Townsend, P., Wedderburn, D., Friis, H., Milhøj, P. and Stenhouwer, J. (1968). "Old People in Three Industrial Societies." Atherton Press, New York; Routledge and Kegan Paul, London

Shanas, E. and Maddox, G. L. (1976). *In* "Handbook of Aging and the Social Sciences." Eds. R. Binstock and E. Shanas. Van Nostrand, New York

Somers, A. R. (1976). *Annals of Internal Medicine* **84**, 466–476

Somers, A. R. and Moore, F. M. (1976). "Homemaker Services: An Essential Option for the Elderly." (Unpublished)

Transcentury Corporation (1975). "Adult Day Care in the US." A Final Report to the US National Center for Health Services Research

US Vital and Health Statistics (1971). "Persons 55 Years and Over Receiving Care at Home, July 1966–June 1968." Series 19: 10

US Vital and Health Statistics (1975*a*). "Current Estimates from the Health Interview Survey, US — 1974." Series 10: 100

US Vital and Health Statistics (1975*b*). "Selected Operating and Financial Characteristics of Nursing Homes, US 1973–74." National Nursing Home Survey. Series 13: 22

Williams, T. F., Hill, J., Fairbanks, M. and Knox, K. (1973). *Journal of the American Medical Association* **226**, 1332–1335

Integration of Components of Health and Social Services

Daphne H Krause
Minneapolis Age and Opportunity Center, Inc,
Minneapolis, Minnesota

Before presenting an extremely brief survey of the many programs and consortium of partners of the Minneapolis Age and Opportunity Center, Inc. (known as MAO), I would like to tell you a story that illustrates graphically the callous disregard towards many of our most helpless elderly, that I believe is one of the root causes of our lack of commitment to them.

It seems there was a country and a time where it was the custom to take the elderly up onto a mountain to die of exposure, when the community felt they were no longer of use. A man, carrying his father up the mountain, felt tears on his neck and asked, "Why are you crying? You know this is the law and you have had many years to grow used to your fate." The father replied, "I am not crying for myself, my son, but for you, and what your son will do to you."

There are many issues this story raises. Is it possible that in our countries and our time, a neglected house, a dingy apartment, or an unnecessary nursing home, are our mountains of obliteration for our unwanted elderly? Certainly very old age is the ultimate death sentence, and I believe it is our unconscious fear of this reality that is behind our agism and neglect.

We must ask ourselves, Are all old people alike? And we will find they are not, and a large percentage are comparatively or completely independent. Are they all a burden on the community? For those who do need our assistance we must ask: Where does our responsibility to help them lie? What types of services do they need and how do we provide them? Indeed, can we even afford to do so with the steadily increasing elderly population? The MAO experience is one answer to these vital questions.

Beginning in 1967, I met with a number of senior citizen leaders and others, to address these questions. The major priority that emerged was a need for an alternative approach, that I called "medi-supportive," for those particular seniors with multiple health and socio-economic problems, needing various levels of medical and social supportive services to help them delay or avoid unneccessary institutionalization.

We analyzed the existing fragmented services, many of which were excellent in themselves, but not sufficient to provide the full range of medical and social supportive services needed by the dependent elderly.

My first thought was to try to coordinate these existing programs and then fill in the gaps. Immediately, I ran into many problems. There were two major stumbling blocks. While most private and governmental agencies talked "coordination," it had to be within the context of their own program's funding survival, and must not impinge on their "self-decided" territory. Their protective reaction was often disguised under the term "duplication of effort", when in reality, you cannot duplicate services that do not exist. I also found that one of the most frequent methods of obstruction was to form endless committees to discuss the problems, without leading anywhere.

The second major obstacle was the lack of Federal or local funding for a comprehensive program, and what funding did exist was channeled through the State and local governmental agencies, which were already committed to their own programs, and to already selected private institutions and agencies. Therefore, because of the limited funds available, they were reluctant to fund a new concept, and their reaction was to question why we needed to put together so many services. Why couldn't we limit our request to a few. I felt this to be wrong, because of the variable needs that had to be met, if we were to truly provide an alternative to institutionalization.

My determination was to proceed with the MAO concept in several ways. First, by attempting to reassure the private agencies and institutions that we were not trying to obtain their funding, that there was room for a variety of programs, and that would leave the door open to those who really wanted to coordinate.

Second, I decided to develop a consortium of partners from local resources, by my analyzing their individual concerns and objectives, then designing programs that would be mutually beneficial. (Some other good precepts to follow in order to gain partners, are always to treat your partners as the senior partners, giving them recognition first before your own agency, see that your partners get full credit for their work, don't waste their time in unnecessary meetings and always respect their autonomy. This is particularly true in your partnerships with voluntary organizations, that may fear being swallowed up by your more visible agency). Finally, we would apply for a variety of federal funds for those services our partners could not provide.

From the beginning some nine years ago, I knew I had to plan and develop a program that was not only humanly effective, but also cost-effective in every possible way. I felt this as a challenge to rethink existing methods, to take nothing for granted, and most important of all, in my planning, I never forgot the woman who told me, "I know I am going to die, but I don't want to die every day."

The "medi-supportive" concept was based on my fundamental belief that health in the future can no longer be considered in terms of medical intervention alone, however important these services are. Equally so are any social supportive services, and that these services must be welded together to meet the diverse problems of the client/patient. Health is also our environmental, nutritional and emotional well-being; really anything that goes to make up the quality of our lives, and the most important services are always the ones based on the individual's particular needs.

I have used a quotation from Carl Sandburg, "Nothing happens unless first a dream", to describe the foundation of MAO. It would not be an overstatement to say that many times I felt that it was an impossible dream.

Finally in 1969, MAO was incorporated as a non-profit organization. The majority of MAO's governing board are senior citizen leaders, representing many major senior citizen organizations. They in turn represent literally thousands of senior members. These senior citizen governors chose others from the community to sit on the governing board, such as the mayor, a state senator, aldermen, hospitals, government agencies, businessmen, including representatives from our partners' organizations, and so on.

There are none of the usual power struggles, because the senior citizen governors retain complete control of MAO through their council structure within the governing board. While the seniors' groups are divergent in the aims of their individual organizations, they are strongly together on MAO's objectives, and publicly supportive of the MAO programs. This is important to understand in terms of MAO's development. Also, it means that MAO has direct access for information and testing the feasibility of any programs we are developing, with an enormous reservoir of knowledge and expertise to draw on.

The following litany of funding demonstrates the time-consuming difficulties of current government sources. We applied for and received various federal funding from the Administration of Aging Title III, the Office of Economic Opportunity, Model Cities, Community Development Block Grant, and Title IVA and Title XX Social Service Programs. It is impossible to convey the trauma of trying to obtain federal funds for a program you believe in. One has to have survived that process in order to understand. This is especially true when trying to fund a new concept for which no designated comprehensive funds exist. It is like setting the cart before the horse — you need to demonstrate the program in order to gain fund appropriations.

Many times you are forced to compete for funds with other good programs, and pit need against need, which is personally heartbreaking. Although I committed myself to serving seniors, it doesn't mean I have no compassion for the young.

I knew about programs that had been defunded; many were rightly terminated. For others, it just didn't make sense, until I realized these programs were often ended because they were only serving a small segment of critical unmet needs, and therefore the government was concerned about the financial liabilities of opening the floodgates. The consequence is, that if you need help, however desperately, you had better be of the correct age, sex, and race, with the right set of eligibility standards, living in the right location at the right time, or you will probably not get the services you need.

But before placing all the blame on the complexity of federal funding sources, let us look to ourselves, and our responsibilities for these fiascos. For far too long, people in public and human services have felt it beneath their professional standing to be concerned with the costs of their programs, unless they were part of the administrative staff responsible for obtaining funding. If we truly care about serving our people and feel strongly that no one should make a "profit business" out of human misery, we must reverse this attitude, and personally hold ourselves accountable fiscally, as well as professionally, and also involve and teach our staffs the same principles before it is too late.

With this in mind, I designed our multiple reporting procedures, not only to meet the various federal guidelines to show accountability of services given, but also to show how much time was spent on each service. Thus, we are able to estimate the direct costs of serving each individual. Of course, this is not enough by itself, so I also built in methods of evaluating the quality and effectiveness of our services.

Some planners feel programs should show "shadow" costs as part of the total unit-cost. I don't agree. These costs must be shown and accounted for separately, as they are not actual federal dollars. However, these records are important in evaluating the ability of the program to draw on its community resources. These resources will probably vary in different areas, and even from senior to senior, depending on the individual's own resources.

I found that true and simple analogies are effective in drawing on local resources and support, by gaining community acceptance of our program. For example, one irate taxpayer called me to complain that he didn't have as good a car as the ones in which we transport our seniors. I pointed out that one senior with mobility problems that we save from slipping and thus avoiding a serious hip fracture would more than pay for one vehicle. It is more difficult to persuade different governmental branches to look at the total picture of costs, or even to accept the notion that most human services can in the long run be cost effective. Our recording systems have become MAO's key in demonstrating this, by citing a variety of individual case histories, showing human effectiveness and comparative cost effectiveness.

Some other examples of problems with federal funding, are guidelines that limit our services chronologically. This can be discriminating, especially when serving the minorities who have a lesser life expectancy. The degree of disability and need should be the determining factor. Also, in trying to ensure quality services, the guidelines at times force a higher level of expensive professional services than is warranted. Yet other services that are essential for this age and disability level are disallowed, such as cervical smears, dental care, and drugs needed to maintain health. There is not much point in providing medical care if the senior cannot afford the prescribed medications. It becomes a waste of medical resources.

Nevertheless, it is the federal funds that enable MAO to provide all its 156 social supportive services paid staff, ranging from attorneys, three levels of counselors, employment specialist, three levels of home care staff, handymen, drivers, home delivered meals, counselors for emotional health, alcoholic and drug dependency and abuse and so on.

MAO's current annual budget from all our federal funding sources is $638 000. We serve approximately 9000 seniors with medi-supportive services. Of these, we serve a recorded average of 2800 individual seniors a month, with an average of 16 000 recorded services a month. About 5000 individual seniors receive medical services from our clinic with Abbott-Northwestern. Through our various voluntary action programs, we are serving a recorded 32 000 individual seniors. We do not keep monthly statistics on our voluntary programs, because of their large volume; however, we do keep basic records on these seniors. All direct services given to our seniors by paid staff and voluntary staff are recorded, plus related data.

MAO's medical partner is the Abbott-Northwestern Hospital, Inc. I chose this hospital because of its proven record of delivering top-quality medical services with, as their president put it, "tender loving care," and because of their visionary and flexible leadership which had already pioneered new outreach programs, such as their regional organization, which provides management, purchasing, consultation and so on to fifty hospitals.

As my relationship with the hospital developed, I learned about the serious financial crises many of our hospitals face, due to a regressive cost reimbursement formula that doesn't adequately allow for capital expenditures, new technology and equipment, or even needed repairs. These problems are further compounded by the percentage of empty beds for peak loads which many hospitals carry, which drive up overhead costs. Yet, I also knew from the seniors that many of them were not seeking critically needed medical services because of their inability to pay the cost above Medicare. Therefore, I asked the hospital to subsidize the uncovered costs for in-patient and out-patient care for low and near poverty income-level seniors. In return, I projected a better utilization of the hospital's resources. Not only did this prove to be true, but in the course of time, the hospital found that with increased utilization, the cost of hospital services to all Medicare patients was reduced by $4.20 per patient day. This saving, together with a rationale and methodology regarding allowable costs as collectable bad debts, has made it possible for the hospital to invest in providing jointly my medi-supportive concepts. Mr Tierney of the Bureau of Health Insurance at the national level and Mr Flavin of Blue Cross/Blue Shield of Minnesota have been most cooperative.

The hospital runs the Abbott-Northwestern Hospital, Inc./Minneapolis Age and Opportunity Center, Inc. Senior Citizens Clinic, providing nurse practitioners, visiting nurses, eight nurses in our clinic, plus nurses for our mini-clinic centers, laboratory technicians, dietitians, a clinical pharmacist and an assistant, and provides our on-site pharmacy, where our seniors can purchase prescription drugs at a substantial saving. The hospital's kitchens provide our meals in the home, including special diets.

Abbott-Northwestern's physicians showed their support of our program by forming the Community Medical Associates, P.A., a private medical practice which provides our five full-time physicians, and nine part-time physicians. Besides staffing our joint clinic, our physicians serve MAO's patients in the hospitals, as in any private practice.

MAO has its own counselors serving within the hospital, as well as in our joint clinic, to provide an unbroken service. The clinic and MAO have a single intake procedure, and our social service records and medical records are kept together in one case history file to further cement the medi-supportive concept to all staff viewing these records. MAO's supportive services and our joint clinic are housed together in an attractive modern building, owned, remodeled, and furnished by Abbott-Northwestern, to meet our methods of delivering medi-supportive services. The space MAO occupies is leased from the hospital. All services are on the ground floor. The atmosphere is warm and welcoming, reflecting the respect we have towards the people we serve. Seniors are never seen in an office atmosphere, but individually in intimate, comfortable and private "mini" sitting rooms, or modern, well-equipped examination rooms.

Besides serving seniors in our center, we bring MAO's services to their homes, and to ten mini-clinic centers scattered throughout the city, with one in the county. Some are housed in schools, churches and other agencies' buildings. We are not charged overheads, and we do not charge for the services provided by our nurses, counselors, attorneys, or whatever other MAO services are needed in that neighborhood. MAO does not charge for any of its services anywhere. Seniors may make a donation if they can and wish to. It is interesting to note that while client donations are given towards direct field services, such as meals, home services, or transportation, rarely are they given for counseling, which is absolutely vital to providing a good client/patient care plan.

In designing a care plan with the senior, whether on an episodic or on-going basis, we use what I call the "wheel" concept. The spokes of the wheel are the various social and medical services provided by MAO and our joint clinic and any other resources that our staff has developed or knows of. These spokes surround the senior and the counselor, who are in the center of the wheel. The pattern, type and frequency of services drawn on, are based on the senior's needs as he sees it and on his acceptance of the services and without the counselor either giving, or asking for, unreal expectations. If a care plan is made that cannot be produced, or that the senior cannot live up to, the senior will "drop out." I believe some of the people who need help the most, are "drop-outs" because medical and/or social services staff set up impossible client/patient care plans that ignore the individual's life-style and willingness or ability to participate in that plan; then on failing, the client/patient doesn't return, so he can avoid the embarrassment of professional disapproval.

The MAO counselor first and always encourages the senior to be as active as possible, and do the things he can for himself, reassuring him that we will definitely come in with the services he needs if he feels tired, is ill or if he cannot continue. Then wherever possible, the counselor involves any family and/or friends who are willing and able to provide assistance, again firmly reassuring them that MAO will come in immediately, if and when they need us, or if they need a "vacation". Finally, MAO provides the rest of the services needed. Rarely do we find a senior we have to do everything for. We have also found that the difference between the senior with many medical and social disabilities, who is able to stay at home with our help, and a senior, perhaps with lesser problems, who properly has to be institutionalized, is their determination and ability to participate in a sensible and reasonable care plan.

We train all our staff to ask for personal information respectfully and delicately, explaining to the senior simply and directly, without professional jargon, why, and what, we need to know in order to serve them. And we remind all our staff from time to time during regular in-service training, to avoid the tendency in interviewing a senior, of it becoming just a "routine", and forgetting that it is not so to the senior who has to bare his personal life to a stranger. Even after a relationship is established, it can break down if the staff person becomes insensitive or careless in his attitude. We ask staff to serve the seniors, as they would wish to be served, pointing out that they don't know what their own old age holds for them.

We pay special attention in training the field staff, because they usually spend the most time with a senior, and their knowledge is extremely valuable in knowing whether we are doing the job, or whether there are other unmet needs. So they are an important part of the "wheel" concept and report regularly to other medical and social service staff.

MAO's offices are on the second floor, and the majority of our various programs' key staff are housed in one large office, so they can easily, without loss of valuable time, consult with each other, or consult as a multi-disciplined team, which may include different levels of medical and social services staff, as well as field staff. In other words, anyone who needs to be there to discuss and coordinate individual cases, no more, and no less, than the essential components.

Staff have volunteers attached directly to them at all levels. I have a voluntary administrative assistant, and one of our three full-time attorneys is a volunteer who came on our staff after he retired. MAO has around two hundred volunteers in our various voluntary action programs, such as operation grandparents. We train our staff to be helpful and attentive to our volunteers, and not treat them as second-rate staff. Our volunteers are offered the same training opportunities, and career ladder development as our paid staff. In fact, some of them eventually become paid staff of MAO.

Besides Abbott-Northwestern, we have several other partners, such as the Junior League of Minneapolis, who provided us with our volunteer coordinator and helped establish our free blood bank, and the Minnesota Restaurant Association, for whom I wrote a program without federal funds, that provides low-cost meals in 140 restaurants during their off-peak hours. Here again, I used the principle of better utilization of resources. Then there is the Lampert Lumber Company, Shedd-Brown, Inc. and Young Presidents' Organization, who are auditing our books without charge and at my request, so they can judge whether their tax dollars are spent effectively. These businesses and this organization, as well as some banks and other businesses, have made contributions to our programs, both fiscally and as volunteers, and St Mary's Friends have provided our crisis funds.

It is not possible here to relate the full story of MAO, its concepts, partners, programs, methods of delivering services, and training. During the last few years, MAO has received over 1260 requests for consultation and training from all over America, from Canada and other countries, and so I have just completed the foundation, which began in 1973, of the MAO National Institute on Aging to share and teach MAO's programs and experiences.

I have spoken of our foundation and this leads to the form and substance of MAO, which is shaped by the realities and the dream. The realities are our people's needs, the dream is how we serve those needs. Hopefully, we have taken the best of the past and dared to attempt the future. We have looked for people not afraid of human emotions, not afraid of words like compassion, dedication and service. Our staff has joyfully entered the field of human services, because they believe in those principles. We know that emotions harnessed to knowledge and direction can be a powerful tool in helping our seniors successfully use the services we provide.

I will continue to seek the advice of our seniors, accept their leadership over us and learn from their experience. In the final analysis, my dream has one major objective: to provide seniors with the services they need, when they need them, and in the manner in which they wish to be served.

The Role of the Physician

Sir Ferguson Anderson
Department of Geriatric Medicine,
University of Glasgow

In 1881, Charcot wrote "the importance of a special study of the diseases of old age would not be contested at the present day. It is agreed, in fact, that if the pathology of childhood requires clinical consideration of a special kind and which it is indispensible to be practically acquainted with, senile pathology too has its difficulties which can only be surmounted by long experience and the profound knowledge of its peculiar characters, and yet this very interesting part of medicine has been long neglected and hardly in our own days has it succeeded in gaining its independence."

As far as the physician is concerned, the first priority in caring for older people can be summed up in the one word "diagnosis".

The doctor must visualize the elderly as individuals with a limited reserve capacity of bodily function when placed under stress, but who, in every-day activity, should look well, feel fit and be in sound mental health. His concern should be for their physical condition, for their mental state including their motivation regarding daily living, and for their social circumstances and their personal interrelationships with relatives, if any, or friends.

Diagnosis

The duty of the physician is to train himself adequately to be able to reach a correct diagnosis or more commonly a list of diagnoses. Certain physiological changes occur as people age; pain sensation is altered, e.g. patients with silent coronary thrombosis or with the relatively painless abdominal emergency; the elderly woman who falls and fractures the femur whose main complaint is inability to move her leg, may make minimal reference to pain. Postural control is upset and this manifests itself in the common initial symptom of a fall. Almost any severe illness in an elderly person can be brought to the notice of the doctor by a fall. Sometimes the traumatic results of the fall are more than adequately treated and yet no investigation is instituted into the cause of the fall in the first place. Temperature regulation is impaired in some older people who may not be aware of the lowering of the ambient temperature in which they are living and, thus, may develop hypothermia. Fever is not as accurate a response to infective illness as in the young or middle-aged. Thirst sensation seems to be diminished in some older individuals who present when ill with a dry, brown tongue, sometimes mental confusion and often faecal impaction.

The common occurrence of many pathological conditions, each single one of which may seem relatively minor, makes correct diagnosis difficult. The woman of 75 years who presents as a patient with senile dementia, went to bed because of painful corns, bunions and onychogryphosis. Already slightly deaf, she became worse due to increased accumulation of wax in her ears and because of inactivity developed faecal impaction. Mental confusion followed in this individual with diminished brain reserve perhaps because of diminished sensory intake due to deafness, and of dehydration because of inability to take fluids. On examination, faecal stained fluid was leaking from the rectum so anti-diarrhoeal agents were commenced. What is the outlook for such a lady unless she is examined carefully and completely? She runs the risk of being labelled "chronic brain syndrome with faecal incontinence" and may well be sedated and so become a chronic invalid. In fact, after around one week of clearing the different and appropriate orifices and attending to her feet, she went home.

The next problem is insidious onset of disease. Fatigue or tiredness as the main presenting symptom like a fall may denote almost any illness and indicate the need for careful clinical examination with a chest X-ray, a haemoglobin estimation, and blood biochemistry. Cardiac failure, anaemia, dietetic potassium deficiency, hyperthyroidism may all present with these symptoms.

Atypical presentation of illness is the bait which lures the clinician to study and enjoy the clinical care of his elderly patient. The golden rule here is that you must believe your patient's story. If you have never heard the like before, then do not diagnose neurosis or neurasthenia; take longer than usual to unravel the history and examine your patient with increased care. The individual with persistent pain in the lower neck or at one point in the back of the chest may, without any pain whatever referable to the gastro-intestinal tract, have a benign lesser curvature gastric ulcer. She will not benefit from massage, neck-stretching or reassurance but from a correct diagnosis and appropriate therapy. The very old, highly intelligent man who has constant desire to micturate and keeps soiling his trousers resents being thought of as mentally deteriorated when he has a large bladder stone. The professor's mother of 87 who felt her history books becoming heavy on her arm on the way home from the library and eventually was unable to stand had not had a stroke, but a dietetic potassium deficiency. Her son, an accurate observer, had noted that this bright lady had suddenly become old. Innumerable examples must occur to everyone and the diagnoses will only be made by careful history-taking, often from a relative as well, by thorough clinical examination and relevant investigation. There are many non-traumatic ways of obtaining accurate information, e.g. the EMI scanner.

Simpson (1974) stressed the changing patterns of diseases in older people, categorizing them as follows:

(a) Those illnesses where the characteristics have not changed, now occur in much older people when previously they were seen more frequently in the middle-aged. Examples given are pernicious anaemia, motor neurone disease, rheumatoid arthritis, acute leukaemia and acute glomerulonephritis.

(b) Illnesses may present in an atypical way in old people; such are tuberculosis, bacterial endocarditis, diabetes mellitus and thyrotoxicosis.

Tuberculosis of the chest may be seen in elderly subjects, diagnosed as chronic bronchitis or unresolved pneumonia because of persistent cough, or may present as a pleural effusion. Cryptic miliary tuberculosis may be discovered in an elderly individual with a pyrexia of unknown origin, malaise and weight-loss (Proudfoot *et al.* 1969). The presence of a heart murmur and obscure pyrexia should make the clinician think of bacterial endocarditis, while a glucose tolerance or two-hour postprandial blood sugar tests are essential in the diagnosis of diabetes mellitus. Old people may be discovered in refractory congestive heart failure or atrial fibrillation, or as apathetic, sometimes confused people, when suffering from thyrotoxicosis.

(c) New diseases are now being found among the elderly. These include polymyalgia rheumatica, cranial arteritis, Waldenström's macroglobulinaemia, primary acquired sideroblastic anaemia, accidental hypothermia and hyperosmolar non-ketotic coma.

It is worth noting that the three common presenting symptoms in the elderly are falls, mental confusion and incontinence.

Ascertainment of Old People in the Community

In the United Kingdom, although there is no financial barrier and everyone has a general practitioner, many older people do not consult their doctors when unwell. Williamson (1966) called this the iceberg of unreported illness and showed that with certain complaints, for example painful feet, difficulty in walking, problems with micturition, anaemia and dementia, the older individual frequently did not seek medical advice. This may be due to the acceptance or fatalism of older people or their relatives, or the fears which some elderly individuals have that they may be put away somewhere, i.e. admitted to some form of institution or hospital. Some of those in the upper age range who have always been fit have the strong instinct that illness will not strike them and do not admit the possibilities of being unwell.

Andrews *et al.* (1971) demonstrated the increase in morbidity with age and revealed that many of the conditions discovered were remediable. In further random sampling of the elderly in their own homes, Akhtar *et al.* (1973) found that major disability, defined as the inability to lead an independent existence, increased dramatically with age. By the age of 85 years, approximately 80% of people suffered from such disability.

In view of these findings, it has been suggested that a Community Nurse (Health Visitor) should visit every individual 70 years and over, fill in a structured proforma and report back to the general practitioner. Anderson (1976) believes this is the only way to make an early diagnosis in the upper age range and to stop disability from worsening.

Mental Health

The physician must be alerted to the inter-relationship between physical and mental disease in the elderly and to the pitfalls of diagnosis in mental illness itself, e.g. the individual with depression presenting as a confused or demented person.

Godber (1975) stresses the importance of psychological stress as a precipitant or complicating factor in physical illness and this is certainly so in the elderly where mental confusion can be compared with convulsion of the infant, and an attempt must be made to reach a correct diagnosis in such cases. Many elderly people with an impaired reserve of mental capacity, perhaps due to loss of neurones, become confused when a younger individual would not suffer from this symptom. Faecal impaction, urinary retention, anaemia, infective illness, dehydration, cardiac failure and uraemia are among the common causes of such confusion. Metabolic disease such as diabetes mellitus, hypothyroidism and hyperthyroidism may present with mental upset, and potassium deficiency among older people may produce depression, apathy, weakness, paranoid ideas and disturbances of sleep rhythm (Judge 1973). Andrews *et al.* (1971) found a prevalence of mental illness in people aged 65 and over of 22.5% of men and 39% of women.

Numerous studies (Stenbäch 1975) have revealed a prevalence of depression from 10 to 30% in older people in the community and the close association between depression and physical disease, while a figure of 3 to 27% is given for the prevalence of dementia in a population aged over 65 (Gilmore 1974).

Perhaps the greatest danger to the physical and mental health of older people today lies in the number of drugs prescribed for them; the mental confusion caused by common drugs appears to be insufficiently realized. Wallace *et al.* (1975) have shown that ability of the plasma of elderly patients to bind drugs falls significantly when subjects are given more than one drug.

The mental attitude of the attending physician must also be borne in mind; the experienced doctor tends to consider first in his diagnosis where the elderly are concerned, an illness of irremediable type. It seems to be imprinted in the doctor's mind that the old person should have a fatal illness. In fact, commonly the disease is treatable, especially if diagnosed early. Care must also be taken not to attribute blame to people who are incontinent, but to use a rational clinical approach, utilizing all necessary investigational methods to make a correct diagnosis. Brocklehurst (1976) has demonstrated the value of adequate investigation in regard to success of therapy.

Continuity of Care

Continuity of care is another part of the physician's duty in regard to old people. The factors which caused the illness initially may recur, so careful watch must be kept on future progress. In addition, not all older people will recover completely and adequate hospital beds of high amenity must be available to the doctor for continuing treatment. This may include rehabilitation or nursing of high skill for terminal care. Here, the physician has perhaps his most important part to play and his most difficult ethical problems. The relief of symptoms which although minor can render life so miserable, the reassurance and support of mental health and the friendship of the doctor are so worthwhile.

Prevention

The physician has also a duty to plan for his older patients — pre-retirement training, to advise on the re-employment of older people who desire part-time paid occupation in retirement, to play a full part in health education and in advising about nutrition.

Teamwork

The physician is one of a team, and must take advantage of the knowledge and skill of others, e.g. the social worker, the nurse and para-medical staff. Preventive, like therapeutic, work with old people depends on successful co-operation and co-ordination, with each individual in the team making an important and especial contribution.

Universities

Universities must concern themselves about this increase in the elderly in our populations. Town planners, architects, social workers, ministers of religion, transport and housing managers are other groups who require knowledge from informed physicians on the diseases and disabilities of older people.

Teaching in geriatric medicine is essential for medical students, in order to inspire them to help their elderly patients. Old people in developed countries are here to stay and will not simply go away. Students, medical, social and para-medical, may feel cheated unless made aware of the type of patient they are likely to see in their daily work. It is inevitable that they will be asked to help many elderly people with long-term clinical illness, and will not in the future be seeing so many of the young with acute disease. This does not mean they will not enjoy their professional life, but indicates the need to educate them for this situation.

The physician, then, has two options; he may regard each older patient as uninteresting clinically, time consuming, and wasteful of his talents, or he can look at the elderly with affection, as presenting a challenge to his clinical and therapeutic skills. He may be helped by bearing in mind that old people would not still be living if not made of good material, and are likely, with correct diagnosis and therapy, to get well.

The elderly have a right to a full place in our society and from the physicians, expect a correct diagnosis when ill, appropriate therapy and continued advice to keep fit. They may well expect more in the future. They will want to avoid disease, to have guidance as to fitness for continued employment and, from the community, opportunity for learning and training for their third career.

References

Akhtar, A. J., Broe, G. A., Crombie, A., McLean, W. M. R., Andrews, G. R. and Caird, F. I. (1973). *Age and Ageing* **2**, 102–111

Anderson, F. (1976). *Journal of the Royal College of Physicians of London* **10**, 161–168

Andrews, C. R., Cowan, N. R. and Anderson, W. F. (1971). *In* "Problems and Progress in Medical Care". Ed. G. McLachlan. 5th Series. Oxford University Press, Oxford: pp 57–86

Brocklehurst, J. (1976). Personal Communication

Charcot, J. M. (1881). "Clinical Lectures on Senile Diseases." The New Sydenham Society, London

Gilmore, A. J. J. (1974). *In* "Geriatric Medicine". Eds. W. F. Anderson and T. G. Judge. Academic Press, London: pp 77–93

Godber, C. (1975). *In* "Specialized Futures (Essays in Honour of Sir George Godber)". Ed. G. McLachlan. Nuffield Provincial Hospital Trust. Oxford University Press, London: pp 155–187

Judge, T. G. (1973). *In* "Textbook of Geriatric Medicine and Gerontology". Ed. J. C. Brocklehurst, Churchill Livingston, Edinburgh: pp 113–121

Proudfoot, A. T., Akhtar, A. J. Douglas, A. C. and Horne, N. W. (1969). *British Medical Journal* **ii**, 273–276

Simpson, R. G. (1974). *British Journal of Hospital Medicine* **12**, 660–677

Stenbäch, A. (1975). *In* "Modern Perspective in the Psychiatry of Old Age". Ed. John G. Howells. Brunner/Mazel, New York

Wallace, S., Whiting, B. and Runcie, J. (1975). *British Journal of Clinical Pharmacology* **3**, 327–330

Williamson, J. (1966). Ageing in Modern Society. Paper presented to the Royal Society of Health

Discussion

Dr Richard Besdine (*Physician in Geriatrics, Boston*) I would like to emphasize a point that Sir Ferguson Anderson made in his talk. We have all been talking about abandoning the inappropriate medical model in long-term care but we should guard against throwing out the baby with the bath water by abandoning the diagnostic accuracy and acumen for which Sir Ferguson so well emphasized the need. In moving away from a medical model it is important not to leave the doctors behind, and have as an outcome the continuing care of people without medical assessment or accurate diagnosis.

Ms Anna Brown (*City of Cleveland Office on Aging*) I think one thing that area agency directors in this country would like to see is a great deal more emphasis at the Federal level on the interchange of departmental information. Very often model projects are being sponsored by the Administration on Aging, and HIBAC and HEW themselves seem not to get the information that would give cost-effective analysis, and also save the tedium of doing research on model projects that have already been completed.

Yesterday Mr Ball mentioned the problem of Medicare and Medicaid and some of the cost issues about those programs. I think he also touched on the problem of the non-compliance of physicians in accepting assignment. On last Monday HIBAC, which is the Advisory Council to the Secretary of HEW, was dealing with that particular problem. And you have to remember that, aside from not taking the assignment, there has to be some ingredient there to give an incentive to physicians to take on the tremendous amount of paper work that our government continues to require, and which only adds to the cost of health care in this country.

Mr William Oriol (*Staff Director, US Senate Committee on Aging*) I would like to ask Professor Grimley Evans how the local assessment boards operate in the British system; and also whether he and Dr Shore could explain the difference between the residential home for old people in the United Kingdom versus the home for the aged in this country.

Professor Grimley Evans To take the second question first; residential homes in Britain are run by local authorities and in theory are for elderly people or others who are unable through disability and social isolation to live in their own homes but who do not require continuous nursing attention. In practice the homes cater for a much wider variety of inmate than this definition suggests, a fact which creates serious problems. The term local assessment board is not one we use in Britain in this context but I take it that you refer to the geriatric assessment unit. My interpretation of the British scene is that this unit is the key to the whole of a geriatric service in an area. It is a unit in a District General or Teaching Hospital, with full access to all the usual diagnostic facilities. It is administered by a consultant physician in geriatric medicine who works as co-ordinator of a multi-disciplinary team including nurses, physiotherapists, social workers, speech therapists and voluntary workers. This unit is fully integrated with what goes on in the community and elsewhere in the service, so that team members receive feedback on the results of what they have done. This means not only does the team learn from its mistakes, but it also reaps the clinical rewards of its successes.

Associated with the unit are out-patient and day-patient facilities to carry out similar programs of diagnosis, assessment and therapy-planning for patients not requiring hospital admission.

Speaker Are older people involved in the feedback in some way?

Professor Grimley Evans We obtain the feedback by visiting patients after they have been discharged, obtaining information either ourselves or more usually by social workers calling on the patients or their relatives, and also in a formal out-patient or day hospital setting if further surveillance is needed. On the other hand if you mean are older people involved in the design and evaluation of a service as a whole there is in my view regrettably little scope for this within the bureaucratic organization of the British system. The recently created Community Health Councils theoretically give a voice to "consumer" opinion but some of them seem to be dominated by local politicians and to provide more of a complaints procedure rather than a platform for suggestions and constructive criticism.

Dr Shore I believe Bill Oriol picked up precisely on the point I was trying to make in the presentation — that when we use a term like institutional care without precision in definition, we are describing a continuum; and that there is massive confusion around what we mean when we say nursing home: are we talking about the levels of care or the levels of licensing; are we talking about free standing independent units that are designed for retirement independent living — or are we talking about a campus arrangement that might cut across independent living to terminal independent care. So what I was trying to point out was that there is a difference between "the nursing home" and "long-term care", in which nursing care is one of a continuum of services. When we want to define policy, we should look at the appropriate use of the facility for the appropriate need, and get a better definition and a more discrete understanding of services appropriate to people at proper times. This avoids the rigid dichotomy of non-institutional vs. institutional care — they each have their place, they each make a contribution if they are each used appropriately.

Dr T Franklin Williams (*University of Rochester, New York*) We have had a demonstration project on evaluation and placement of people, mostly elderly, facing the need for long-term care for several years now, which has shown very clearly that a careful medical/nursing/social assessment can achieve a much greater degree of appropriateness of care, including maintenance of people at home or at whatever level of care is needed, than was going on in this community by the usual, rather unplanned approaches. We operate this largely as an out-patient service. I recognize the value of admitting patients, as apparently goes on more in England, under certain circumstances for even more thorough assessment when needed, but I simply wanted to point out that it is possible to set up an out-patient service for many people to accomplish the same things. Now our greatest problem is with the Federal and State governments, in that they are not willing to pay for this as a service. We have been able to finance it through project funds, but it has not yet been acceptable as an authorized service under Medicare or Medicaid, and therefore stands little chance of continuing beyond the support of special project funds.

Dr William Hall (*Lutheran Hospital of Maryland*) I am Chief of Staff at a small 200-bed hospital in Baltimore, and I am trying to persuade the Board of Governors and the Board of Managers to create a pure geriatrics department in the hospital. I want to ask one question which relates to education. From numerous talks that I have given in the community I have found that it is not only the elderly that need to be educated, it is the middle-aged and the young also. We have to bring about what I call integration of the ages, and make everybody aware of the aging process. The news media have been very neglectful in this aspect, simply because most of the programs that are on television are on the UH frequency and most people can't get these channels. The articles that are in the newspapers are put in a section of the paper that nobody reads; they should be placed on the first page. I would like to know how we are going to educate the masses to make them more sympathetic to the problems of the elderly, because the most important thing is that you've got to love older people. I think this is where we have to make our big impact, because if we don't make people sympathetic to the needs and the problems of the elderly, how are we ever going to get any Federal, municipal or local support?

Professor John Brocklehurst I would like to bring up one other point which hasn't been dealt with in the questions but which Grimley Evans mentioned, and that is the question of housing and particularly of sheltered housing. Grimley Evans referred to the debate as to whether we should invest more in sheltered housing or more in additional residential care. I personally have no hestitation in saying that sheltered housing is where our money should go at the moment. It ensures independence for people in a protected environment, and I think there are many people in residential homes who could quite well be living in sheltered housing. I wasn't clear what you have in the US — to what extent you have sheltered housing — and I would be interested to know. But the point that I especially wanted to make was that the costs of creating sheltered housing could very well be saved if we could get a better disposition of the housing stock. We heard from Margot Jefferys yesterday that in the UK about 20% of old people live in municipal housing. One knows from one's visits to these people that, by and large, old people live in housing which is entirely unsuitable; they live in houses with three or four bedrooms which they have occupied since they were young and married. If we could try to move towards a better redistribution of housing stock, we would then allow families to move into these larger houses, we would not have to spend so much money on rehousing families, and we could spend more money on providing sheltered housing for the old people who are struggling, very often in difficult circumstances, because they are living in houses that are far too big for them.

Mrs Elaine Brody We don't call them sheltered housing in the United States, but we have developed a great number of highrise buildings for the elderly in the past fifteen years particularly. But we have not only the highrise buildings, there are all sorts of other arrangements — retirement communities, and so on. The figures on how many people occupy these kinds of houses are very hard to come by, but the best estimates I have heard is that roughly 5% of all older people live in apartment buildings or in age-segregated housing. Of course, these houses have a varying pattern of services; some of them have practically no services, some have one or more services, such as one main meal or some recreation services. There are a few that provide significantly more services, such as two main meals, and so on. There is also a trend towards developing a range of innovative kinds of housing. For example, we have at the Philadelphia Geriatric Center something we call community housing, which are semi-detached homes in which each house was renovated to create three apartments with a kitchenette, a bathroom, a bed-sitting room, and a common living room shared by three tenants. There are various plans afoot and some in varying stages of development that come close to that while they don't quite replicate it — buying old houses to renovate them, looking into things such as group living of older people, and so on. I think, in general, the answer to the question is that we are experimenting with a very wide range of possibly innovative kinds of housing; apart from the highrise apartment buildings, they are primarily, at this date, on an experimental basis. The highrises have been studied very extensively, primarily by Dr Lawton, and it was his finding that I reported in my paper yesterday, that the service-rich houses tend to attract people who are less competent; in other words, people find their own level and go where the level of their service needs can be met. It is generally agreed also that there are too few housing units of that type for older people. The issue of age segregation vs. age integration has proved to be a false issue since it depends on which group of older people one is talking about. Some like to live with other older people and some prefer to live in age-integrated neighborhoods. And since we have such a heterogeneous population, we need a very wide spectrum of options for older people.

Mrs Daphne Krause All of those options that Elaine Brody mentioned of course are excellent. But I become very concerned when we start making plans for people without consulting them. Some years ago we went into this extensively with the seniors who were still living in their homes. They utterly oppose leaving those homes, and leaving their neighborhoods. The house itself is familiar to them, and they adapt to it as their problems increase. I am not saying it is desirable, I am just saying this is how the seniors feel about it; and any time you remove something from them you make them aware of the deteriorating process that they are moving towards. One of the things that we created with the seniors is what we called live in/live out services, where a younger person would live in the home with the senior and, in return for doing chores around the house and taking care of it, they would get a lower rent or no rent at all. What I am saying is, preserve the options.

Dr Robinson As one final comment, I want to mention a point that Dr Shore made this morning about antibiotics and the antidepressants and other drugs leading in part to the large number of patients who have now become geriatric patients and institutionalized patients by their effort in prolonging life. I believe that the antidepressants and the other drugs developed for mental health, and certainly the antibiotics and particularly those that have been efficacious in the treatment of chronic disease, have reduced the number of beds that are occupied in our institutions.

This afternoon we shall discuss aspects of research on aging. Several times yesterday we briefly talked about the importance of research and its effect in delaying and preventing the onset of illnesses that lead to debilitation and hospitalization of the aged. In looking at our research priorities we must keep in mind the importance of stimulating and helping research that is concerned with such entities as hypertension, atherosclerosis, osteoporosis and other important diseases with the aim of delaying the onset of illness and fostering a population of elderly individuals who are in good health.

Research Developments and Implications

Developments in and Implications of Research in Gerontology

D Bellamy*
Department of Zoology,
University College, Cardiff

Lack of Strategic Planning

Research on aging in Britain suffers, like many other areas of applied medical and biological research from the absence of strategic planning to achieve desired aims. In particular, there is no generally accepted view by which objectives, policies and programmes may be integrated into a cohesive whole. This situation arises because the British Science Research Council, although it may maintain tight operating controls over the detailed activities of individuals who receive project grants, does not have an overall view of aging. It therefore cannot draw the motivational and resource commitments of all functional groups and geographical centres into a cohesive whole. Unless a central research body devoted to the furtherance of gerontological research exists, which is able to oversee the integration and balancing of subordinate plans and commitments, the individual holders of project grants are unlikely to use their joint resources to optimum advantage.

Since special budgeted funds administered by a special agency are not available from either private or government organizations of gerontological research in Britain, there can be no marshalling and allocation of scientific resources to attain major goals. Therefore, in terms of conventional strategic planning we have no clear objectives which state what is to be achieved and when results are to be expected. Consequently, there are no definitions of rules or guidelines which express the limits within which research should occur to achieve worthwhile objectives and there are no proposed sequential experimental investigations designed to achieve major objectives. On the other hand, it cannot be said that money made available to gerontological research from general scentific funds is being wasted because so little is being spent in this area.

* *In absentia*, read by Dr Michael Green.

Through attempting to assess goals, limiting factors and research prospects, this paper aims to provide a basis for the formulation of a plan for experimental gerontology. By reflecting on it, hopefully, we may be able to evaluate our current position in relation to future needs, and so design alternative courses of action and appropriate objectives, policies and programmes.

Problem Areas and Goals

Experimental gerontology is essentially a laboratory-based subject with experimental material drawn from the entire living world. It may be contrasted with geriatrics where the emphasis is upon the study of old people in either a clinical or social context.

It therefore has a much wider scope than medicine. Its lines of research extend deeply into biology, and in terms of both the terminal loss of fitness and the species' specific lifespan, the field of aging research rests firmly on evolutionary theory. From this standpoint, the overall aim of the experimental gerontologist is to discover how it comes about that different organisms have characteristic lifespans, which involves a study of the past history of the species, as well as its present life-cycle. Within this general area of enquiry, there are two important subsidiary aims: to examine the possible connection between development and aging; and to seek methods of pharmacological, dietary and environmental regulation in order to improve the quality of human life in the later decades. It is in this very broad sense that gerontology is a unified body of knowledge with clear guide-lines of principle.

We *do* need to study the principles of gerontology in depth for sound academic and social reasons. At the academic level, aging may be seen as an inevitable outcome of life being organized as an interlocking system of unstable chemicals and sequential chemical reactions that tend to drift towards disorder. From this viewpoint, life may be viewed as an evolutionary strategy to overcome aging. This places the study of chemical deterioration at the centre of biochemistry and molecular biology. The fact that up until now, gerontology has made little impact on biochemical thought is simply due to the historical development of both subject areas, and is not due to any fundamental disharmony in subject matter. In this context, the viewpoint of the gerontologist is likely to be of great importance to the future development of biochemistry and molecular biology in that it provides additional scope for formulating new concepts and increasing fundamental knowledge of living chemical systems.

It is already apparent that a need to understand the temporal deterioration of living systems is beginning to arise from fundamental biochemical work. Also, since time is the most important aspect in the late manifestation of many biological phenomena, such as cancerous growth and the failure of reproduction, gerontological investigations are clearly of general academic relevance to the fields of physiology and behaviour.

The two examples of temporal change just given above have important medico-social implications and are also obviously on the borderline between the academic and practical goals of gerontology. The future practical rewards of research on aging will be gained from efforts to accommodate successfully the extra years of human life won by medical research over the past century. This work will depend on fundamental knowledge, as well as clinical investigations.

It must be stressed that the only justifiable social goal of gerontology is to enable people to reach their natural lifespan with the minimum mental and physical disability. The deliberate search for an "elixir of life" or general rejuvenating treatment, with the aim of giving men the freedom to alter drastically their individual aging process, should *not* be a primary motivation in gerontological research. This constraint is necessary because of the catastrophic social upheaval that would follow success. It is also clear that past research orientated only towards the prolongation of life has been responsible for our present unbalanced fund of knowledge about aging. Indeed, as we come to know more about aging it appears less likely that human lifespan is capable of practical extension as a balanced physiological system.

Obstacles to Progress

In terms of the complicated factors that limit its growth, gerontology appears to be unique amongst the various branches of science. The present low level of support for gerontological investigations in Britain is partly due to the way in which gerontology developed within medicine from what was the low status field of geriatrics, and also to the absence of aging as a well-defined body of knowledge in most British medical and biological curricula. In this respect there is a lack of appreciation of long-standing laboratory studies on the part of many geriatricians. To these historical reasons may be added a current bias against research proposals arising from ignorance on the part of those in competing fields; the high cost of maintaining stocks of experimental animals of known pedigree into old age; and the difficulties that many specialists encounter in moving into what is essentially an inter-disciplinary area of research. There are also impediments to the movement of research personnel between disciplines arising largely from the dominant influence of specialism in promotions within the medical and scientific establishment. To these impediments might be added an important, but largely unassessed, factor arising from the fears of many scientists who could potentially contribute to gerontology, that the study of aging might provide a way of greatly prolonging human life and so add to our many present intractable social problems. In this context, in a healthy society, we can neither stop the questions of fundamental research being asked, nor disallow the acquisition of a certain kind of fundamental knowledge because of possible social consequences arising from future exploitation. Control should be exerted at the level of the technological resources that have to be mobilized in order to capitalize on laboratory studies. Also, knowledge which has a bearing on aging derives from many diverse fields which also have application to the well-being of younger age groups, such as immunology, endocrinology and cancer research, making it impossible to impose restrictions on work concerned with aging in practice.

Removal of some of these obstacles is a simple matter involving the allocation of more funds to the maintenance and supply of old animals, the organization of the teaching of gerontology on an interdisciplinary basis and the introduction of fellowships to enable workers to move freely from other fields into gerontological laboratories. Others are bound up with the socio-scientific aspects of research and are going to be with us for some time to come.

Research Prospects

Experimental Medicine

Taking the general definition of aging as a loss of adaptability resulting from a decline in tissue and functional reserves, human aging is first manifest at the behavioural level of biological organization. It is at this level that future clinical gerontologists must work on a wider scale collecting data by cross-sectional or longitudinal analysis, which is subsequently classified to provide a description of gerontological phenomena. This may suggest an appropriate treatment for an undesirable condition and the analysis of the results of the treatment provides information about the nature of the phenomenon as originally observed.

There is also great scope for descriptive analysis of aging in laboratory animals. This complementary approach to clinical problems has the advantage that the various phenomena described may be subjected to detailed experimental analysis.

Although past research has produced many descriptive studies of human aging, these investigations have tended to delineate the group rather than the individual. There is also some confusion about the term "normal" as applied to group data, because it is used to cover both a statistical entity, i.e. the standard or representative value for a given age group as well as the value for those individuals without abnormality or free from pathology. This difficulty is at the root of all cross-sectional studies of population aging. Despite the great logistical difficulties in organizing longitudinal studies, we may expect great rewards to come from this alternative methodology in the future, with its emphasis upon individual variability.

From the point of view of adaptability to environment, future clinical research will, no doubt, be concerned with the age-related loss of immunological and neuro-endocrine coordination with the associated metabolic disorders. This area of study includes the loss of cognitive function, as well as sensory and motor failures. Alongside this stand all complementary investigations of trauma resulting from poor adaptability to cold, malnutrition, accidents and infection.

From their contribution to human death rates, heart and vascular disabilities may be singled out for special consideration. In particular, cerebrovascular disorders, although only the third most frequent cause of death in Great Britain, give rise to a considerable amount of chronic invalidism which commands a large proportion of the country's nursing resources. With regard to vascular changes of the atherosclerotic type, the view is gradually gaining ground that this is a pathological aspect of aging with a multifactorial aetiology. In this respect, it has been generalized that multiple pathology is the rule and not the exception in later life. Nevertheless, these conditions, including many forms of cancer, appear to have a well-defined age incidence indicative of an underlying cellular failure, which it is the future aim of the gerontologist to identify.

Suitable research strategies based on clinical problems would involve the study of the appropriate sensory input, the neuro-endocrine system, the motor system and the short-distance intercellular regulation that is responsible for the maintenance of cellular populations in those organs involved in the disability. A particular difficulty in implementing this approach is that clinical problems arising when the body fails to meet demand and the points of physiological failure appear to be multiple. For example, old people fail to respond adequately to cold through a failure in detection, endocrine secretion and the lack of functional capacity in liver and muscle. To the extent that any one organ dominates a particular environmental response, that organ will also appear to dominate aging of the response.

It must also be remembered that successful adaptation of old people occurs through the matching of the home environment to declining physiological capabilities. From this aspect a good practical solution to problems of cold stress would be to provide the elderly with cheap fuel and free fur coats. In terms of practical goals it could be argued that money should be devoted to this end rather than to fundamental work into thyroid function.

Research in Model Systems

In searching for fundamental mechanisms the experimental gerontologist cannot handle the complex, multifactorial aspects of whole organism aging and so must resort to simple systems that are amenable to experiment. This means that the research worker should select various models of whole body aging largely for convenience and ease of study. Models in gerontology may be defined as systems that are taken as being representative of major factors of aging and which, by their very nature, open up the possibility of generating new data and ideas. These models fall into two categories of mathematical models and biological ones. Because the choice of a model means that the real problem is not being studied in all its aspects the results will not be generally applicable to the real problem. The extreme viewpoint of the biological modeller is a theoretical one. Various theories about the fundamental nature of aging are posed in terms of the available knowledge and tested with the simplest convenient system. At the moment major theories are posed in terms of the two simplest ways of viewing aging at the chemical level; as a deterioration of individual molecules and as the deterioration of systems of enzymes responsible for metabolism.

Deterioration of molecules is inevitable as they interact with their immediate chemical environment. If such sensitive molecules cannot be replaced, or if the product cannot be removed, there will be a gradual loss of chemical efficiency.

Deterioration of enzyme systems could occur either by loss of genetic information (i.e. mutations) or by errors in the use of genetic information. Errors in the use of genetic information would result from *mistakes* in assembly of the component macromolecules, the nucleic acids and proteins, and from random changes in the *rate of flow* of information, particularly if this had a feedback component to irreversibly alter information flow.

(*a*) *Mathematical models.* Mathematical models may be subdivided into those used for the prediction of mortality rates and those that indicate possible mechanisms of aging. Examples of prediction models are the equations derived from population data in human blood cholesterol and subsequent lifespan which have a good prediction value in relating present blood cholesterol to future mortality.

Illustrations of mathematical models devised to support particular mechanisms of aging are given by the Gompertz equations, which are all derived from mortality curves and usually contain functions pointing to the importance of "speed of living", "loss of stability" and cumulative "random errors" of the underlying systems.

(*b*) *Biological models*. Many living and non-living systems have been used in aging research because they appeared to offer advantageous properties for solving a particular problem. No doubt many more such models will become available in the future. It is therefore difficult to deal predictively with the future potential of biological research, particularly as many past models have not been adequately exploited. Therefore, what follows is merely an attempt to show the diversity of models available with only in some cases an assessment of their future potential.

Micro-organisms, plants and lower animals. Micro-organisms and some common invertebrates and plants have been much used as biological models because of their dependence on an external environment that can be defined and controlled, despite the fact that the living system used may differ greatly from that of the human body.

If it is assumed that all living things are built to a common plan, questions arising from studies on aging micro-organisms have an important bearing on aging of higher animals. What are the mechanisms by which cells with a common mitotic lineage, cultivated in a constant environment, develop an orderly sequence of phenotypes? Also, how does nuclear reorganization halt the process of aging and transform a degenerating cell into a totipotent individual? Other models relevant to the study of these questions may be found in the dedifferentiation of planarians, the conversion of iris epithelial cells to lens cells in vertebrate embryos and, in plants, the apparent conversion of leaf epidermis cells into non-aging meristematic tissue. This list serves to illustrate how problems of aging may have a bearing on those of development.

A number of the smaller invertebrates possess properties particularly advantageous in the study of whole organism aging. Insects, for example, have a wide diversity of habits; free living and parasitic, cryptic and aerial. They can also cope with habitats from arctic to tropics. Many are characterized by a short life, a high fecundity and may be inbred in the laboratory, and the smaller ones may be maintained at low cost in small containers. It is also possible to select other invertebrate types with the above characteristics that have very short lifespans of the order of days to months enabling the researcher to obtain results quickly.

Higher animals. Vertebrate animals do not offer much scope as general models for studying environmental and genetic effects on lifespan because of the long periods that must be devoted to experiments and the great expense involved in their upkeep. There is also the important problem, common to all whole animal studies, of interpreting effects on lifespan in terms of effects on the rate of aging. However, particularly with regard to rats and mice, they are the nearest approach to human organisms possible in an experimental setting and are arguably the best specific models for human aging.

A general deficiency of whole animal models is that all data are open to criticism on the grounds that lifespan is very much dependent on nutritional status. Very careful control of dietary factors and total energy intake is required in setting up whole animal models to ensure that the effects of a particular form of treatment are not due to changes in food intake.

Organ systems. At the level of organs, many systems have been examined because they show marked age-changes, and several of these changes have led to particular theories of aging. A large proportion of these organ models have the shortcoming that they are not capable of experimental manipulation, and the theories are not vulnerable to experiment.

Amongst the more striking, but invulnerable, models may be placed the age-pigment system of nervous and muscular tissue, which still defies precise interpretation in biochemical and physiological terms. It is difficult, however, because of the dramatic accumulation of age-pigment in a range of human and animal organs, to dismiss this substance from consideration.

Generally, organ models suffer from the disadvantages that they are composed of diverse cellular elements that may age in different ways, and they do not lend themselves readily to experimentation, particularly *in vitro.* Despite the poor experimental returns from many organ models, however, there is still much scope for research, particularly using models concerned with the important phenomenon of organ involution. Tissues such as ovary and adrenal cortex which change with age dramatically at the histological level were intensively studied by early gerontologists, and it is encouraging to see work beginning with these tissues into cellular involution at the biochemical level. These models may also be expected to throw light on the failure of endocrine control.

Other, complex models with a so far limited application to problems of aging, are annually senescing leaves and stored seeds with the associated random loss of viability. *In vitro* aging of eggs and sperm also offers scope for setting up models to test epigenetic theories with the advantage that aging amphibian eggs are already used as models for cancer research.

Another badly neglected area with promise for the future, is transplantation research. Ovary and skin transplants have been important in establishing the principle of multi-factorial aging, and transplant models have scope for furthering research into new theoretical areas of gerontology. Transplant models will clearly yield much new information about the modifiability of age changes in differentiated cells with regard to both intrinsic alterations and systemic influences.

Cell cultures and transfers. Protozoan models clearly illustrate the temporal effects of continuous cell division, but a better human model for the aging of mitotic cells is given by vertebrate cells maintained in tissue culture. Fibroblast cell strains are currently opening new fields of knowledge concerning several theories of aging, as they relate to the limited division potential of mitotic cells.

It is now well-established that populations of diploid human fibroblasts can proliferate in culture for only finite periods of time. Typically, after explantation, there is a period of rapid proliferation during which the cultures can be subcultured very often. This is followed by a period of declining proliferative capacity, when the cells become granular, debris accumulates within the cells, division ceases and the cells die out. It has been demonstrated that these changes are not related in any simple way to toxicity of the medium. Fibroblast cultures derived from tissues from young individuals undergo more doublings before dying out compared with cells from old tissues.

Similarly, an inverse correlation exists between the age of the donor and the doubling potential of skin cultures. The suggestion that aging changes are reflected in various properties of tissue cultures is not new. For example, it has long been known, since the early 1920s, that age-associated phenomena occurring in plasma can inhibit cell growth *in vitro*. In addition, early work showed that the time elapsing prior to cell migration from explanted tissues increases with increasing age of the tissue.

One of the most important questions concerning the validity of the cell-culture model deals with the possibility that the phenomenon of limited lifespan is a test-tube artifact. From a theoretical viewpoint, cells within the body may divide either tangentially or logarithmically. In a tangential or symmetric division system, where a stem cell multiplies to produce another stem cell and one differentiated cell, then many more divisions would be necessary to maintain a population than if a logarithmic mode of division occurs in which all offspring divide before differentiating. At the moment it is difficult to assess the relative importance of these two modes of proliferation in the body.

We can expect more *in vivo* and *in vitro* models composed of proliferating cells to be used for gerontological research in the future. Also, as many of the techniques come from the rapidly expanding field of immunology and as the loss of the immune response is an important feature of human aging, there should be a constant interchange of ideas between immunologists and gerontologists in this area.

Biochemical and Molecular Models

So far most biochemical studies have been largely descriptive of whole animal aging and have not been carried down to the test-tube level for detailed analysis of mechanism. Nevertheless, at the biochemical level, there is much scope for setting up models of complex enzyme systems under test-tube conditions, where it is possible to test for the failure of different components by substituting young components for old and vice versa.

On the whole, molecular models have been little used in gerontological research, despite the pioneering work of Verzar on the molecular changes in collagen. Rat-tail collagen has yielded much valuable information on the relationship between chemical constitution and physical properties, but the age-changes in structure of collagen are probably of less general significance for the aging of other macromolecules than was once thought. Each type of macromolecule will have to be studied separately. There is also scope for investigating the potential of natural and artificial polymers many of which have already been studied from the point of view of synthesizing a structure that resists chemical deterioration.

The Need for Inter-disciplinary Studies

Enough samples have been covered to show the great scope for experiment in the field of gerontology. The great range of models that have been used also emphasizes that gerontology has its roots in many different disciplines. This is its strength as a body of knowledge, yet there is a general lack of appreciation of the gerontologist's viewpoint in these different disciplines and this is perhaps the most important factor limiting the accumulation of knowledge relevant to the aging process.

All the models referred to so far have been posed in relation to aging of humans in our artifically protected urban environment. Hardly any models have been set up to deal with aging in natural animal populations, despite the fact that such models would be expected to throw light on the evolution of rates of aging. They would also be expected to illuminate aging in the human population because diversity in genotype is a common feature. This immediately highlights the present barrier between ecology and gerontology. So far, ecologists have not been concerned with the physiological aspects of mortality in the wild. Age-dependent mortality is certainly an ecological fact but it will need the future collaboration between those familiar with ecological methods in order to delineate the gerontological basis of natural selection operating through failures in homeostasis. In this context gerontology impinges upon one of the most urgent problems of contemporary biology concerned with the nature of the mechanism that regulates the transition from a given state of the cellular genome to the pattern of the active genes responsible for the next stage of development. This problem is central to development, but it is also clearly related to aging. In many organisms, especially plants and insects, aging is typically a morphogenetic process which leads to death almost immediately after reproduction. The prevention of sexual reproduction, for example by the elimination of flowers in monocarpic plants, can significantly increase the lifespan, but only by slowing down the rate at which the morphogenetic programme is realized. In this context the morphogenetic programme operates in all organisms with selection occurring on internal mechanisms that build up the largest numbers of efficient organisms within a narrowly defined period after fertilization. What we need to understand is whether aging simply results from the steady decrease in the selective value of survivors as natural populations lose individuals through accidents and predation, or whether terminal deterioration is a consequence of earlier advantageous developmental programmes. From either point of view, aging may be seen as an evolutionary inevitability, and men cannot aspire to immortality. On the other hand, these considerations point to the importance of genetical analysis and more breeding experiments should be carried out in the future, particularly among lower organisms with short lifespans.

Conclusions

From the above classification of experimentation it is clear that there are many research methods available to the gerontologist which overlap considerably both within gerontology and with related disciplines. From the medical viewpoint we need to systematize the relevant detailed work. In order to achieve this end, appropriate general objectives for gerontology would be to determine the fundamental chemical basis of the major causes of disability in old age with the aim of providing effective medical treatment. The corresponding policies would delineate the types of experimental models to be used for each disability. The relevant research programmes would specify the sequence of experimentation necessary to relate behavioral or physiological findings to the biochemical controls that govern particular deleterious changes in the human life-cycle. Only in this way can we establish a rational basis for dietary and pharmacological treatment that has direct relevance to the care of the elderly. How then do we evaluate the work of the non-clinical gerontologist? To answer this question, it is informative to classify research according to the day-to-day questions that are the real motivation for individual workers. When this is done it appears that there are three main motivational questions that govern the pattern of gerontological research: How do organisms come to have different lifespans? What is the chemical basis of aging? How can we alleviate the undesirable aspects of human old age?

Each one of these questions is the province of a special category of research worker — in sequence, of the Darwinian biologist, the chemical biologist, and the medical biologist or clinical research worker. These extreme viewpoints are defined by particular fields of enquiry which together with concomitant research strategies are outlined in a highly generalized way in Tables 1, 2 and 3. With regard to the implications of these various strategies, there is often heated discussion between the different types of practitioner which culminates in

Table 1

Classification of gerontological research in the area of Darwinian biology

Leading question:	How do organisms come to have different life-spans?
Fields of enquiry:	Comparative gerontology Genetics Phenology Environmental physiology Behavioural gerontology Ecology
Research strategy:	Examine species and strains for functional correlations with lifespan Investigate influence of early development on lifespan Examine possible connections between environment and lifespan

Table 2

Classification of gerontological research in the area of chemical biology

Leading question:	What is the chemical basis of aging?	
Fields of enquiry:	Theoretical biology Cellular physiology Biochemistry Molecular biology	
Research strategy:	*Reductionist approach*	*Holistic approach*
	Formulate a chemical theory based on current knowledge of cellular function Select best living or non-living system to test theory	Formulate a chemical theory to account for a particular widespread feature of aging Select simplest system exhibiting phenomena to test theory

confrontation between pure and applied research. This kind of conflict is non-productive because no single viewpoint will give a full understanding of the aging process. All research proceeds on the basis that increased knowledge has a cultural value. With regard to aging, research also carries the implication of ultimate control over those aspects of aging which result from a simple chemical process that can be inhibited or reversed. In our present state of knowledge there is no way of predicting accurately which approach is more likely to yield this practical key.

Table 3
Classification of gerontological research in the area of medical biology

Leading question:	How can we alleviate the undesirable aspects of human old age?	
Fields of enquiry:	Clinical medicine Bio-medical research Most of the fields in Tables 1 and 2	
Research strategies:	*Laboratory-based*	*Clinical-based*
	Determine the chemical basis of aging Devise the most convenient general treatments to counteract the important processes of aging	Delineate serious disabilities that are widespread in old people and which lead to a need for a high level of care Determine the physiological basis of each disability Analyse the relevant physiological systems for age-dependent limiting factors Devise specific treatments in an effort to support the failing system with a view to reducing dependance on hospitals and welfare services

Some clear evidence of fundamental progress towards improvement in the care of the elderly is appearing in the field of neuropharmacology. This area relies on fundamental knowledge of the biochemical basis of conduction, which aids rational drug design, as well as on the clinical classification of brain disorders in the elderly. This is a powerful illustration of the complementary nature of two research strategies. It also indicates that fundamental data relevant to aging often come from areas of science where the temporal aspects are not an important motivation and highlight our current task which is to devise an appropriate division of resources to ensure that we have the broadest possible biological base for the interpretation of the clinical work. In Britain, at the present time, taking into account support from the Health Service, Department of Health, the Drug Companies and the Medical Research Council the partition of resources specifically for research on aging is about 50:1 in favour of clinical research which is arguably too great a ratio for a well-balanced strategy.

Developments in Research on the Biological and Behavioral Aspects of Aging and their Implications

James E Birren and V Jayne Renner
University of Southern California

There has been a considerable increase in research on the processes of aging at all levels from the cellular and molecular to the clinical and societal. In the process of preparing three handbooks on aging, about 50 000 references on aging were identified as being published between the years 1959 and 1974. The conceptual state of the field is such that a wide range of particulars are difficult to assess because there are few general principles. While chronological age is a powerful index to many important facts, the common element of chronological age is not sufficient in itself to bring together useful information.

In the face of so much literature it is of course presumptuous to review all recent research on aging, let along to attempt it in one brief paper. Partly the task has just been done. Present reviews on specific topics are the three 1976 handbooks, "Handbook of the Biology of Aging", C Finch and L Hayflick, eds.; "Handbook of the Psychology of Aging", J E Birren and K W Schaie, eds.; and "Handbook of Aging and the Social Science", R Binstock and E Shanas, eds.

In view of these considerations what can be a reasonable purpose for this paper? It can examine those issues which cut across problem areas and also try to give a perspective on the more portentous areas. More colloquially put, an attempt will be made, admittedly biased, to suggest the "hot areas" in gerontology from which many developments might come.

Before doing this, however, we should consider the issue of why the field of aging appears to be a vast area of unorganized information. This partly derives from the use of age as an index. Because a tremendous number of processes are correlated with age and may be filed and accessed by the term age, nothing is implied about the communality or relatedness of processes. For example, the probability of dying goes up with age as does the probability of cerebrovascular disease and cancer, but merely because phenomena are jointly indexed by age does not imply a common cause.

One concept of aging that would fit the state of the literature is that the individual organism moves forward in time with simultaneous but independent processes going on, many of which have the potential for limiting the individual lifespan. The search for contingencies among the probabilities of events occurring with increasing age of the organism is precisely the issue in assessing the information about aging. The handbooks show that there are some clusters of functions that are related to age and which appear to be tentatively explicable in terms of causal relationships. This kind of determinacy is what the natural scientist looks for so that age can be replaced by other variables in explanation. An analogy can be drawn to the atomic clock in which the disintegration of atoms with time is so regular that the age of the sample, or dating of an object can be inferred from the measurement of change. No great amount of interest need be expressed in which atom disintegrates, whereas in the human situation we are interested in the disintegration of the individual organism and the nature of the processes which lead to it. Presumably there are some common processes which are shared not only by individuals within a species, but are shared across species as well.

Insofar as one looks for processes of aging that are shared across species, one is attempting to explain something different than if one examines individual differences within a species. This leads to the principle that there does not appear to be one single factor governing aging but there are many. There is also the point that mankind, as a species, is genetically heterogeneous which makes for diversity and presumably patterns of aging reflect that diversity. Such considerations make it incumbent upon us to state explicitly what aspects of aging we are addressing and which we hope to explain.

There seems a gradient from the biological sciences to the social sciences in the effectiveness of dealing with the natural phenomena of aging, with psychology being intermediate between biology and sociology. Partly this is due to the length of time the disciplines have been devoting to research on the subject. But more than that it has to do with the conceptual basis of the science. Biology uses the metric system in its explanations and uses concepts and theories from evolution, genetics, and biochemistry. Also, most biologists implicitly attempt to explain either what controls the longevity of a species or the length of life of individual members of a species. Psychologists are occasionally interested in the behavioral correlates of longevity, but in addition may be interested in changes with age in selected behavior which may be only remotely regulated by biological factors controlling length of life. Indeed, some behavior may improve with age unlike biological processes which generally degrade with time and lead to an accelerated probability of dying. One may have a wise old person dying from a disease which leaves the intellectual processes spared until death. The lifespan process of incremental acquisition of experience which is stored in the nervous system for either routing or creative retrieval, must to some extent be independent of factors leading to life limiting failure of an organ system. If, at the biological level, all organ systems followed an independent course with age, then there would be no contingent probabilities of organ failure and the half-life of the organs could be studied in a totally independent manner. In a sense the old organism always dies as a result of some accident, self-induced or otherwise, but the organism is prone to that accident, i.e. the state of the older organism makes it vulnerable to the consequences of environmental interactions.

Generally, American physiologists and psychologists, until very recently, have not been disposed to thinking about the nervous system or the neuroendocrine system as instigators of effects we might identify as aging. The Russians, by contrast, because of the Pavlovian tradition have, and are more apt to cast the nervous system in the role of a pacemaker or initiator of influences. To the regulatory role of the nervous and neuroendocrine systems should be added the immune system, for like the nervous system, it has a capacity for memory and when its memory fails the organism as a whole deteriorates. While the organism may fail terminally in death because of some organ failure, this failure has often been prepared for by changes in the nervous system or in the immune system. Growing out of this perspective this paper will consider the following areas for discussion: rhythmic activity in the central nervous system, arousal and the central and autonomic nervous systems, the neuroendocrine system and change in levels of neurotransmitters circadian rhythms, stress, and some phenomena of the immune system itself which are coming to be significant in the field of aging.

Evolutionary Perspective

If one compares the longevity of various species one cannot help but be impressed by the fact that the longevity seems to remain relatively fixed. One infers that there is some determinate character for the characteristic longevity of a species and that it rests upon a genetic basis. One of the logical problems that arises is how there came to be genetic control over longevity since the trait of longevity does not appear until after the age of reproduction has passed. One explanation of the control over late life events is that there is a counterpart relationship between the selected early life characteristics and their expression in late life (Birren 1960). Thus, how a species ages is a function of the pattern that was selected, presumably a sloth will age differently than a hummingbird.

While the ultimate causes of the features of aging are not clearly predicted from early development, encouragement is given to the expectation that mechanisms of aging can be identified. Since aging is a somewhat ambiguous outcome of the genetics of development, to identify mechanisms is more difficult than that of studying the pre-reproductive development of an organism. While this gives cautious hope to research on aging, hopes of identifying the ultimate causation of aging in the evolutionary sense may not be satisfying to the investigator of humans who might hope to ease the stresses on aging adults. While seeking the remote causes of aging that arose in the long time of evolution, more proximal variables to the problems of human aging also warrant attention. This view is also justified since the major genetic controls have evolved over a long time from the selection of which individuals survived and propagated in particular environments. Exposing organisms to environments different from those in which they were selected can lead to unexpected results; for example, putting prairie dogs in a wood or polar bears at the equator.

A prime example of evolutionary selection is circadian rhythms which must provide some survival advantage, yet one might query what would be the outcome if an animal were moved into a foreign environment with regard to light–dark cycles or seasonal changes. Mankind does this by flying across many time zones in a 24-hour period and there is concern that thereby regulatory processes are disturbed and we are less able, if not to negotiate an international treaty, at least to eat and sleep in a familiar relaxed manner. This suggests an experimental tool, for one can take animals of different ages and expose them to environmental conditions that deliberately throw circadian rhythms off cycle. Latency, duration and pattern of recovery of the normal cycle can be observed. Such observations will provide a basis for inferences about the effectiveness of the regulatory processes, how they might change with age and in adjusting the environmental circumstances of human aging to advantage.

In the case of mankind, we know little about the environments under which our genetic traits were remotely selected but it must be obvious that our characteristics were not selected under conditions where sedentary cerebration was a prime factor in survival. The stress diseases of aging adults living in urban society strike one as being the result of an interaction of a genetic program and an environment foreign to earlier forces of selection. Such considerations dictate that in the study of aging, biologists and psychologists should have both a genetic and evolutionary orientation as well as a functional orientation to the present environments of aging organisms.

Rhythmic Electrical Activity of the Brain

Electrical activity of the brain can be recorded from the fetus and thereafter show changes with age. The most discussed electroencephalogram, EEG, frequency is the alpha in the range of 8–13 Hz. Even in subjects selected for good health, there is a drift toward lower amplitude and slower alpha frequencies with age, and also, alpha frequencies are observed for a shorter period or percentage of the recording. An increase in waves slower than alpha, between 1 and 7 Hz, has also been reported as occurring more commonly in the very old subject (Marsh and Thompson 1976). This diffuse slow wave activity is not as universal as the drift toward slow alphas. The basis of the diffuse slow wave activity of the aged remains basically unknown in contrast to focal slow wave activity in which vascular insufficiency is regarded as a prime factor (Obrist and Busse 1965).

One of the best developed of explanations of CNS change with age is that of reduced blood flow due to arteriosclerosis. As a consequence regional ischemia develops with the results that neurons die and limitation of functions becomes apparent. One can hardly deny the plausibility of the reduced blood flow explanation of certain of the EEG changes with advancing age or of cognitive deficit. The question is, how much of the change in electrical activity of the brain in later life can reasonably be attributed to the reduction in blood flow?

Obrist (1964) claimed that mild increases in blood pressure may be essential to the maintenance of cerebral circulation. Also, Wilkie and Eisdorfer (1971) found that mild elevation in blood pressure in early senescence resulted in no change in intellectual functioning or was related to slight improvement in performance. Presumably however, one is observing a compensatory effect in individuals with some increase in vascular resistance, such as in atherosclerosis.

The discontinuity hypothesis was advanced by Birren *et al.* (1963) and Birren (1964) to indicate that over a broad range of physiological variations in such variables as blood flow and oxygen, how much is available doesn't determine the level of functioning of the nervous system. The reasoning is that the brain is buffered against the variations of the physiological environment and in this manner the nervous system can execute its task of regulating vegetative functions and behavior with stable limits. It would be a strange system indeed if by increasing the blood flow to the brain we could become geniuses. Rather, by reduction of blood flow there are critical limits below which further reductions in blood flow to the brain as a whole or to regions will result in disruptions in function.

A major study of the electroencephalogram was reported by Busse and Obrist (1965) on 424 community volunteers. There was a change with age in the percentage of records judged to be normal: 85% between ages 20 and 39; 65% between 40 and 59 years of age; and 51% between ages 60 and 70 years. In middle-aged and older adults, females showed a significantly greater percentage of records that showed fast EEG activity. In the oldest age range, it was 4% for males and 23% for females. With age, too, dysrhythmic activity was found in the anterior temporal region in about 36% of the elderly subjects and about 20% of the middle aged group. There were no sex differences in this feature. The authors reported that such anterior temporal lobe disturbance in the EEG does not seem to have any obvious correlation with behavioral functions. The authors believe there is little evidence to suggest that the temporal discharges in these otherwise normal subjects are related to ischemia due to reduced blood flow.

At Duke University, 182 of 260 volunteers over age 59 returned 3 to 4 years later for follow-up examinations. The mean occipital EEG frequency was significantly lower in 55 subjects selected from the 182 on the basis of freedom from evidence of cardiac, pulmonary, or nervous system disease. The data led the authors to "... hypothesize that the occipital frequency in healthy old people is closely related to 'physiological aging', and that the relationship between these two variables may be altered by the presence of various pathological conditions affecting the central nervous system" (Wang and Busse 1974).

The EEG seems to have value in helping to assess CNS disease associated with advanced age but not in showing clear relationships with other physiological functions or behavioural changes. More research activity, at the moment, is expressed in studying the processes of aging in the electrical responses to sensory stimulation. The average evoked potential (AEP) is derived from an analysis of many cortical responses to sensory stimuli. Several studies have reported differences with age in the amplitude and latency of the sensory evoked potential. Of particular interest are the changes in amplitude and latency of the late components of the evoked potential which have been linked to processing sensory information (Schenkenberg 1976, Harkins *et al.* 1976, Smith *et al.* 1976). Smith *et al.* reported that the early components of the AEP did not differ in latency, though late components did, and it took longer for the older subjects to return to their baseline. Also, a significantly longer response of dishabituation to a novel tone was observed in older subjects. This offers the prospect of doing important research on the behavioral correlates of electrophysiological changes with age, particularly changes in speed of information processes.

Straumanis *et al.* (1965) studied amplitude and latency of evoked cerebral responses to visual stimulation in 20 patients with intellectual deterioration thought to be due to cerebral arteriosclerosis: 18 older controls, and 18 healthy young adults. "Patients' responses differed from those of old controls mainly in events occurring after 100 msec.; their latencies were prolonged and rhythmic after-activity was markedly reduced. Differences associated with age were found mainly in the portions of the response occurring before 100 msec.; latencies tended to be prolonged and amplitudes greater in the older *Ss*" (p 505). Since the differences in brain syndromes were similar to those observed in acute delirium and sleep, they were interpreted as concomitants of altered sensorium. The authors favored a view that individual responses in amplitude became larger in older subjects, due to a diminished inhibitory activity.

A recent addition to the gathering evidence on electrophysiological changes of aging is on contingent negative variation, an electrical correlate of anticipating a second stimulus following a first. Older subjects show a lesser anticipatory response to a second signal in the late portions of the anticipatory interval. More effort should be directed toward determining how much of the changes in expectancies or set, reported to be age related, are coupled to features of the CNV.

Wang and Busse (1974) reported a faster EEG frequency and higher amplitude in older females than in older males. Also, sensory evoked potentials show a sex difference, with boys showing a larger potential up to puberty and females showing a larger response in adolescence through old age (Beck *et al.* 1975). Given the fact that females have a greater life expectancy, sex differences in a variety of CNS, ANS, immune and behavioral measures can be examined for those that favor females in the later years. The large sex difference in life expectancy warrants further study, since simplistic explanations in terms of the favorable effects of the presence of the X chromosome or estrogens in the female mammal do not seem adequate. Castrate human males live longer than non-castrate and intact females (Hamilton 1948). Also, castrate male cats live longer than intact male (Hamilton 1965).

Surwillo (1963, 1968) suggested that there was a causal relationship between the slowing of the alpha frequency with age and the speed of simple reaction time. He found a very high correlation between the EEG period and reaction time and suggested that the EED alpha rhythm was the master timing mechanism in behavior. Surwillo (1964) was not successful in modifying the EEG frequency with a photic driving method so as to produce different frequencies and thereby test the consequences for reaction time.

Woodruff (1972) carried out an experiment in which she attempted to reverse the slowed alpha frequency seen in older adults by biofeedback conditioning. She had young and old adult subjects conditioned to increase or decrease the mean frequency of the alpha waves. Older subjects were able to increase the production of alpha frequencies higher than their usual average, implying that the older nervous system has retained at least some limited amount of plasticity. Since the correlations within individuals between alpha frequency and reaction time were not statistically significant, it does not support the hypothesis that the EEG is the master timing mechanism, though the research does establish the point that EEG frequency and speed of response are related if through an intermediary mechanism yet to be identified. These results, together with those of Dru (1974) on recovery of visual function in old and young rats, suggests that one can expect that this area of research will produce further optimistic findings. In this way, even where there is tissue loss, the older organism can be brought to a higher level of functioning by appropriate conditioning, learning, or patterns of use.

One should not overlook the possibility of primary neural changes with age (Ordy and Brizzee 1975). Bondareff and Geinisman (1976) found a 27% decline in synaptic density in rats 25 months old compared with 3-month-old rats. The findings were based upon a quantitative electronmicroscope study of the dental gyrus. At yet another level, DNA repair was studied in cerebellar neurons of beagles following radiation induced damage. The investigators reported no age related decrease in the ability of cells to rejoin single strand DNA breaks but did observe a decline with age in the size of the DNA molecule (Wheeler and Lett 1974).

Sensorimotor slowing has been observed in many studies of healthy older adults (Birren 1964, 1965). Furthermore, slowness of reaction time does not stand alone but shows correlations with other cognitive functions (Birren 1971, Schaie and Strother 1968, Dirken 1972). The emergence of a general reduction in speed of response with age that has high correlations with speed of information processing of all types, does not exclude other influences as well. In addition to a slowness of response that may rest upon changes in the neurophysiology of the aging nervous system, older adults may be cautious and take longer to decide upon their choices.

Botwinick (1966) studied cautiousness with age by requiring subjects to make a choice in two alternatives about real life situations, one implying a rewarding but high risk alternative, and the other one a less rewarding but more safe alternative. Elderly subjects were more cautious in their decisions. Decisions about problems of the aged were made less cautiously than corresponding decisions regarding the problems of younger adults. This was true for both age groups of *S*s, but more so for the elderly. Apparently older subjects require more certainty in the outcomes of their decisions before risky alternatives are chosen.

It is of interest that slowness of behavior has been observed even in subjects well selected for high education and health. Schaie and Strother (1968) studied a superior group of men and women who were retired university faculty members or retired academic and professional workers. The most common physical findings were problems of vision and hearing which existed in most of the subjects, almost 90%, and cardiovascular problems which existed in about 20%. The means of performance on the Tests of Primary Mental Ability indicated that the group was at about the level of a 17-year-old population, with women performing significantly better on the verbal tests and men better on the spatial tests. Decreased psychomotor speed was noted and the mean was about ½ to 1 standard deviation below that expected in middle age.

Since psychomotor speed was the largest decremental factor it was correlated with cognitive measures. Surprising is the fact that psychomotor speed correlated 0.68 with verbal meaning and 0.67 with reasoning. These correlations were higher than those between a composite memory score and the same variables. The authors concluded, "The results of our physical and social studies suggest that this obvious decrement from peak performance is most likely related to a physiological decrement, particularly of a sensory nature, and probably to the general slowing down of response speed as well" (Schaie and Strother 1968, p 307). With regard to the possibility of disuse factors, significant positive correlations were found between the verbal meaning score and an index of environmental interaction as well as between verbal meaning, reasoning, and number with amount of leisure activity. It would indeed be useful to know to what extent one can by a volitional plan follow a course of higher interactions with the environment and participate in leisure activities with the result of maintaining or expanding particular intellectual abilities.

The quickness of discrimination responses to visual information has been studied by Rabbitt (1965) by having the subject search for relevant items among a field of irrelevant items, and make differential responses to the relevant items, but exclude all irrelevant items as a group. The subjects were required to search for either 2 or for 8 letters of the alphabet among the varying numbers of irrelevant letters. Response times were little affected in young subjects by increasing the number of items and the sets between which they must discriminate. In both conditions older *S*s took longer than young to discriminate between relevant and irrelevant letters. The speed with which the subjects ignored irrelevant information varied with the number of items being searched. Rabbitt suggests that older adults sample letters in smaller groups than do the young subjects. He held that if the size of the perceptual sample diminishes with age, old people are at a disadvantage in many perceptual skills, for example, reading.

While reaction time in young subjects remains a relatively isolated factor when correlated with other psychological measures, in old subjects the correlation is much higher, indicating that it becomes a general factor which perhaps begins to influence the level of other functions. Reflex processes are slowed with age but not as much as are simple reaction times. Furthermore, complex reaction times are disproportionately slow compared with simple reaction times. The higher the level of the nervous system that is processing the information, and perhaps the greater the number of synapses involved, the greater the slowing. Thus slowing is not essentially a peripheral phenomenon but one intimately involved with the properties of the aging nervous system. Association of slowness of response speed with physiological variables is therefore of considerable interest, since the findings have the prospect of having broad implications for understanding the organization of aging and the behavior of the older nervous system. One current research interest is concerned with age changes in the arousal of the central and autonomic nervous systems in relation to behavior and a change in the relative levels of excitation and inhibition.

Arousal of the Central and Autonomic Nervous Systems

Changes in the regulatory capacities of the CNS are accompanied by changes in the ANS as recently reviewed by Frolkis (1976) (*see also* Frolkis 1966). There appears to be a general weakening of sympathetic and parasympathetic nervous system influences as degenerative changes in sympathetic and parasympathetic ganglia, in the postganglionic nerve endings and perhaps most dramatically in the hypothalamus where impairment will reduce the effectiveness of homeostatic control. Such hypothalamic impairment is considered to take the form of increased excitability in the anterior and posterior hypothalamus and decreased excitability in the medial hypothalamus. In addition to affecting regulation of homeostatic control, the range of responsivity in the ANS is also decreased, and there is increased sensitivity of the hypothalamus to physiologically active substances such as the catecholamines, serotonin, acetylcholine and a number of hormones, for example, the steroids, thyroxine and insulin. Thus, administration of small doses of these physiologically active agents will cause greater shifts in blood pressure, heart rate and other hemodynamic features in the old as compared with the young. This not only subjects the aging organism to increased susceptibility to disease, but hemodynamic changes and altered bioelectric activity will cause altered and even pathological disturbances of metabolism and function in the aging organism. The relation of these physiological variables to the subject of attention and arousal has now become one of the focal points in the gerontological literature.

In terms of the ANS there are two schools of thought. There are those who claim that with age the ANS is under-aroused and those that claim that the ANS is over-aroused. In interpreting the research evidence March and Thompson (1976) emphasize that arousal may not be a unitary process and studies are quoted in which at the onset of a task which requires attention there may be increased activity in either the parasympathetic or sympathetic nervous system or both, depending on the nature of the task. In addition, arousal cannot be seen only in terms of the ANS, for there are also changes in the CNS which affect arousal. From evidence of changes in the AEP Shenkenberg (1970) suggests that in the aged there may be diminished effectiveness in the ascending reticular activating system. This, from our knowledge of this system, would lead to a diminished level of generalized diffuse activity over the cortex.

Of the research supporting the under-arousal hypothesis with increasing age, the following studies are described to illustrate their theoretical and empirical position. These are also reviewed by Thompson and Marsh (1973) and Marsh and Thompson (1976) . In general, these studies have used a conditioning paradigm, taking shock as the unconditioned stimulus. The GSR has been used as the physiological dependent variable, with the assumption that it is a measure of sympathetic activity and an index of the subject's general level of activation or reactivity.

Using a tone as the conditioned stimulus, and a shock to the fingers as the unconditioned stimulus, Botwinick and Kornetsky (1959, 1960) used volunteer male subjects in two age groups. Their results showed that older subjects conditioned more slowly and extinguished more rapidly, although it should be noted that there were large individual variations in spite of the significant age differences. In terms of the normal aging process the results support the authors' contention that the elderly have a lower reactivity level than the young.

To support the under-arousal hypothesis, Shmavonian *et al.* (1965), with a similar conditioning paradigm to the one above, produced results which demonstrated that the general level of activation as indicated by basal measurements was higher for young subjects. Higher levels were maintained by the young throughout the conditioning and extinction procedures. The GSR and vasomotor levels of response were at a lower level in the elderly, and the total activity of the EEG was higher in the older age group. Analysis of the EEG data showed no significant differences between the young and old on the delta and alpha rhythms but there was three times as much beta activity in the older group. Urinary catecholamines were also measured and although they are a rather crude index of either brain or peripheral tissue amine levels, they do describe possible trends. Both groups showed a decline during the conditioning procedure in norepinephrine levels, but whereas the young showed a significant increase in urinary adrenalin levels, the old showed a significant decline. On pre- and post-measures of the two catecholamines, the elderly had significantly higher levels, which implied that initially, before testing, the older group was more aroused, but during the conditioning experiment these higher levels were not maintained indicating that the older group was less aroused. Shmavonian *et al.* (1965) offered 3 interpretations for their data. First, that peripheral factors affecting sympathetic nervous system responses "such as arteriosclerosis, drying of the skin and disruptions in sweat gland activity" (p 255) play a significant role in these changes but are not exclusively responsible. Secondly, the hypothesis was put forward that excitation decreases with age and inhibitory processes increase. The aged subjects are said to display not only autonomic inhibition in conditioning situations, but from the EEG data it is thought that the fast beta activity of the old is also of an inhibitory nature. Thus, increased beta activity in the older group during conditioning trials is conceived of as reflecting increased inhibitory processes which in turn inhibit conditioning. In contrast the young who showed a decrease in fast beta activity during conditioning may reflect the onset of excitatory processes which facilitate learning. Thirdly, Shmavonian *et al.* (1965) postulate that the autonomic nervous system (ANS) inhibition is "partly due to hypothalamic degeneration which not only produces autonomic inhibition but may also produce biochemical reactions disproportionate to the situation" (p 256).

A further study by Shmavonian and his colleagues (Shmavonian *et al.* 1968, 1970) produced a similar pattern of results to their earlier experiments. In a discrimination conditioning task older males and females both showed significantly less reactivity than younger subjects. Although no significant age difference could be found with respect to a consistent pattern of cardio-deceleration during the experiment, the older male and female subjects showed no systematic cardiac variability to either the unconditioned or conditioned stimulus during the adaptation period and essentially exhibited accelerated heart rate during conditioning. In contrast, the young males and females showed much greater reactivity during the adaptation period, although the young females failed to show either vasomotor conditioning or cardiac deceleration, whereas the young males exhibited the former and approached the latter condition. Consistently low voltage fast EEG waves in the older groups were related to the cardiovascular responses. The authors suggest that explanations of their results could be made by considering carotid sinus mechanisms in that deceleration of heart rate could be the result of the carotid sinus reflex, whereby heart rate is slowed following peripheral vasoconstriction. This seems plausible in view of the fact that the baroreceptor reflex mechanisms become less effective with age and would explain why the phenomenon of cardiac deceleration is not found in the majority of older people in many of these experiments, including the arousal experiments on reaction time tasks (*see* Thompson and Nowlin 1973).

The under-arousal hypothesis is also supported by studies of autonomic reactivity during vigilance tasks. In a study done by Surwillo (1966) age differences were not found in either heart rate or GSR or skin potential during a vigilance task which involved monitoring a Mackworth clock, but significant age differences were found, during the last 45 minutes of the task, in skin temperature which declined progressively during this time for young subjects, but not so for the older group where it remained unchanged. Surwillo argued that since a decrease in skin temperature is associated with active cognitive behavior or stress, his results imply that the older subjects decline more rapidly in attention or arousal levels during vigilance tasks.

Studies supporting over-arousal in the ANS have relied heavily on biochemical measures which related to sympathetic function, particularly measures of free fatty acids (FFA). Increased levels of ANS activity are believed to be accompanied by elevated plasma levels of FFA due to increased mobilization of these acids from storage sites. Neither mobilization nor peripheral disposition of lipids appears to be affected by age (Eisdorfer *et al.* 1965). Earlier experiments in this area such as Powell *et al.* (1964) and Troyer *et al.* (1966), showed that during serial learning and vigilance tasks, the elderly as compared to the young had higher FFA levels before the task, during the task, and after the task, suggesting that older subjects are more highly aroused than the young on tasks which involve them cognitively. From such experimental evidence Eisdorfer (1967, 1968) suggested that not only may the performance decrement seen in older people during learning tasks be due to autonomic over-arousal, but that in general older subjects are in a state of high arousal. Response inhibition on learning tasks is then due to very high levels of internal arousal reflecting high levels of autonomic activity. Eisdorfer (1968) in a series of studies done on young and old males, showed that the older adults learn less readily and make more errors of both omission and commission. He suggests that this may be due to a failing ability in end organs to suppress response, changes in the feedback system and/or a loss of tolerance in older people to cope with high levels of arousal, all of which would lead to decremental changes.

Earlier research had emphasized that age differences in learning under paced conditions where subjects were exposed to short intervals, were due to errors of omission which were greater in the older group. However, as shown in an excellent review by Arenberg and Robertson (1976), there are a number of studies which indicate that older adults also make more errors of commission, i.e. incorrect responses. Eisdorfer (1968) as did Troyer *et al.* (1966) found that although the number of omission errors decreased with an increased stimulus interval, the errors of commission did not change in any significant way. Thus, the improvement in learning in the older groups seen under conditions of lengthened stimulus exposure is not just due to the time allowed to view the stimulus. Troyer *et al.* (1966) and Eisdorfer (1968) found that if the subjects are familiarized with the experimental conditions so that the effects of arousal and stress are minimal, performance is improved. Learning under paced and stressful conditions without allowing older subjects to adapt will result in a large number of inhibited responses, whereas under the same conditions where subjects have been familiarized with the situation and allowed to adapt, the number of inhibited responses from older people significantly decreased. In addition, these studies showed that task complexity contributed to the poor performance of the older group, since when the task was simplified, responses and apparent learning increased. Troyer *et al.* (1966) and Eisdorfer (1968) also found that even after adaptation has taken place those subjects who are put under a rapid regime for learning will show significantly more errors than those under slower pacing conditions. The latter group exhibit high post-test FFA levels, whereas those in the faster paced group return to low FFA levels suggesting "that FFA level is related to work levels rather than to the level of arousal generated by the pace of the task" (Eisdorfer 1968, p 207). If the task is seen by older adults as being too difficult, response suppression or inhibition will occur as the subject withdraws and his level of arousal drops. Such disengagement is suggested as "a valuable stabilizing mechanism in the interaction of aged persons who feel unable to master their environment" (Troyer *et al.* 1966, p 418).

Eisdorfer *et al.* (1970) argued that the over-arousal of the ANS was not merely a reflection of an activated CNS during learning or mental activity. Rather, a major factor in performance decrement may be due to feedback to the CNS from the peripheral reactions to over-arousal. Thus, by partially blocking the beta receptors in the ANS, learning should be improved. Using two groups of older men, where one group was given propranolol, which partially blocks beta-adrenergic end organ responses, and the other group was given a placebo, it was found that the experimental group exhibited lower FFA levels, slower heart rate, a tendency for a lower GSR (although this last measure was not statistically significant) and significantly better performances on a serial learning task. Of importance, too, is the fact that the placebo group did better than groups in other studies where neither drugs nor placebo agents were used indicating the significance of placebo effects. The authors conclude that not only can learning be improved in older adults with pharmacological intervention, but that learning deficits in older people are due to "a state of heightened rather than depressed automatic end-organ arousal" (Eisdorfer *et al.* 1970, p 1329).

Eisdorfer (1970) predicts greater use of the adrenergic blockers in modifying ANS reactivity and thus facilitating sustained levels of interest and activity. As the present authors point out in a later section, there is more recent data which tends to contradict the 1970 findings of Eisdorfer *et al.* and a compromising solution is given.

At first glance there would appear to be severe discrepancies between the under-arousal and over-arousal positions. Large methodological differences used make comparisons between these two schools of thought difficult or impossible. Those supporting the ANS under-arousal hypothesis have used bioelectric measures whereas the ANS over-arousal camp have used biochemical measures related to sympathetic activity. Thompson and Marsh (1973) and Marsh and Thompson (1976) suggest that the different end-organs under ANS control may change differentially with age which would reflect itself in the divergent results we have presented, and that the change in these end organs is such that they do not accurately reflect the state of arousal on either the CNS or ANS. Thus, according to this hypothesis, under conditions of stress or intensive stimulation such as that which occurs during cognitive tasks, discharges from the CNS will not be reflected in all peripheral ANS systems. Those systems where deterioration may have taken place, such as those reflected in cardiovascular, vasomotor and GSR responses will show apparent under-arousal, while those which remain intact reflect the distortion of CNS–ANS feedback relationships by manifesting over-arousal. As a consequence, performance is impaired. The present authors would also suggest that the ANS as such is not a unique entity, but rather a collection of discrete units which although interconnected with each other and with the CNS, can function independently, just as the CNS may also be looked upon as a series of organs which, although related are relatively discrete units. This would become more apparent during the aging process as the different units change at different rates.

Finally, difficulties in interpreting the two schools is also due to the fact that very different tasks have been used. Those supporting the under-arousal theory have used shock as the unconditioned stimulus or the monotonous tasks of monitoring as a vigilance task. Neither task puts the subject under any great cognitive stress. In contrast those supporting over-arousal explanations for the decline in performance with age, have placed the subject under comparatively more cognitive stress during the trials where learning is assessed, and this may be of more significance to older groups.

Earlier, the present authors discussed studies which indicated that the CNS is under-aroused. Slowness in response with age reflects the general lowering of activation levels in the CNS and it is possible that this central process is closely associated with changes in the ascending reticular arousal system (Birren 1974). There have been numerous studies done to illustrate the age changes which occur in speed of behavior together with the physiological correlates (*see* Birren 1965, Birren and Spieth 1962, Hicks and Birren 1970). Thompson and Nowlin (1973) suggested that there was an inter-relationship between the CNS and ANS which explained differences in behavior in terms of the physiological evidence. They pointed out that while age differences in the CNS may appear minimal when subjects are behaviorally or cognitively active, marked age differences may occur in the ANS. They speculated that not only were high levels of performance dependent upon a balanced alignment between CNS and ANS activity, but that the loss of this balance which may occur in the elderly would be related to performance decrement.

This becomes increasingly plausible when we observe the difficulties that elderly subjects have in formulating preparatory sets within specified time limits. Birren (1974) cites evidence that shows the older individual to be better at incidental learning as compared to directed or intentional learning with which he has difficulty. In this paper, Birren suggests that older subjects are less adept "in controlling attention or set" (p 812), and that taking in too much information makes the older person unable to concentrate his attention on the most relevant cues.

Thompson and Nowlin (1973) were able to confirm their hypothesis of loss of congruence between the ANS and CNS with age. They showed that a decline in reaction time tasks in older adults was associated with a lack of relationship between the ANS and CNS. For their ANS changes they used heart rate changes. Internally directed arousal or attention is associated with heart rate deceleration whereas externally directed attention is related to acceleration of heart rate. In a reaction time task Thompson and Nowlin did not obtain any significant age differences in the electrocortical measures used, namely the amplitude of the CNV which became larger with increased attentive states required for the fast reaction times. In both age groups there was a significant heart rate deceleration in the preparatory interval but it was significantly lower in the older age group. In addition, whereas there was a relationship between heart rate decleration and reaction times in the young such that the faster the reaction time the greater the heart rate deceleration, no such relationship was found in the older group. Although the cortical measures indicated that the aged were as aroused and as attentive as the young, this was not reflected in performance since the elderly had significantly longer reaction times. In comparison the amplitude of the CNV was related to performance speed in the young group. Thus, in addition to a loss of relationship between CNV and reaction time the elderly group also failed to show the related cardiovascular responses found in younger groups in reaction time tasks. Thompson and Nowlin conclude that their evidence indicates an uncoupling of the CNS–ANS linkage which leads to slower performances.

A study done by Froehling (1974) did not support the results of Thompson and Nowlin. Three groups of elderly subjects were used: those given propranolol administered intravenously, those given a saline injection and those who had no medication at all. Froehling found no significant differences in learning across the three conditions, a result which, incidentally, is contrary to that found by Eisdorfer *et al.* (1970), but as Marsh and Thompson (1976) point out the results are not directly comparable since drug dosages were different. On Froehling's other physiological measures of heart rate, FFA levels and GSR measures, the expected decline in heart rate and FFA levels was found in the propranolol treated group, such changes being significantly different in the treated group, and no changes in the GSR. However, in addition, she found that there was a significant relationship between speed of response and amount of heart rate deceleration in her elderly subjects as well as between amplitude of the CNV and reaction time. Marsh and Thompson (1976) point out that Froehling's subjects were carefully screened for medical fitness and suggest that her sample may have had a younger biological age than those subjects in other experiments.

Harkins *et al.* (1976) found further support for Froehling's findings in a group of biologically fit men. They found that: (a) propranolol has no effect on cardiac deceleration, CNV, or reaction time, suggesting that heart rate deceleration is largely independent of heart rate and that the anxiety reducing effects of beta adrenergic blockers may be due to peripheral changes which reduce the ANS feedback to the CNS. Certainly in this experiment propranolol had no effect on CNS activation. (b) The CNV and heart rate deceleration are both related to psychomotor performance as measured on reaction time tasks in healthy elderly males. Fast reaction time trials were significantly more related to greater CNVs and heart rate decelerations than were the slow reaction time trials. The authors suggest that the general loss of concordance between the ANS and the CNS is not lost in old healthy people and that the minimal deceleration found in previous studies of older groups may be due to a decline in these individuals' inhibitory and selective responses so that they are unable to repress irrelevant muscle activity (*see also* Birren 1959, 1970). Thus the prediction made by Eisdorfer (1970) of a future greater use to be made of adrenergic blocking agents in pharmacological intervention for elderly populations may still have applicability. All this evidence does, however, emphasize to the medical and para-medical professions the necessity of meticulously and accurately assessing the health and biological age of older individuals before prescribing treatment.

Other Neural and Endocrinal Considerations

The question of drug treatments applicable to the elderly has considerable pertinence in view of recent research indicating the changes which occur in the neuroendocrinological system and changes in the levels of neurotransmitters and their enzyme systems. The recent evidence has been well reviewed (*see* Frolkis 1966, 1976, Andres and Tobin 1976, Finch 1976*a*, *b*). Generally there is a weakening of neuroendocrinological control which may be one of the leading regulatory mechanisms in aging. Thus, though there is a decrease in the amounts of steroids produced by the adrenal cortex and gonads with age, to take one well-researched example, the controlling factor in reproductive senescence in females at least, is attributable to a deficit in the mechanism which regulates the cyclic discharge of the gonadotrophin releasing factors from the hypothalamus which controls the output of the gonadotrophins in the anterior pituitary (Finch 1976*a*, *b*). Finch reviews experimental evidence which shows that a hypothalamic deficit in the mechanisms of catecholamine synthesis and metabolism may be responsible for the loss of the cyclical behavior. Injection of adrenalin, a catecholamine, L-Dopa which is converted to the monoamines dopamine and norepinephrine, and iproniazide which inhibits the hydrolytic enzyme monoamine oxidase (thought to increase with age, at least in rat heart and human brains), restores the reproductive cycle in rodents for an indeterminate time.

We now know that with age there are shifts in the state of cholinergic and at least some adrenergic receptors, and that the concentration of neurotransmitters, such as acetylcholine and the catecholamines changes with age. This may be due to changes in many of the enzyme systems, for example, a reduction in cholinesterase and coenzyme A activity (Frolkis 1966, 1976) which leads to less acetylcholine with age in different organs; and a decrease in neuronal catecholamine synthesis, at least in the basal ganglia of humans and rodents which is thought to be due to loss of activity in the rate limiting enzyme tyrosine hydroxylase which is responsible for catalyzing the reaction to synthesize dopa (the precursor of dopamine) (*see* Finch 1976*b*). Finch (1976*b*) cautions against making broad generalizations from discrete neural cell populations to the brain as a whole, for such individual neuronal regions may change independently with age. Finch emphasizes that more needs to be known about the function of distinct pathways and cell groups to understand more fully the effect of aging on the brain. Such clarification would then allow us to discern more clearly the relation of physiological correlates to the behavioral changes which occur with age, thus facilitating the search for effective intervening agents and/or measures. But our present knowledge does reinforce the necessity to query the sometimes questionable over-prescribing of pharmacological agents to the elderly populations, since drugs will affect many neuronal and metabolic processes. For example, due to altered catecholamine metabolism and reduced uptake mechanisms, the threshold level is lowered for those drugs which are antagonists of the catecholamines, such as the phenothiazines, so that Parkinson-like symptoms are more easily induced in those older patients taking these drugs (Finch 1976*a*).

The mechanisms of hormonal action on tissues and end organs also changes with age, such that the ability of hormones to bind to tissues may be reduced in later life. For example, the sensitivity of the adrenal cortex to ACTH is reduced with age (Andres and Tobin 1976). In addition, the change with age in levels of hormonal substances and the neurotransmitters may differ in the plasma and the CNS.

Ziegler and Lake (1976) report that in a study of a group of healthy normotensive subjects, aged 10 to 65 years, the mean norepinephrine levels in blood plasma were twice as high in the oldest compared with the youngest subjects. This applied whether the subjects were lying down, standing or doing an isometric exercise. Cardiovascular responses, such as blood pressure and heart rate did not correlate with age, so the authors concluded that the higher levels of norepinephrine reflect the necessity of increased output of norepinephrine with age in order to maintain similar cardiovascular responses found in the young. This necessity for increased output is probably due to decreased target organ sensitivity.

Reis *et al.* (1976) report that in rodents there is an increase in certain of the catecholamine synthesizing enzymes in the superior cervical ganglia and adrenal medulla. The activities of tyrosine hydroxylase which gives rise to the amino acid dihydroxyphenylalanine (Dopa) from the amino acid, tyrosine, increased with age by 186%, and there was an increase of 220% in the level of Dopa decarboxylase which converts Dopa to the catecholamine, dopamine. Significantly, there was no change with age in dopamine-beta-hydroxylase which converts dopamine to norepinephrine, and the levels of phenylethanolamine-Nmethyl transferase (PNMT) responsible for the methylation of norepinephrine to form epinephrine, are reduced by 60% in the adrenal medullas of old rats. Changes of these enzymes in the brain were minimal. These investigators concluded that with age the increased capacity for peripheral biosynthesis of dopamine is associated with a concomitant decrease in the ability to synthesize norepinephrine and epinephrine in the peripheral tissues.

In order to integrate the findings of the last two experiments described, the present authors offer the following speculation. If norepinephrine and epinephrine synthesis is decreased with age in the peripheral tissues and yet the concentration of catecholamines in the blood stream is increased with age (assuming there are no species differences in these parameters) then it is possible that the catecholamine hydrolytic enzymes in the peripheral tissues have reduced synthesis and/or activity in old age.

Against such a background it is perhaps not so surprising that with age there is a change in our metabolic and circadian rhythms.

Circadian Rhythms

A study of diurnal blood concentrations of a number of metabolites during normal activity, feeding patterns and sleep was done by Rowe *et al.* (1974) on 24 non-diabetic patients aged 25 to 95. They found that the mean concentration level for all of the substrates measured increased with age and that fluctuation in concentration of each of these metabolites also increased with age. This suggests that the regulatory homeostatic mechanisms controlling metabolism decreased in efficiency with advanced age. Rowe *et al.* suggest that such information provides a useful framework in elucidating the metabolic mechanisms involved in disease, which increases in terms of susceptibility with age.

Reduced and less efficient metabolism with age may help to explain the change with age in sleep and activity patterns and possibly in other circadian rhythms. Control of circadian rhythms would appear to be centered in the hypothalamus (Sampson and Jenner 1975), particularly the ventromedial portion.

Nisbett *et al.* (1975) cite evidence where animals with lesions of the ventromedial hypothalamus show disrupted or deteriorated circadian rhythms as reflected in eating and activity behavior. Such animals also show a significant weight gain, increased emotionality, and increased sensitivity to taste. Nisbett *et al.* (1975) studied old and young rats of both sexes to determine whether a similar profile of behavior emerged with increased age. Circadian rhythms, as measured by eating patterns during light/dark cycles were found to deteriorate for both sexes with age, increased emotionality and irritability increased with age only in males, while taste responsivity increased in both sexes. Such results, Nisbett *et al.* conclude, indicate lower levels of ventromedial hypothalamic function with age.

Reduction in sleep and activity patterns in aging humans also reflects that disruptions of circadian rhythms occur as the organism gets older. Total sleep is reduced in humans with age and this reflects the decrease in REM (rapid eye movement) and stage 4 or slow wave (SW) sleep (Berger 1975, Marsh and Thompson 1976). Both stages are thought to be necessary in maintaining effective cognitive functioning. Indeed Berger (1975) claims that such studies indicate that a disruption in established circadian rhythms of the sleep-wakefulness cycle will impair waking mood behavior and performance, irrespective of the amount of total sleep obtained. He concludes that "the integrity of waking functions may depend not so much on an absolute amount of sleep as on the maintenance of a regular sleep-wakefulness rhythm" (p 100).

The sleep–wake cycle is correlated with adrenal function which has its own circadian rhythm. A study by Serio *et al.* (1970) showed that there was a shift in the rhythmicity with age as reflected in plasma cortisol levels. Of particular importance was the finding that there was no difference in the rhythms in the two groups of old subjects (70 years and over), (1) normal aged and (2) aged suffering from insomnia. The latter group, although apparently awake for a considerable part of the night, did remain in bed in darkness, and during the experiment were not permitted to sleep during the day but took part in the same activities as the normal aged, and thus they were not subject to an inversion of rhythmic activities which may alter cortisol and other circadian rhythms.

Research has been reported on electroencephalographic changes in mice. Eleftheriou *et al.* (1975), used the electroencephalographic pattern associated with sleep and wakefulness to study age changes in the central nervous system activity in two strains of mice. As in humans, slow-wave sleep declines with age, as does REM sleep. Older male mice spend more time in the waking state. The trend with age was much more apparent in the strain DBA/2J than in the strain C57BL/6J. No rapid eye movement sleep was observed in the 23.5-months-old mice of the DBA/2J strain. This led the authors to suggest that there may be genetic influences on sleep patterns in the process of aging but caution that other studies need to be done on the genetic mechanisms of sleep and aging before generalizations can be made. In this experiment these genotype differences between the two strains resulted in more accelerated biological aging in the DBA/2J strain as compared with the C57BL/6J strain.

That change in circadian rhythms may explain the aging process is suggested by Berger (1975) who puts forward the hypothesis that a decrease in metabolism with age may be reflected in a decreased need for sleep, especially stage 4 sleep during which metabolism is at its lowest level. He suggests that not only may aging be in itself a rhythm but that "artificial disruption of the body's rhythms may reflect back onto the basic aging processes so as to change its period" (p 101). That the sleep–wake changes with age reflect basic changes in circadian rhythms, again has medical implications, particularly in terms of the pharmacological agents used on the elderly. Most hypnotics and barbiturates used with patients with insomnia eliminate REM sleep, the implication being that since this stage of sleep decreases with age, psychological disturbances, including that of disorientation (often seen in elderly patients taking such drugs), may be accentuated with such strategies of treatment in older people.

Susceptibility to mental illness increases with advancing age (Birren and Renner 1968*a*), and with the above cited evidence that desynchronization of circadian rhythms reduces mental efficiency, the studies described by Sampson and Jenner (1975) suggesting that some types of mental illnesses may reflect disturbances of these rhythms, takes on new import when we consider the pathology involved in the psychiatric illnesses of later life. In this connection a brief mention should be made of the relationship of stress to aging and disease since stress may accelerate aging or precipitate certain diseases.

Stress

This subject matter has been recently reviewed by Eisdorfer and Wilkie (1976). They relate stress and performance to levels of arousal showing that either high or low arousal will produce performance decrements, and hypothesize that persistent stress and arousal in the ANS will result in disease. This possibility is further strengthened when one considers that the range and rate of responsivity also declines so the older individual with a smaller repertoire of adaptive responses in stressful situations and slower reactions, is more prone to disease, particularly of a cardiovascular nature.

Henry (1976) reviews the pathophysiology of hypertension relating it to psychosocial factors. Although genetic factors, such as degree of sensitivity and early experiences play a role, Henry presents evidence to show that prolonged and repeated stress which produces anxiety and/or depression will affect either the sympathetic adrenal medullary system or the pituitary adrenal cortical system, depending on which component of the neuroendocrine system dominates, which will finally result in disturbances in the feedback mechanisms which regulate blood pressure. Not only will hypertension result, but susceptibility to cerebral-vascular accidents and myocardial or renal failure is greatly increased.

From a social psychological perspective, stress is also reflected in increased susceptibility of the old towards anomie or alienation (Martin 1971), in a rapidly changing society where values are apparently changing at a rate too rapid for many elderly people to cope with. Henry and Ely (1976) use the term "culture canon" to refer to norms, standards and general principles which are accepted by the group as their fundamental value systems, and constitute the basic components of a stable society. Henry and Ely suggest these symbol systems are formed from activities which are emotionally significant. Thus loss of a group's cultural canon, which involves cultural changes, is stressful. They cite evidence which links the loss of the cultural canon to physiological responses, namely that loss of the culture canon, reflecting a loss of a stable society, means that the individuals lose an important defense to control neuroendocrinological arousal. In our youth-oriented society the aged are much more prone to subjectively experience these alienating stressful situations.

The Immune System

Brief mention should be made of the recent research findings in the immunological field. These have recently been reviewed by Makinodan (1976) and the behavioral correlates which may be associated with a decline in immune function are discussed by Birren and Renner (1976*b*). The immunological system has a memory in that during development it learns to remember deleterious molecules to which it has been exposed and to reject them by marshalling its immune defenses, i.e. the lymphocytes and plasma cells. The memory of the system becomes less efficient with age. Not only does the immune system lose its ability to tolerate antigenic once familiar substances, but the antigenic-antibody response itself also loses its effectiveness. This means that the antibodies may not only fail to react to unfamiliar foreign substances or antigenic molecules, but may react against or reject some of its own body constituents. Perhaps the changes that occur in this system with age can be best described by saying that the aging immune system becomes absent-minded. Reaction against its own body constituents results in an increased incidence of autoimmune disease with age. Autoimmune disease may also be due to a genetic change which occurs in the somatic cells during aging, so that they become antigenic, stimulating the production of antibodies. Other diseases which increase in incidence with age, related with a decline in immune function, are infections and cancer. That the age-related increase in cancer may also be linked with a decline in immune functions is emphasized by Makinodan (1976) when he points out that the normal immune system may also protect the body by recognizing neoplastic somatic cells and destroying them. The frequency of cancer is also higher in organisms with reduced immune functions than in those with normal immune systems.

Concomitant with these changes in immune function, there is a slight increase with age in the level of circulating immunoglobulins (Ig). In humans, this is due to an increase in the levels of IgG and IgA. A study by Roseman and Buckley (1975) investigated the relationship of these changes to changes in intelligence scores with age.

Two longitudinal studies done on a large number of healthy subjects aged 45 years and over revealed that there was a negative correlation between serum immunoglobulin levels and intelligence scores as measured by the Wechsler Adult Intelligence Scale. IgG and IgA were found to contribute to the elevated immunoglobulin levels but not IgM. The investigators concluded that elevated immunoglobulin levels were associated with a decline in cognitive abilities, a relationship which was age-related. The variability in the intelligence scores also increased with age. This was found to be related to higher IgG levels. Although the mechanisms for this were not identified, one possibility suggested by Roseman and Buckley is that since brain reactive antibodies increase with age these may contribute to the intellectual decline.

That there may be a link between age, the decline in the immune system and the deteriorative changes that occur in the CNS, has been indicated in studies which have looked at the accumulation of brain reactive antibodies with age and the binding of these antibodies to neurons. Ingram *et al.* (1974) studied this in a large number of subjects over a wide age range. Serum taken from these subjects were tested against young and old brains removed from patients who had died without any neurological involvement. Although some degree of binding of the sera occurred in all age groups demonstrating the presence of these anti-neuron antibodies which had neuron binding specificity, the incidence of this increased markedly with age. This gamma-globulin component, as it was identified, or antibody, bound itself to the cytoplasmic constituents of the neurons. If present, these antibodies complexed with either the young or old substrate and Ingram *et al.* suggest that possibly in the aging living organism there is a breakdown in the blood–brain barrier.

Nandy *et al.* (1975) investigated the specificity of brain-reactive antibodies in old mice, having already established that these antibodies were present in the sera of old mice but not in the sera of young animals. These investigators found that the brain-reactive antibodies are specific to neuronal antigens of the brain which they found to be present in both the cytoplasm and the nucleus. The blood–brain barrier normally prevents these circulating antibodies from migrating into neural tissue and with age this blood–brain barrier may become less efficient. In the presence of degenerating or damaged neurons there are not specific brain-reactive antibody–neuronal antigen reacttions which suggests that neuronal cell death is not the reason why these anti-brain antibodies develop (Nandy 1975). Through the use of isotype studies, Nandy (1975) did find that a slow migration of these antibodies did occur across the blood–brain barrier and suggested that this may explain why there is a slow and scattered loss of neuronal cells in the brains of old mice.

The link between the nervous system, the immune system and a decline in certain behavioral patterns, particularly those involving cognitive tasks, represents an important step forward in understanding the aging process. It now remains to be seen whether these physiological processes are reversible and, if so, whether there are appropriate intervention steps that could be taken to prevent them.

Perspectives on Research

In addition to the remote causes of the genetic patterns of aging there are the proximal causes of disease, disuse, and the outcomes of genetic–environmental interactions. These four major classes of causes must be broken down further in such considerations as the consequences of disuse for the cardiovascular system, muscle, connective tissue, and other organ systems. Chronic disuse over many years of the adult lifespan can clearly simulate a pattern of aging. Whether one can discern general principles that underlie disuse, i.e. whether effects are generalized across organ systems, remains for research to establish. Research does give promise that clusters of relations closely linked with age can be identified and one may soon begin to speak of a longevity factor, a familial vigor factor, a cognitive disuse factor, a physical disuse factor, a species aging factor, and a series of age-related disease factors. Given the identification of many clusters of variables that group together with age there is the inevitable question about the residual plasticity of the organ system involved. With an increase in use, for example, can an individual recover function or increase functional capacity? In some cases disuse or disease related to age may result in relatively irreversible loss of function; in others there may be considerable plasticity in the system to recover function or to compensate for loss. In the case of the nervous system the potentials for recovery of function or compensation may be much greater than we have thought possible.

Summary and Conclusions

1. The purpose of this paper was to describe a limited number of developments in biological and behavioral research on aging. While the literature on aging has grown enormously in the last decade it is not well organized from a conceptual point of view and largely remains a vast body of particulate information indexed by the common variables of chronological age. To a considerable extent this is due to the widely varying definitions of aging whether explicit or implicit, and the many different dependent variables studied. Also the purpose was to isolate a few important areas of research and to examine significant findings and their implications in recent biological and behavioral research in aging.

2. From a scientific perspective one ought to adopt an evolutionary view, that biological controls over length of life have evolved during the slow time of natural selection. While the factors that limit our ultimate life span are undoubtedly genetic, the expression of genetic control varies with the environment. For humans this is particularly relevant since it is most unlikely that the environments which civilized man has created resemble the environments in which the process of selection occurred. Given uncertainty about the outcomes of genetic interactions with the environment, there must be many compensatory physiological and psychological mechanisms available to moderate deteriorative changes associated with advancing age.

3. Of the various organs and systems of the human organism, emphasis should be given to the role of the regulatory systems in aging. In particular, the central nervous system, the autonomic nervous system and the immune system are coming to the fore as leading areas of research. The loss of neurons and dysfunction of the nervous system with age can have consequences for remote cells and organs of the body. The susceptibility of neurons to DNA damage and decrease in molecular size, and the decrease in synaptic density carries with it prospects for a slower response to stimulation and alterations in the recovery phases of activity. Similarly, the autonomic nervous system in controlling vital vegetative functions of the body can disseminate influences undesirable for optimum functioning if its characteristics for arousal and delayed recovery are changed with age. For both the central nervous system and the autonomic nervous system recent reports of changes with age in neurotransmitters are very significant. The neuroendocrines are also being implicated as a source of changes during aging such as menopause.

4. One sign of altered function of the central nervous system with age is a decline in rhythmic electrical activity. The electroencephalogram shows a decline with age in the mean alpha frequency.

Further, electrical responses to sensory stimulation have been reported to show longer latencies and lower amplitudes. The slowness in electrical activity has been correlated with slowness of behavioral processes including cognitive processes. Slowness of behavioral response is closely linked to advancing age and appears to occur in healthy older adults. On the one hand research has sought to relate the slowing to disease such as reduced blood flow and on the other to consequences for higher thought processes. The discontinuity hypothesis was proposed to account for the fact that the brain is a highly buffered organ and its functions are stable against environmental variations. For this reason such variables as blood flow, oxygen, glucose and other essentials are thought to be limiting variables only after some critical limits are exceeded in which case they become the major determinants of level of functioning. For this reason discrepancies may exist between the clinical studies of aging which obtain correlations of, for example, blood flow and intellectual performance which are not obtained in relatively healthy community residents. One of the key issues to be resolved with regard to the functioning of the older CNS is whether with age there is a tendency to lowered inhibition or increased inhibition.

5. The possibility that the sympathetic division of the ANS shows heightened activity with age is important not only in itself, since continued high levels of activity may lead to exhaustion of an organ, but also because sympathetic arousal can influence the central nervous system. The common example of anxiety and its effects suffices to attest to the importance of high arousal. In this area of research there clearly seem significant changes with age, but the pattern is not clear. Partly this is because the various investigators have used different measures of arousal. The evidence from observation of CNS functioning, EEG, AEP, and reaction time suggests that the CNS is under-aroused with age, whereas the ANS is alternately over-aroused or under-aroused. One group of investigators has proposed that there is a lack of concordance between the CNS and the ANS with age, and that such lack of alignment would imply an increasing inefficiency in regulatory control with age with consequences for encouraging the development of stress related disease. In this regard perhaps age changes in the level of neurotransmitters may directly influence the level of activity and the time course of mobilization and recovery.

6. Neuroendocrine changes with age are coming to be identified. Monoamines decline in the brain. There appears to be a rise in norepinephrine in plasma with age. In the peripheral tissues certain of the catecholamine synthesizing enzymes such as dopa decarboxylase increase with age, while others such as that giving rise to adrenalin, decrease. Interpreting these changes is difficult but again it suggests

that there is a lack of parallelism between the CNS and peripheral target tissues which are important in mediating stress responses.

7. Among the more interesting phenomena beginning to be linked to aging are changes in circadian rhythms. Such changes definitely implicate the regulatory effectiveness of the nervous system. Often observed in humans is a change in sleep pattern with advancing age. With age there is less deep or stage 4 sleep, and less rapid eye movement sleep. Regular sleep patterns are thought to be essential for effective cognitive functioning. Mental disorders are also thought to accompany disturbance of circadian rhythms. Circadian rhythms can be used as an important experimental tool, for by altering the rhythms in young and old animals one can study the disrupting effects and the length of time required to re-establish rhythmic activity.

8. Changes in the regulatory capacity of the aging neuroendocrine and autonomic nervous systems are clearly important in mediating stress responses such as changes in blood pressure and cardiac output. Evidence is not yet definitive and one may form a picture of increased activity of these systems with age or a decrease. Loss of stable values and alienation are thought to be significant social stresses having physiological consequences.

9. The immune system is now beginning to loom as a vital area of research on aging because not only do immune responses seem to decline with age, but also the organism may develop antibodies against its own proteins promoting further progressive degradation of function. The possibility that the organism may immunize itself against its own substances gives rise to an increasing prevalence of autoimmune disease with age. Important is the fact that autoimmune processes may involve the brain and thereby disruption of behavioral processes can ensue. The rise in the probability of cancer with age has always been a perplexing issue. While cancer specialists have been most concerned with the nature of the disease itself, important issues lie in the changes in the aging host which predisposes it to the development of malignancy.

10. Given the perspective that the central nervous system, the autonomic nervous system and the immune system change with age it is likely that gains in health by resistance to disease could be improved particularly for the middle-aged population. Reduction in the stress-related diseases are the most encouraging prospect. For the present, controlling the environment to reduce stress and living a life of low caloric intake, high exercise, and regular habits seems a desirable cultural prescription. It offers a reasonable approach while the more remote genetic pathways to aging are being traced. At present there are many pathways to longevity and freedom from age related disease. Clearly some of this variation is related to species characteristics,

unique individual heredity, and the nature of the physical, psychological and cultural environment in which the individual grows up and grows old. Delineation of these pathways constitutes much of the research of the future. One can expect that familial factors will be identified as well as various classes of disease. The worst form of disease would be not to think about aging and not to gather information to better control our own destinies.

References

Andres, R. and Tobin, J. D. (1976). *In* "Handbook of the Biology of Aging". Eds. C. E. Finch and L. Hayflick. Van Nostrand Reinhold, New York

Arenberg, D. and Robertson, E. A. (1976). *In* "Handbook of the Psychology of Aging". Eds. J. E. Birren and K. W. Schaie. Van Nostrand Reinhold, New York

Beck, E. C., Dustman, R. E. and Schdenberg, T. (1975). *In* "Neurobiology of Aging". Eds. J. M. Ordy and K. R. Brizzee. Plenum Press, New York; pp 175–192

Berger, R. J. (1975). *Federation Proceedings* **34**, 97–102

Binstock, R. and Shanas, E. (1976). "Handbook of Aging and the Social Sciences." Von Nostrand Reinhold, New York

Birren, J. E. (1959). *In* "The Process of Aging in the Nervous System". Eds. J. E. Birren, H. A. Imus and W. F. Windle. Thomas, Springfield, Ill.; pp 143–165

Birren, J. E. (1960). *In* "Aging: Some Social and Biological Aspects". Ed. N. W. Shock. American Association for the Advancement of Science, Washington, DC; pp 305–332

Birren, J. E. (1964). "Psychology of Aging." Prentice-Hall, Englewood Cliffs, New Jersey

Birren, J. E. (1965). *In* "Behavior, Aging and the Nervous System". Eds. A. T. Welford and J. E. Birren. Thomas, Springfield, Ill.; pp 191–216

Birren, J. E. (1970). *American Psychologist* **25**, 124–135

Birren, J. E. (1971). *American Psychologist* **29**, 808–815

Birren, J. E., Butler, R. N., Greenhouse, W. S., Sokoloff, L. and Yarrow, M. R. (Eds.) (1963). "Human Aging." U.S. Government Printing Office, Washington, DC

Birren, J. E. and Renner, V. J. (1968*a*). "A Brief History of Mental Health and Aging." National Institute of Mental Health, Washington, DC

Birren, J. E. and Renner, V. J. (1976*b*). *In* "Handbook of the Psychology of Aging". Eds. J. E. Birren and K. W. Schaie. Van Nostrand Reinhold, New York

Birren, J. E. and Schaie, K. W. (Eds.) (1976). "Handbook of the Psychology of Aging." Van Nostrand Rheinhold, New York

Birren, J. E. and Spieth, W. (1962). *Journal of Gerontology* **17**, 390–391

Bondareff, W. and Geinisman, Y. (1976). *American Journal of Anatomy* **145**, 129–136

Botwinick, J. (1966). *Journal of Gerontology* **21**, 347–353

Botwinick, J. and Kornetsky, C. (1959). *Journal of Gerontology* **14**, 503

Botwinick, J. and Kornetsky, C. (1960). *Journal of Gerontology* **15**, 83–84

Busse, E. W. and Obrist, W. D. (1965). *Journal of Gerontology* **20**, 315–320

Dirken, J. D. (ed.) (1972). "Functional Age of Industrial Workers." Wolters-Noordhoff, Groningen, Netherlands

Dru, D. (1974). Ph.D. Dissertation. University of Southern California

Eisdorfer, C. (1967). *The Gerontologist* **7**, 14–18

Eisdorfer, C. (1968). *In* "Human Aging and Behavior". Ed. G. A. Talland. Academic Press, New York; pp 189–216

Eisdorfer, C. (1970). *The Gerontologist* **10**, 62–67

Eisdorfer, C., Nowlin, J. and Wilkie, F. (1970). *Science* **170**, 1327–1329

Eisdorfer, C., Powell, A. H., Silverman, G. and Bogdonoff, M. D. (1965). *Journal of Gerontology* **20**, 511–514

Eisdorfer, C. and Wilkie, F. (1976). *In* "Handbook of the Psychology of Aging". Eds. J. E. Birren and K. W. Schaie. Van Nostrand Reinhold, New York

Eleftheriou, B. E., Zolovick, A. J. and Elias, M. C. (1975). *Gerontologia* **21**, 21–30

Finch, C. E. (1976*a*). *Quarterly Review of Biology* (in press)

Finch, C. E. (1976*b*). *In* "Handbook of the Biology of Aging". Eds. C. E. Finch and L. Hayflick. Van Nostrand Reinhold, New York

Finch, C. E. and Hayflick, L. (Eds.) (1976). "Handbook of the Biology of Aging." Van Nostrand Reinhold, New York

Froehling, S. D. (1974). Ph.D. Dissertation, University of Miami, Florida

Frolkis, V. V. (1966). *Journal of Gerontology* **21**, 161–167

Frolkis, V. V. (1976). *In* "Handbook of the Psychology of Aging". Eds. J. E. Birren and K. W. Schaie. Van Nostrand Reinhold, New York

Hamilton, J. B. (1948). *In* "Recent Progress in Hormone Research". Ed. G. Pincus. Academic Press, New York and London; pp 257–322

Hamilton, J. B. (1965). *Journal of Gerontology* **20**, 96–104

Harkins, S. W., Froehling-Moss, S. and Thompson, L. W. (1976). Relationship between central and autonomic nervous system states: attention and psychomotor performance in the elderly. (Paper presented at Western Psychological Association, Los Angeles)

Henry, J. P. (1976). *Geriatrics* **31**, 59–72

Henry, J. P. and Ely, G. L. (1976). *In* "Biological Foundations of Psychiatry". Society of Biological Society. Raven Press, New York (in press)

Hicks, L. H. and Birren, J. E. (1970). *Psychological Bulletin* **74**, 377–396

Ingram, C. R., Phegan, K. J. and Blumenthal, H. T. (1974). *Journal of Gerontology* **29**, 20–27

Makinodan, T. (1976). *In* "Handbook of the Psychology of Aging". Eds. C. E. Finch and L. Hayflick. Van Nostrand Reinhold, New York

Marsh, G. R. and Thompson, L. W. (1976). *In* "Handbook of the Psychology of Aging". Eds. J. E. Birren and K. W. Schaie. Van Nostrand Reinhold, New York

Martin, W. C. (1971). Ph.D. Dissertation, University of Southern California

Nandy, K. (1975). *Journal of Gerontology* **30**, 412–416

Nandy, K., Fritz, R. B. and Threatt, J. (1975). *Journal of Gerontology* **30**, 269–274

Nisbett, R. E., Braver, A., Jusela, G. and Kezur, D. (1975). *Journal of Comparative and Physiological Psychology* **88**, 735–746

Obrist, W. D. (1964). *In* "Cerebral Ischemia". Eds. E. Simonson and T. A. McGavack. Thomas, Springfield, Ill.; pp 71–98

Obrist, W. D. and Busse, E. W. (1965). *In* "Applications of Electroencephalography in Psychiatry". Ed. W. P. Wilson. Duke University Press, Durham, NC

Ordy, J. M. and Brizzee, K. R. (Eds.) (1975). "Neurobiology of Aging." Plenum Press, New York

Powell, A. H., Eisdorfer, C. and Bogdonoff, M. D. (1964). *Archives of General Psychiatry* **10**, 192–195

Rabbitt, P. (1965). *Journal of Gerontology* **20**, 233–238

Reis, D. J., Ross, R. A., Brodsky, M., Specht, L. and Joh, T. (1976). *Federation Proceedings* **35**, 486

Roseman, J. M. and Buckley, C. E. (1975). *Nature, London* **254**, 55–56

Rowe, A. S., Dornhorst, A. and Alberti, K. G. M. M. (1974). *Clinical Science and Molecular Medicine* **47**, 15 p

Sampson, G. A. and Jenner, F. A. (1975). *Psychological Medicine* **5**, 4–8

Schaie, K. W. and Strother, C. R. (1968). *In* "Human Aging and Behavior". Ed. G. A. Talland. Academic Press, New York and London; pp 281–308

Schenkenberg, T. (1970. Ph.D. Dissertation, University of Utah

Schenkenberg, T. (1976). "Normative data on the cortical evoked potential and aging." (Paper presented at the Western Psychological Association, Los Angeles)

Serio, M., Piolanti, P., Romano, S., De Magistris, L. and Gusti, G. (1970). *Journal of Gerontology* **25**, 95–97

Shmavonian, B. M., Miller, L. H. and Cohen, S. I. (1968). *Psychophysiology* **5**, 119–131

Shmavonian, B. M., Miller, L. H. and Cohen, S. I. (1970). *Journal of Gerontology* **25**, 87–94

Shmavonian, B. M., Yarmat, A. J. and Cohen, S. I. (1965). *In* "Behavior, Aging and the Nervous System". Eds. A. T. Welford and J. E. Birren. Thomas, Springfield, Ill.; pp 235–258

Smith, D. B. D., Tom, C. E., Brent, G. A. and Ohta, R. J. (1976). "Attention evoked potentials and aging." (Paper presented at the Western Psychological Association, Los Angles

Straumanis, J. J., Sheass, C. and Schwartz, M. (1965). *Journal of Gerontology* **20**, 498–506

Surwillo, W. W. (1963). *Electroencephalography and Clinical Neurophysiology* **15**, 105–114

Surwillo, W. W. (1964). *Electroencephalography and Clinical Neurophysiology* **17**, 194–198

Surwillo, W. W. (1966). *Journal of Gerontology* **21**, 257–260

Surwillo, W. W. (1968). *In* "Human Aging and Behavior". Ed. G. A. Talland. Academic Press, New York and London; pp 1–35

Talland, G. A. (1968). "Human Aging and Behavior." Academic Press, New York and London

Thompson, L. W. and Marsh, G. R. (1973). *In* "The Psychology of Adult Development and Aging". Eds. C. Eisdorfer and M. P. Lawton. American Psychological Association, Washington, DC; pp 112–148

Thompson, L. W. and Nowlin, J. B. (1973). *In* "Intellectual Functioning in Adults". Eds. L. F. Narvik, C. Eisdorfer and J. E. Blum. Springer, New York; pp 107–172

Troyer, W. G., Eisdorfer, C., Wilkie, F. and Bogdonoff, M. D. (1966). *Journal of Gerontology* **21**, 415–419

Wang, H. S. and Busse, E. W. (1974). *In* "Normal Aging II". Ed. E. Palmore. Duke University Press, Durham, NC; pp 126–140

Welford, A. T. and Birren, J. E. (Eds.). "Behavior, Aging and the Nervous System." Thomas, Springfield, Ill.

Wheeler, K. T. and Lett, J. T. (1974). *Proceedings of the National Academy of Sciences of the United States of America* **71**, 1862–1865

Wilkie, F. and Eisdorfer, C. (1972). *Science* **172**, 959–962

Woodruff, D. S. (1972). Ph.D. Dissertation, University of Southern California

Ziegler, M. G. and Lake, C. R. (1976). *Federation Proceedings* **35**, 446

Education and Training

Manpower Needs

Martin Sicker
Office of Research, Demonstrations and Manpower Resources, DHEW, Washington DC 20201

In a background paper on training prepared for the 1971 White House Conference on Aging, several issues were raised which were designed to provoke thoughtful discussion and consideration. Those same issues, none of which has been definitively resolved, are of great relevance to the theme of this conference. If we are to meet, competently and humanely, the challenge of dependency presented by the elderly, we cannot but confront the fundamental questions of how to insure that the necessary manpower for the task is available and suitably prepared, what kinds of education and training are needed, who should be trained, who should assume the burden for such training, and how should significant decisions on these matters be reached.

It would be useful to review some of the few bits of data available to gain some perspective on the dimensions of the problem before us. A study of the demand for personnel and training in the field of aging completed in 1968 offered some tentative estimates on manpower supply and demand in programs serving older persons exclusively or primarily. For the period 1967–68 an estimated one-third of a million professional and technical personnel were so engaged. Approximately 290 000 of these were employed in nursing and shelter homes. Of this number 177 000 were identified as nurse's aides, 30 000 as registered nurses, 40 000 as licensed practical nurses, and 24 000 as administrators of nursing and personal care homes. At that time nursing and personal care home capacity was approximately 800 000 beds (Administration on Aging 1969). While we do not have any data on the number of older persons participating in such non-institutional programs or the extent to which demand exceeded supply, we feel safe in suggesting that the population of some 20 000 000 persons over age 65 received very little programmatic attention.

A study of manpower needs in the nursing-home industry completed in 1975 on behalf of the Administration on Aging by the Bureau of Labor Statistics, indicated that in 1973, health service workers alone, which includes nurse's aides and practical nurses, numbered more than 311 000 and are projected to number 466 000 by 1980 and 535 000 by 1985. The requirement for therapists is expected to increase from 4700 in 1973 to 12 000 in 1985. The demand for recreation workers is expected to rise from 2300 in 1973 to 4700 in 1985 (Administration on Aging 1975). Again, we have no data on demands for personnel for programs serving the non-institutionalized elderly. However, an indication of the latter may be gleaned from the situation of the Administration on Aging whose programs are focused on the non-institutionalized dependent elderly. The network of state, area and nutrition project agencies supported by the Administration on Aging alone employs some 10 000 professionals and para-professionals and utilizes some 50 000 service volunteers.

These gross statistics do not present the full dimensions of the training problem. For that we must also consider the annual turnover rate. For example, current annual projections for the nursing-home industry estimate an annual growth of 13 000 job vacancies for nursing aides and orderlies, supplemental by 18 200 replacements; an annual replacement of 2700 registered nurses, an annual replacement of 1800 health administrators, and an annual replacement of 5800 practical nurses (Administration on Aging 1975). The numbers of personnel requiring training to meet the demands of service to dependent elderly may thus be seen to be substantially greater than the total number employed at any point in time.

Given these figures, it seems reasonably safe to say that by 1985 there will be at least one million people fully involved on a professional or para-professional basis in the field of aging with a substantial annual replacement rate in addition to growth resulting from demand.

If we take a close look at the kinds of training and education that this vast amount of people involved in services to the aging requires, it will be seen that the needs vary quite widely, from very sophisticated education on the highest academic levels to rather modest kinds of training covering a broad spectrum of subject matter. It is possible to identify some two hundred skills or occupations that are pertinent to the field of aging. For purposes of analysis, we can array those skill and occupational categories along an employment-training pyramid. This pyramid would display a general relationship between the level of training required and the numbers of persons in the various occupations for whom the training should be provided. By identifying those occupations or skills that represent the highest numbers of persons working in the field, and ranging them along the incline of the pyramid, we begin to get some image of the implications of these relationships. We find, as one might expect, that there is clearly an inverse relationship between the prevalence of an occupation and the level of training in aging required. The very few people arrayed at the pinnacle of the pyramid require a great deal of training while the much greater numbers of people arrayed at the lower levels of the pyramid require substantially less training. One could also make a case for arguing that the pyramid also frequently reflects an inverse relationship between educational level and degree of personal contact with older persons. That is, geriatricians, researchers, and teachers, who are clearly at the top of the employment-training pyramid, may have far less ongoing daily contact with older persons than those who deal with their more prosaic needs. For example, the aide who regularly turns a patient in bed, and who is given less training than may be desirable in order to show proper understanding and sensitivity to the needs and problems of older persons.

Given the spread of professions and occupations as well as the estimates of personnel working in the field of aging, manpower planning becomes very complex and problematic, a situation that is further compounded by relatively high employment turnover rates. Educational institutions focusing on training in aging are confronted by a major challenge in not only being prepared to provide training to a student population expanding at a rate consistent with the growth rate of the older population and the numbers of trained personnel required to meet their needs, but also in training and retraining those personnel who are already working in the field. The latter is crucial if we are to assure that the care older persons are receiving in long-term care institutions and the services and facilities designed to keep older persons from inappropriate institutionalization, are at the qualitative levels that society should insist on. This is clearly a monumental task.

Currently efforts to deal with the indicated problems are impeded by a number of inter-related factors. The field of aging has been plagued by difficulties in recruitment of adequately trained and motivated personnel. Despite significant advances in recent years, the field continues to be characterized by comparatively low salaries reflecting to a large degree low status. There are few career ladders in services to the aged, particularly in the relatively low-skill but high personal contact occupations such as homemaker/home health aides. Without prospects for advancement, a self-selection process takes place which leaves little incentive for a person with ambition and potential to remain in the field very long. These problems, in turn, contribute to that of excessive turnover reflected in a very high personnel replacement rate. However, in addition to the very serious matters of unattractive salary scales and low advancement prospects, there is the difficulty of making a good match between the job to be done and the individual recruited to do it. There seems to be a tendency for many persons to feel overqualified for the positions they occupy. This is particularly true of college graduates entering para-professional or semi-professional fields which do not require degrees or other substantial academic qualifications. Such persons will typically accept such a position only to provide some income while seeking something else that is more attractive for them.

As one progresses up the employment-training pyramid, a whole array of barriers to effective manpower recruitment, training, and utilization is encountered. Institutional barriers such as civil service regulations and personal policies often disqualify the best trained for a particular position in favor of those with longer but often irrelevant work experience. Because of this we encounter the anomaly of highly trained graduates of federally supported university programs in gerontology being unable to obtain positions of substance in federally supported service programs, programs which are thirsty for the very skills and knowledge that those same graduates possess. Inflexibility in the hiring process further exacerbates the problem, by imposing requirements for combination of skills and experience that simply are not available or are not really needed. For example, in one state, the civil service commission required that all nutritionists hired to plan and direct the congregate meals and meals-on-wheels program had to have a medical background. In this case, it seemed fairly evident that hospital experience as a nutritionist was not necessarily the best or most useful background for a community-based services program. There is also a tendency for sponsors of services to attempt to keep costs down by establishing standard rates of compensation. This involves a built-in bias against in-service training of personnel designed to upgrade the quality of services provided. Increased skill proficiencies and competence levels also increase worker dissatisfaction with the existing advancement and salary constraints and thereby contribute to the high annual turnover of personnel. Finally, there is the problem of vested professional interests. A new non-traditionally defined field such as aging is especially vulnerable to the pressures of conservative professionalism. Gerontology, which tends to be multidisciplinary by its very nature, runs counter to the present categorization of professions and specialities, and has so far evoked only modest interest from the traditional disciplines. Professional groups structured around these disciplines have vested interests in maintaining traditional modes of services and service delivery systems. Perhaps one of the more serious consequences of this is that there is not one chair of geriatric medicine in the United States even though half of the annual \$100 billion health bill goes for chronic diseases (Butler 1975). As a result, the restructuring of occupations to accommodate the needs of the field of aging is discouraged. This coupled with the general inertia of such organizations, has had serious effects on the ability of those concerned with the problems of the elderly to build the institutions and mechanisms most appropriate to meeting their diverse needs. The capacity to initiate new and innovative programs has been impaired, and an inordinate amount of the time and energies of those leading professionals who have ventured into the field has been consumed in attempting to overcome these impediments to the development of adequate manpower and training programs in aging.

The paucity of hard data on the manpower needs of the field is matched by an equivalent absence of solid information on current efforts to train manpower for the field. This should not be surprising given the relative newness of an identified field of aging and the lack of any national social accounting ledger in which the desired data would readily be found. However, some feel for the magnitude of current training in aging may be obtained from a review of the present federal investment in the area. Here again the data is incomplete and should be taken as indicative rather than definitive.

In Fiscal Year 1975, as best as we can determine, approximately $12 million was expended by the federal government on training specifically focused on aging. Of this amount, approximately $4 million went for the training for a variety of professionals in the fields of social science, social work, and public administration. Another $4 million was expended on a wide variety of in-service non-medically related short-term training programs, and $2 million on short-term training for staff of long-term care nursing facilities. Finally, approximately $2 million was invested in the training of researchers in the field of aging. To the best of our knowledge, no federal funds were directly expended on the training of medical professionals for work with the aging. This is not to imply that there is no such training taking place, but simply that there is no significant investment of public resources for that purpose.

Efforts are currently under way to obtain better information on the status of gerontological education and training in the United States, but it will be several years before the picture becomes very clear. As is well known, the body count approach to assessing program effectiveness does not yield very reliable information. For example, we do know that under the Administration on Aging's career training program in 1975, which provided partial institutional support to some fifty university programs, more than 560 courses in aging were offered with more than 16 000 enrolled students. However, we would hesitate to conclude therefrom that more than 500 of those enrolled students were preparing for a career in the field of aging. Nonetheless, it can be asserted that we are witnessing a significant order of magnitude increase of interest in the field on the part of persons preparing for professional first and second careers. One indicator of this upsurge of interest is the number of doctoral dissertations undertaken in aging.

A study of doctoral training in gerontology for the years 1934–69 indicated that in 1968, the peak year for dissertations on the problems of aging, 89 dissertations were produced in all disciplines. Of these, 55 were in social and psychological sciences (Moore and Birren 1971). It is worth noting that in 1975, the first year that the Administration on Aging announced a special small grant program for the support of dissertation research in social gerontology, more than 100 applications were received from students who already had dissertation committee approval for their topics in social and psychological sciences. An additional 100 such applications for the 1976 program are currently being sent to reviewers. Considering the professional and institutional barriers to status for careers in aging mentioned earlier, this is indeed a significant development.

Given the dimensions of the manpower/training problems confronting the field of aging and the current societal response to those problems, what courses of action are open to repair the obvious imbalance? An initial reaction might be to suggest that the problems can be overcome by substantial increases in the resources allocated for manpower development in aging. While we would not take issue with the benefits to be realized from judicious increases in the resource levels allocated for this purpose, we do not believe that the problems will be solved by throwing money at them. There are some fundamental issues that need to be resolved if current and potential resources are to be used in an optimum manner. These are the issues that were alluded to at the outset of this paper.

To assure that the supply of properly trained competent personnel needed to meet the needs of the dependent elderly is adequate for that purpose, the triple problem of recruitment, turnover, and institutional barriers must be confronted and solved. This is unlikely to be accomplished without the concerted efforts of all concerned with the field of aging and the well-being of older persons. Unless the notion of "quality of life" is translated from a euphemistic rhetorical flourish into an operational value, the conditions necessary for dramatic changes in the field will probably not be realized. Somehow, the idea of quality must gain entrance into the cost versus benefit calculations, and not continue to come into consideration as an additional thought only after the quantitative analysis is completed. This is a major educational problem. Textbook notions of what represents "economy" and what "diseconomy" must be challenged, as well as other allegedly "value-free" notions which are in reality heavily value-laden. An increase in concern for the quality of care as an essential element of a service on the part of service providers would serve as a key to begin to unlock the problem from within. We have little confidence that it can be done from without. Recognition of the need to constantly improve the quality of services, rather than merely maintain them at a socially acceptable level, would set a premium on employee competence and qualifications. In conjunction with this, the problem of job advancement must be addressed if the turnover rate is to be reduced.

One possible approach to establishing career ladders in the field of services to the elderly would be through a radical revision of the methods by which in-service training is provided. The current pattern is largely that of contracting for the delivery of discrete training packages focused on limited training objectives. Perhaps what is needed is an aging services training center, institutionally based, either free-standing or located within an existing community-based post-secondary educational institution, and which would provide a wide range of training opportunities for persons working or planning to work in the field of aging at a sub-professional or para-professional level. Indeed a recent study suggested establishing a field of para-gerontology offering degrees at the associate level (Korim 1974). Coupled with requirements for some sort of certification of qualifications and training for those working in services to the elderly, it can readily be seen how a career ladder could come into being.

The problem of vested professional interests is one which may be addressed more effectively by co-option rather than confrontation. There are signs that some of the traditional bastions of resistance to recognizing that there is a legitimate professional field of aging are beginning to weaken. We are witnessing this now in the field of law and are beginning to see cracks in the wall protecting dentistry from the elderly. This year, for the first time, the Administration on Aging will be considering proposals for support for medical schools for gerontology programs. While this effort, because of limited resources, cannot but be most modest, it will nonetheless represent what may be the first direct federal support for training of physicians in the problems of the aging. Perhaps the day is not too far off when some medical school will establish a chair of geriatrics (even if it has to be a "soft" chair for a while).

The issues of what kinds and what levels of education and training are needed in the field of aging are in many respects more difficult to deal with, at least conceptually. It is one thing to argue that a professional dealing with the problems of the elderly in one or more aspects would benefit from a broad exposure to the literature of the field and the particular insights that different disciplines bring to it. It is difficult to raise an objection against education as such. It is quite another thing to argue that such a broad exposure, which goes beyond the minimum tools and knowledge that a professional *needs* to function competently, merits the same priority for allocation and use of resources as the latter. As we move down the employment-training pyramid, our difficulties in this regard become more complex. How much exposure to the issues in the psychology of aging does a nurse's aide require to provide services at an acceptable qualitative level? It is with regard to these issues that the resources allocation problem becomes acute. Particularly with regard to public resources, how does one calculate the trade-offs between support of continuing professional education and in-service training, between professional and para-professional training, between social workers and public administrators, between doctorates and baccalaureates, and a host of other necessary choices? Unfortunately, we have no simple answers to these rather formidable questions. Resource allocators tend to "fly by the seats of their pants," their judgements conditioned by their own exposure to the manifold aspects of the problem. Perhaps some research and experimentation are in order.

The corollary issue of who should be trained is a relatively new one, one which is just now coming to be recognized as very real, given the demographic projections, calculations of dependency ratios and related factors, along with the concurrent transition from an industrial to a service economy. Should resources allocated for the training of personnel to serve the elderly continue to be expended as at present, or should an increasing share be allocated to the training and retraining of older persons to provide services to other older persons? The under-utilization if not the waste of the skills and professional talents and competencies of our older population is well known, and there is an ever-increasing pressure to allow those who have been excluded from the traditional labor market to participate in the delivery of services to their peers. This issue is not yet one that is receiving a great deal of attention. However, it is one that will have to be dealt with soon.

The issue of who should assume the burden of providing for such training as may be necessary is one that is certainly not unique to the field of aging. It is a fundamental issue of public policy contingent upon perceptions of the proper role of governments and non-governmental institutions' pluralist society. It is essentially a political issue rather than a professional one.

The related issue of how significant decisions on the matters under discussion should be reached is both political and professional. It is worth recalling here that a formally legislated structure, the Federal Council on Aging comprised of presidentially appointed members representing a broad spectrum of the community concerned with the problems of the elderly, is in place and operating with a broad mandate for recommending priorities in the field of aging. It is beginning to focus its attention on the issues of manpower and training in the field of aging. However, many aspects of the issues raised here are matters of professional judgement and it is difficult to imagine how these can be resolved without substantive contributions from the professional community. To date, the professional community as well as the national organizations of older persons have been very effective advocates for programs in aging and their efforts have borne tangible fruit in the form of increased appropriations. However, their record in terms of contributions to the formation of policies through recommendations on how best to utilize those resources is rather bland. This is in part true because of deep divisions within the professional community over the issues calling for resolution. This has in turn created a situation where those who cannot avoid making decisions do so on their best individual judgement. We are confident that, on the whole, those judgements have been sound. They have not, however, resolved the fundamental issues which have for the most part been simply deferred, such that the issues we are considering today are the same as those raised five years ago and are no closer to resolution now than they were then. In this respect, it appears that the professional community has not shown the leadership we believe it capable of demonstrating.

We believe that the times are propitious for a closer collaboration between the professional community and the governmental establishment; not necessarily in the sense of formal advisory bodies, but rather through active communications and open deliberation of issues of concern to all. It is probably a truism to state that the financial resources for education and training in the field of aging that are currently available, or that will be made available in the future, will never be enough to cover all identifiable needs. In face of this prospect, it becomes increasingly essential that we take stock of what we are doing, what we are planning to do, and, perhaps most importantly, explore approaches that may be more productive. We are currently witnessing a very rapid proliferation of training programs in aging, the relative benefits of which are unclear. Large-scale diffusion of training resources will not necessarily result in better care and services for the dependent elderly, particularly where there is little connection between the expenditure of such resources and the needs of the services' industries and those they serve. More dollars and more programs do not necessarily produce more quality. Quality may actually be lowered unless steps are taken to develop standards of excellence against which resources may be applied.

As is evident, there is no master plan for resolving the numerous issues confronting us, nor is it clear that a master plan is desirable. What is needed is some hard thinking and exploration of these issues in an atmosphere of closer collaboration between public resource allocators and the professional and educational communities. Without such active collaboration, there is indeed little prospect for resolving or alleviating on a society-wide basis those problems of the dependent aged and aging which require the skills and undertaking of the properly trained hand and mind.

References

Administration of Aging (1969). "The Demand for Personnel and Training in the Field of Aging." Administration on Aging, Washington; No. 270. (1975). "Manpower Needs in the Field of Aging." Administration on Aging, Washington

Butler, R. M. (1975). "Society's Responsibilities to the Elderly." Government Printing Office, Washington

Korim, A. S. (1974). "Older Americans and Community Colleges: A Guide for Program Implementation." American Association of Community and Junior Colleges, Washington

Moore, J. L. and Birren, J. E. (1971). *Journal of Gerontology* **26**, pp 249–257

White House Conference on Aging (1971). Background and Issues: Training. Washington

Inculcation of Appropriate Attitudes and Skills

J C Brocklehurst
Department of Geriatric Medicine,
University Hospital of South Manchester,
Manchester

In defining attitudes and skills required in the care of the elderly I am obliged (and delighted) to try and define the whole field of care of the elderly; for the skills are those things that must be done — and attitudes the way we approach them. In Great Britain, as a geriatrician, I am constantly being asked what is a geriatric patient, what is there about geriatric care that singles it out from other forms of medical practice? In essence, geriatrics is a form of caring and the special skills that it requires are not those in the practical sense, as with cardiac catheterization or gastroscopy, but in the development and deployment of a special system of care and in the understanding of complex and unique problems. A geriatrician is an organizer of geriatric care, a co-ordinator of community and medical resources, an educator (both of his colleagues and of his patients), an innovator, something of a epidemiologist, an expert in rehabilitation, as well as being (and this is his essential basis) a competent clinician.

The geriatric nurse has many similar skills — above all, to be able to give support and foster independence simultaneously. She must also be able to recognize and prevent the host of associated problems which may so easily and insidiously develop in disabled old people. The breakdown itself is compounded of many problems, but usually precipitated by one, that is by an acute medical or social disorder. The associated problems include pressure sores, constipation, incontinence, dehydration, apathy, depression, frustration, anger, shame and a host of others.

The therapist must adapt her skills to the context of deceptive frailty which old people show — deceptive both as to its underlying resilience and also to its hidden risks. She must know the basis of these risks — sensory deprivation (especially hearing and vision) — insecure balance and fear of falling, inattention and memory difficulties and many others: she must take account of these in her work. At the same time she must realize that living dangerously with independence is sometimes better than being cocooned in an institution.

The social worker must be supportive without being coercive; helpful without being patronizing, in the patient deployment of her skills. The resources she develops will always be in short supply and she must be able to adjust for this.

The manager of an old persons' home or warden of sheltered housing must be reliable, confidential, able to recognize incipient breakdown, but willing to allow participation and involvement by the old people she serves. Above all she must realize that the happiness of a group of human souls lies in her hands: it is very largely up to her whether they are straitened, fearsome and querulous — or free and relaxed.

Some of these things are skills, some are attitudes and it is not always easy to discover the boundaries of each.

The most important attitude of all is that old people matter — their lives are (or can be) full and rich, that they have a right to a full share of resources (based on wealth that they themselves will have created); that old age is as sentient and satisfying a part of life as any other. An attitude so admirably expressed by Browning:

> "Grow old along with me.
> The best is yet to be
> The last of life for which the first was made".

The amazing thing about care of the elderly is that once people become involved they become enthusiasts. It is an exciting and satisfying way of life — and for most of us needs no contrasting specialty to set it off.

The problem lies with our colleagues — in every sphere. To them old age seems dull, negative and unworthy of specialization. The old person is no longer a wage earner; chronic disease no longer curable; and this combination makes medicine in old age seem irrelevant to many physicians. For too long has medical education inculcated that cure is all and care — including the maintaining of independence in old age — of no importance. It is our colleagues that we must educate, whose attitudes we must seek to change. This can only be done if we begin when they are students and still free of prejudice.

May I therefore outline the educational programme as I see it (and try to practise it in Manchester), which we must deploy as we attempt to inculcate the appropriate skills and attitudes towards care of the elderly.

I shall outline these from the point of view of a university teacher of medical students, realizing of course that while a good deal of what I am describing is necessary also for students in nursing, social work, therapy and general care, there are bound to be alterations in emphasis in relation to each of these. However, the complete undergraduate teaching programme in geriatrics should contain, at least in part, all the ingredients necessary in the whole field of care of the elderly.

Aging

Gerontology has three fundamental strands; biological, sociological and psychological, and the medical student should know something of each. In his pre-clinical years he should receive some teaching from a gerontologist about age-changes in organs, tissues and cells, in the metabolic consequences of these and in the major theories of their causation. At this stage also, he should consider the social implications of aging, particularly of retirement, of family relationships, problems of institutional care and of the consequences of all of these in the use of national and world resources. The gerontologist who is a psychologist should teach of society's attitudes to old people and the reasons for these. The old person's attitude to himself, the way in which people age according to their varying personalities, their aspirations and fears, are important ingredients of gerontology. Also the effect of aging on memory, learning and work in an industrial setting, theories of disengagement and those which have superseded them and the use of psychological tests in assessing age-change, should all be taught.

This whole core of knowledge about gerontology will form an essential basis for subsequent medical training — and it should figure very prominently in the curriculum as part of the teaching of cell biology, biochemistry, psychology and sociology. Gerontologists — perhaps from a central institute of gerontology, linked with a university department of geriatric medicine — should have honorary appointments in these parent departments and participate in their teaching programme.

Once the student has reached his early clinical years and has learned the simple skills of history taking and examination and something of pathology and therapeutics, he should then consider the following:

Demography in relation to an aging population. Population trends, now and in the future, where old people live, their dependency, the effects of retirement migration, family support and so on, have profound implications for the practice of medicine. The student at this stage should consider these both from the point of view of society and of himself as a future doctor.

Age effects on body functions. Senescent changes affect the *milieu intérieur*, individual organs, cells and metabolism. These reflect both on the natural history of disease and also on the sensitivity of the old person to drugs.

The special features of medicine in old age and particularly multiple pathology and socio-medical interdependency. These highlight the need to think in terms of total disability, compounded of both of these factors when dealing with illness in old people. There are very few "pure" social problems in old age. Breakdown is multi-factorial and complex, requiring the most careful analysis of all factors, both medical and social, by the physician. It is, *par excellence*, the medicine of the whole man. With an informed approach and infinite care the frail old person can usually maintain some form of independent living until almost the very end of his life.

The altered presentation of disease in old age. Illness presents particularly with an absence of pain and other classical features. The best known examples are myocardial infarction, peritonitis, sub-acute bacterial endocarditis and thyrotoxicosis, but the whole spectrum of disease is involved.

In addition there are four major presenting symptoms of disease in the elderly. These are quite different from the main presenting symptoms in younger people. Moreover they are symptoms and not diseases and require as full an elucidation and differential diagnosis, followed by specific therapy, as do any other symptoms. They are:

incontinence
mental confusion
postural instability and falls
immobility

These form the whole basis of geriatric medical practice.

The structure of the geriatric service. This, of course, will vary according to the country in which the doctor is practising. In great Britain there is an almost universal specialist geriatric service. The medical student must learn how it is structured, what are the functions of its various parts, how he may refer patients to it and what he may expect of it. The geriatric service includes in-patient care which is generally in the form of progressive patient care embracing acute wards, rehabilitation wards and continuing care in long-stay wards. It involves the use of planned short-stay admission (and re-admission), both for investigation and for the relief of strain on relatives. It involves the use of the day hospital and the out-patient consultative clinic. The closest liaison with a psychogeriatric service on the one hand and social services on the other is required and very often there is a system of a pre-admission assessment of patients in their own homes who are referred by general practitioners.

The existence and extent of unreported illness in the elderly. The student must consider both the extent of unreported illness and to what extent the physician has a responsibility to set out to discover as much of this as is remediable. There are various ways in which this may be undertaken as, for instance, by the use of health visitors attached to general practices and working from the basis of the age–sex register of that general practice. There is, of course, a unique opportunity to do this in Great Britain, since 98% of the population are registered with a general practitioner of their choice. The economic consequences have to be thought about. Since most medical students at the present time are destined to become general practitioners the seed of this idea should be well sown in their minds.

Miscellanea. There is a group of conditions, not unique to old people, but about which the geriatrician in a teaching hospital often finds himself taking the only initiative as far as medical student education is concerned. This includes care of the dying and effects of bereavement, rehabilitation of patients with stroke, prevention and management of pressure sores and medical ethics.

This, then, is the basis on which rests the education of medical students in care of the elderly. Such teaching will involve many techniques, some didactic, others using bedside teaching, case conferences, seminars and visits. Case conferences should include the review of patients undergoing in-patient rehabilitation, and those attending the day hospital from their own homes. In these the whole geriatric team would participate. Socio-medical case presentations based on a single patient unfolding the progress of his illness in relation to the history of his life, offers a fruitful basis for small group discussion. Clinicopathological case conferences — showing histology in relation to aging and disability — also capture students' imaginations and inform them of the relevance of multiple morbidity.

During these seminars and case conferences the students will observe the attitude of the geriatrician to his patients and the working together of the geriatric team. It will be a poor teaching department which does not inspire some enthusiasm for the subject.

The amount of time devoted to such teaching in the medical curriculum will be limited because of the constant desire of every department in the Faculty for more teaching time. In Great Britain a maximum level now reached is in the region of sixty hours for each medical student (of obligatory teaching). This would seem to be a good minimum level to set — it does allow a reasonable exposition of the subject. In addition there should be optional elective periods of study for those with a particular interest — who are likely to become the geriatricians of the future.

One point which unfortunately cannot be forgotten is the importance of examinations in moulding students' attitudes. Inclusion in the examination seems to give a subject on the curriculum respectability and credence. This is a sad fact but one which cannot be neglected. Questions must be asked, therefore, both in undergraduate and postgraduate examinations, from within the special field of medicine in old age.

It is only in the last four or five years that geriatric medicine has had any real place in the undergraduate curriculum and still it affects only about half the medical schools in Great Britain. The importance of postgraduate education in this subject will, therefore, be apparent. Indeed, most general practitioners are well aware of the defects in their knowledge and education as they deal with the increasing number of elderly people on practice lists. Half-day, weekend and, indeed, week-long residential courses in the medicine of old age are popular and well-attended. The subject-matter and structure of such courses will differ little from that of the undergraduate.

Thirdly, there is the question of vocational training for the specialty of geriatric medicine or of a career in geriatric medicine combined with internal medicine. The Joint Committee of the Royal Colleges of Great Britain which is concerned with higher medical training, lays down a training programme for physicians wishing to specialize in geriatric medicine in the same way as it does for other specialties. This includes (after registration) a period of general professional training of three to four years. A large part of this is likely to be spent in appointments in internal medicine, but it may also include appointments in medical specialties including geriatrics or in pathology, psychiatry or general practice. During this time the diploma of Membership of one of the Royal Colleges (MRCP) should be obtained. The second period of training which follows this is specialist training, and is usually open only to doctors who have obtained the MRCP. This specialized training lasts for two to four years and is carried out mainly or completely within geriatric departments. If the physician wishes to practise general medicine with a special interest in geriatric medicine then at least two out of the four years would have to be spent in further training within internal medicine.

At the present time the whole question of vocational training is under discussion within the European Economic Community. The matter is urgent since reciprocity of specialist qualifications throughout Europe has to be implemented by the end of 1976. At the present time three of the eight EEC countries have a recognized specialty of Geriatric Medicine (Great Britain, Eire and Denmark). The content and form of specialist training has yet to be agreed.

Nurses require the same basic knowledge as medical students, but with different emphasis. They must be taught to ensure that the fact of hospitalization does not do positive harm to an elderly patient. They must therefore be skilled in preventing pressure sores, incontinence and constipation and knowledgeable about the various special types of equipment and of furniture which are available for the comfortable management of old and ill people. This extends to clothing, dishes and cutlery as well as more technical equipment such as water beds and walking aids. In hospital geriatric practice the nurse is the key figure and her attitude and understanding will probably be the greatest single factor in the success of geriatric care. Unfortunately, most nurses receive very little training in geriatric nursing and, indeed, there has been very little research to date into this subject. However, there has been very little nursing research at all and the application of research methods to nursing, at least in Great Britain, has been particularly pioneered in the geriatric field by nurses such as Doreen Norton and Thelma Wells. To make good this deficiency in nurse training the Joint Board of Clinical Nursing Studies in England has produced a national post-registration course at two levels: one is a six-month course and the other a two-week course (Curriculum obtainable from Adam House, 1 Fitzroy Square, London W1P 6DS). Both have been designed with the greatest care to develop the appropriate skills and attitudes. Both are equally applicable for nurses in hospital and those working in the community.

Social workers, too, require special teaching in the problems of old age and their education will be developed by attending case conferences in geriatric departments. Once again, the attitudes and skills are related to those already discussed and once again, the amount of teaching that most of them receive at the present time is equally nebulous.

Other care-giving professionals include manageresses in homes, wardens of sheltered housing, home helps and voluntary service organizers. Here day-release courses of training will be important and once again, it is this type of worker whose attitude will be all-powerful in producing happiness or misery in the life of their elderly client.

Finally, let us not forget old people themselves and those who work with and for them on a voluntary basis. In Great Britain, Age Concern is a major national organization through which voluntary service for old people is channelled and a significant part of the work of Age Concern is involved with the education of volunteers. It is sometimes thought that an educational programme is incompatible with the role of the volunteer, but this is not so. An understanding of the problems, of the services available and of the needs of the old people they serve will give the volunteer more confidence and allow her to see her role more broadly and positively.

Education for people themselves involves both pre-retirement courses, of which many are now established in Great Britain on a day-release basis for industrial workers during the ages of 55 to 60, and also the health education of old people themselves.

The teacher has been portrayed from every possible point of view in literature. One of my favourites is Robert Burns' epitaph on Willie Mechie, a teacher, which is as follows:

"Here lie Willie Mechie's banes,[1]
Satan when ye tak' him,
Gie him the schuling of your weanes,[2]
For clever de'ils he'll mak' them".

The teacher must impart knowledge and even produce "clever de'ils", but the most important function of education is surely to produce enjoyment. It is only as a result of education that most people enjoy the things that are generally regarded as being most worthwhile, for instance opera, the paintings of Matisse and Picasso and Havana cigars.

In education for care of the elderly, therefore, it is enjoyment and satisfaction in the care-giver (as well as the old person) for which we should aim. If we achieve this then the attitudes and skills that have been inculcated will almost certainly be the right ones.

References

Brocklehurst, J. C. (1974). *Age and Ageing* **3**, 3–11

Cohen, C. (1968). *Gerontologia clinica* **10**, 108–115

Pathy, M. S. (1974). *Gerontologia clinica* **16**, 179–184

World Health Organization (1973). "Education and Training in Longterm and Geriatric Care." World Health Organization, Copenhagen

[1] Bones
[2] Children

Discussion

Dr Robinson We now have about 30 minutes for discussion and questions.

Dr T Franklin Williams (*University of Rochester, New York*) I have a comment and a question. Efforts at teaching about aging and chronic ilness in this country are at least beginning. I can vouch for one in Rochester, where we now have an impact on all medical students and essentially all house officers through a university program in a chronic illness facility. There is also a recently published summary of work in this country by the Fogarty International Center, "Teaching of Chronic Illness and Aging", a symposium that was held a couple of years ago. Just beginning efforts, but at least I think it shows that it is possible to get started.

I have a question for Dr Sicker whose comments I thought were very instructive. I wanted to ask about support for continuing education. I heard recently of one setting in which it was shown that, because of continuing education of nursing supervisory personnel, the turnover of other nursing personnel had been considerably reduced. This touched on your question about turnover. Also, as one of the efforts in Rochester, we have been trying to develop a medical directors' group organization, through which we hope to achieve more competence and quality of performance by the physicians who take on the medical director's roles now required in all nursing homes. The key to this is continuing education, and I just wondered whether Dr Sicker could say anything further about potential support — or his views about the role of continuing education and potential support for it in the aging field for various professionals.

Dr Sicker I think that the point is certainly a very valid one, and clearly I think there are means of getting support for continuing professional education. The problem is that our main emphasis has been on beginning-career programs. The question of how you allocate resources — whether on continuing professional education or on primary professional education — is the kind of issue that needs to be resolved by the professionals who are operating in the field. There is nothing to preclude a major emphasis, in resources that are currently available, on continuing professional education than there is on new education. That just has not been the pattern; there is no reason why it could not be.

Dr Jerry Solon (*National Institute on Aging, NIH*) The contrast between the last two presentations could not be sharper in bringing to bear before us how we stand in the United States, as contrasted with the United Kingdom. Dr Sicker indicated several times over that we don't have any chair of geriatric medicine in the United States, in the medical schools. I do think we may have two or three, although they may not be in that form. There is some geriatric education presence, I understand, in two or three schools; I have heard Nebraska, North Dakota, and Hawaii mentioned. But at any rate, to hear Dr Brocklehurst, apologetically of all things, saying that only half of the medical schools in the United Kingdom have departments of geriatric medicine, is stunning to us in this country. Theirs is a vast development from our point of view. I think the major issue that faces us in this country is how we should in the several years ahead prompt and guide the development of geriatric training in the medical schools. There are different forms and models that this might take.

I found something in the program that I would like to inquire about. Dr Exton-Smith and Dr Brocklehurst and Sir Ferguson Anderson have the titles of Professor of Geriatric Medicine. But Dr Evans is listed as Professor of Medicine, parentheses, Geriatrics. I would like to inquire as to whether this reflects some difference in the way the geriatric presence in the medical school is structured.

Professor Grimley Evans There are three threads in the current development of geriatric medicine as an academic discipline in Britain. On the one hand, we have the pre-existing pattern, going back 25 years in which geriatricians were second-line specialists receiving other people's therapeutic failures. This pattern does continue in parts of Britain, although I think it is perhaps becoming less prevalent. The second thread is the idea that geriatrics should be an age-defined specialty — taking either the age 65 or 75 — with the idea that geriatricians should receive and look after all people above that particular age. This is often regarded as being analogous to pediatrics; one might call this the separatist model. And then, rather out on a limb, is the Newcastle pattern, of which, I hasten to assure you, I am an inheritor and not an architect. According to this pattern, geriatric medicine is an area of special interest and, above all else, special responsibility within general medicine. And therefore, in Newcastle, the academic title is of Medicine, brackets, Geriatrics; and all the consultants in geriatric medicine in Newcastle hold appointments as consultants in general medicine as well. My oldest patient at the moment is 102; the youngest is 15½.

It is an area of debate as to which of these three approaches is going to turn out to be the best for the elderly, because this is what it is really all about. It is very important that we don't sacrifice the elderly on the altar of some medical ideology or another. I want to emphasize that I personally have a very open mind about which of these patterns will eventually turn out to be more commonly the best.

We are disturbed about the first pattern, the therapeutic failure pattern, because we think it does not give good care to the elderly if they only meet experts and people interested in their problems, as it were, at second throw. We also feel that this will not give good recruitment to the specialty, because it will really only call upon those with missionary zeal. I don't know whether the American medical profession is better than ours at producing missionaries, but I should be surprised if it were.

The second pattern, of the separatist or parallel system, is conceivably wasteful of resources. If you have to have two coronary care units, one for the over 65s and one for the under 65s, there would seem to be scope for rationalization. And also, we dislike the idea in Newcastle because it seems to be biologically unsound. Pediatrics, a specialty with which the analogy is drawn, is not an age-defined specialty; it is defined by a biological discontinuity, that of puberty. There is no similar change at the other end of life. The problems that people face at 65, 75, or 85 are only exaggerations of similar problems that they face elsewhere in their life.

We think that the third pattern justifies itself in being explored further — and I would emphasize that we are only exploring it; we are not fully committed to it forever. We think it is better for education because we have access to all the nurses and the doctors whether or not they take further post-graduate training in geriatrics. The big difficulty about it, which worries many of those of us who remember British medicine 10 or 15 years ago, is that there was a time when a lot of dual appointments were made between geriatric and general medicine, and in many of these cases the men appointed turned away from their geriatric commitments and spent all their time in so-called general medicine. This was at a time when there were a lot of manpower difficulties, and a lot of the people at that time had, as it were, been dragooned into geriatric medicine commitments because of difficulty in finding posts. I think that phase has now passed, because the Department of Health and Social Security has a more rational manpower policy; so that those of us who have come into geriatrics in recent years are volunteers and not conscripts.

Dr Mary Harper (*Center for the Study of Mental Health and Aging, National Institute for Mental Health*) I have two or three kinds of comments to make. I want to comment first about personnel turnover. I was with the Veterans Administration for 30 years and, we had one of the largest institutionalized populations of over 65 people. Turnover is not only costly in terms of quality of care, but also in terms of employment, salaries, and the like. I did a study on causes of turnover, and found that we were teaching one thing in the classroom setting, but this was not being implemented in the clinical setting. This is the dichotomy that we must take into consideration.

I think that when we talk about dependency, institutional administrative procedures and policies can foster dependency. Let me give you an example. I found, again, that what was taught in the classroom was not being implemented. The head nurse has the pressures of having things ready for grand rounds at ten o'clock in the morning. There is not enough time then to teach the patient, or have the family assist, because there is such a pressure to have everything nice, clean and neat for rounds in the morning. As long as the administration has one set of criteria in terms of what is an efficiently operated ward, and the head nurse has a different set, patient care is going to suffer. Also on dependency, I think it is very important, first, to teach the patient to do those things for himself that he can and is willing to do; second, to teach the staff to do only what the patient can't do. The patient, the family, and the staff must be vitally involved in prevention of dependency.

Edith Robins (*Division of Long-Term Care, Public Health Service*) I wanted to respond to Dr Williams' comments about training. I might give credit where credit is due: the Public Health Service has, since 1971, invested $1.8 million a year in short-term training programs for professionals and para-professionals and for the development of curricula for specialists such as physicians, medical directors, social workers, para-professionals. But I think it is rather significant that at a meeting like this there was no formal representative from The Public Health Service speaking. I can understand it, because the Public Health Service, except for the basic research and the research aspects, has been rather remiss as far as aging goes. But we have a new term in which aging can fit: long-term care. Broadly defined, it takes care of the aging, takes care of the medical and social needs; it also includes the other age groups.

Phyllis Schultz (*Medical Care and Research Foundation, Denver, Colorado*) I was going to comment on the considerable interest and recognition of the role that nursing has to play in the care of the older person; and yet we do not have a significant paper from nursing in the two-and-a-half days of this seminar. That is probably to our deprivation, because there are a number of nurse researchers and nurse educators with a focus on the geriatric patient. Nursing has taken considerable leadership in the study of gerontology, and we have a number of programs in this country now training nurses to deliver primary care to the elderly population — the Geriatric Nurse Practitioner programs. One of the first was at the University of Colorado in Denver, another was at Texas Women's University, and I think a similar program exists in Rochester. And although the federal establishment has seen fit to fund these programs in education, they have not seen fit to fund the appropriate reimbursement mechanism by which nurses delivering primary care can be supported to do that work.

One of the most significant nurse researchers and practitioners in the field of aging is a wonderful lady named Irene Mortonson Burnside, who has just published her most recent book on nursing care of the aged. She has a particular theme that I have yet to hear very much from the speakers in this conference, with the possible exception of Sir Ferguson Anderson and Daphne Krause. And that is that we must learn from the elderly themselves; they will teach us about how to live and grow old both gracefully and intelligently and with vigor. They will teach us about dying and loss and grief, about adaptation, about change. It is with their help that we will teach our professional caregivers.

Dr Robinson Thank you very much. As you pointed out, Daphne Krause did mention the importance of learning from the elderly.

Martin Loeb (*Director of Faye McBeath Institute on Aging and Adult Life, University of Wisconsin, Madison*) Of all the things that I shall take away from this meeting, the most vivid will be what I shall call the Brocklehurst Dream. I spend a good deal of my time trying to get my collegues in the medical school to do something — anything, as a matter of fact — about aging. What I hear mostly has to do with the medical school curriculum. I have been studying professional curricula for many years, and the medical curriculum has its own very special in-bred concerns. I don't know how you get anything added to it at all. What has happened over the last 25 years is that every little piece of the curriculum has been crammed full and nothing has ever been thrown out. And so, the notion that there should be in the undergraduate medical curriculum 60 hours in the field of aging — if I were to take that back to Wisconsin I would be greeted with the wildest gasps that I can imagine. They have, I think, agreed to about six hours of human development — but 60 hours! Well anyway, I will take back this dream.

One other comment: as one looks over the Western world, at least, one notices that the specialty of geriatrics arises almost simultaneously with the innovation of comprehensive health insurance. I think that this comes about because under comprehensive health insurance patients can't be dissuaded from coming. Nowadays, in most medical practices in this country, the elderly patients are dissuaded from using their physicians, not just for financial reasons but because physicians don't know enough and don't like it. The best way of dissuading an elderly patient is to keep on saying, I know it hurts but you are all right for your age. After two or three of those, you don't really come back; or it reasonably isn't worthwhile to come back. But if you have to see them, as national health insurance programs require, then the doctor becomes more interested in how on earth he can make his own life a little better because he knows what to do. And I am pretty sure of this correlation between health insurance and the development of geriatrics.

I have one question, largely to those from the United Kingdom. I want to know why it is that the physician should, in addition to being concerned with the direct health care of his patients, also be an expert in the organization of services and the administration of various pieces of it. It seems to me that that is itself a specialized area, and that we are just burdening the physician with responsibilities that other people could just as well take on; and, if we got someone else to do it, it would leave the physician to the more direct practice of medicine.

Dr Robinson I might ask if Dr Brocklehurst would respond to that.

Professor Brocklehurst I think the last point is a very real one. I think the reason why geriatricians at the moment in Great Britain do have this role, or have taken to themselves this role, of organizing their own unit is because the whole evolution of geriatric medicine in the last 25 years has been one of wielding resources which have very often been diverse, very often inadequate, and trying to create a unified department. I think none of us would have trusted anybody else to do this. Now that we are getting to the stage where we are reasonably established and where there are two and sometimes three and more geriatricians to any particular unit, the question of administration tends to become one person's responsibility rather than that of two or three consultants. Maybe, as time goes by, we will be sufficiently trusting to allow an administrator to take this over. But we are, from our background I think, highly suspicious of everybody, and so we like to do things ourselves.

If I may just say one word about the curriculum, we do in fact teach 60 hours — this past year. The curriculum, although I do agree with you that it is a battleground for establishments and for pressures, nevertheless I think it does evolve slowly. And I think one of the things that happened in Manchester is that we now have so many students that the powers that be are quite happy to share the teaching around, because it is getting almost more than the established teachers in most of the other subjects can cope with.

Dr Robinson Thank you very much. Dr Green, I guess you have the last comment.

Dr Green We have found the way to approach geriatric teaching is not to say we want X hours, but to challenge the whole philosophy of five or six years' training; to say that, for instance, a student should deliver a baby in a taxi better than a taxi driver, but he doesn't need three months of obstetrics. The anatomists and physiologists have reluctantly given up time because they concede that anatomy doesn't need as much dissection at that level. They haven't given it up to the geriatricians, but they have given it up, in a sense, to try and improve the overall curriculum. We have gone together with that, and in fact teach in the first year, with the anatomist if possible; and the students see an elderly person when they are 19. And then for the rest of their time they realize that perhaps this is part of medicine, even if they don't get enough geriatric clinical teaching.

Dr Robinson Thank you very much, Dr Green; and I wish again to thank all the speakers for wonderful presentations.

Introduction to Final Session

Chairmen: Dr David A Hamburg
President, Institute of Medicine

Sir Gordon Wolstenholme
President, Royal Society of Medicine

Dr Hamburg We have had two very interesting, informative and stimulating days. Now we are at that point in the program when we hope to relate the events of the past two days to the formulation and implementation of public policy. As Robert Ball noted in his opening address, there is no sharp focus in the policies of the Federal Government in this country on the problems faced by the three to four million dependent elderly. Instead we have concentrated our attention on guaranteeing at least a minimal income to all elderly persons.

In Great Britain, Margot Jefferys pointed out that it was only recently that special consideration of the elderly emerged in the provision of health and social services. Before that there had been a policy of equal access to the national health service irrespective of age or life situation.

Our increasing knowledge as reflected in the research reports about the genetic and environmental factors relevant to the severe decline in functional ability among that special group of elderly persons who become highly dependent on others to perform the tasks of daily living is helpful in practical ways in the setting of realistic goals. Adopting Dr Birren's and Dr Bellamy's suggestion to view aging from an evolutionary perspective, it is clear that we cannot confidently expect to make substantial inroads on the basic aging process within our lifetime; yet there is clearly a ferment in this research. Clinically and socially we can formulate responses in light of the growing information on the physiology and the psychology of aging, rather than merely reacting negatively to the decline in abilities so stereotypically depicted in the past.

As Drs Brody, Butler and Neugarten have written, the attitudinal component of our policies toward old people reflects a negative reaction to the condition of being old and chronically dependent on others for care. This orientation to the problem really must be drastically modified, and one senses here at this meeting the possibility of doing so.

Along with the necessary reliance on statistics and cost figures to tell us about old dependent people and the services they require, we are fundamentally talking about a value issue. As Dr Maddox told us, looking at the cost of services alone is not a sufficient means of assessing alternatives to our current approaches, because community and home care may be more costly, yet more effective, in maintaining people at a higher level of functioning than would be the case if they were institutionalized. We may have to decide that it is worth it to us to devote more resources to old people in order to improve the qualities of their lives. This is not to say that we should by any means abandon efforts to utilize the existing community services in a creative and low cost way, as evidenced by the work of Mrs Krause at the Minneapolis Age and Opportunity Center.

Nor is it to say that institutional care for the very old and the very sick is inappropriate. We have seen a number of useful distinctions made among that truly heterogeneous population, the elderly, moving away from stereotypes. Rather we should be able to make long-term care, where it is necessary, truly supportive and interactive, stimulating people to preserve whatever independence and coping skills they possess at the point of intervention, and indeed, utilizing learning capacities that have so often been underestimated in the elderly.

This approach represents a remarkable shift from the all too familiar view that long-term care must be merely custodial. To do this sort of thing, to make these changes, it will be necessary to create coalitions among many different groups and care providers in the community. The problem is much larger than any one professional group. No one has a patent on it. It goes beyond any single social institution. If the demographic patterns are a window into the future, the problem can only get worse unless we turn the situation around through innovative public policy initiatives and sustained leadership.

Let us hope that this conference, the ensuing book that will come out of the conference, and our continuing contacts, some of which are shaping up in the course of informal discussions here, can help to provide that kind of leadership.

It now gives me great pleasure to introduce a distinguished participant who has made important contributions to this field over many years. He was recently appointed the first Director of the newest institute at the National Institutes of Health, the National Institute on Aging. Just two or three weeks ago he was awarded a Pulitzer Prize for his book, "Why Survive? Being Old in America", a very critical and constructive policy analysis.

Dr Robert N Butler (*Director of the National Institute on Aging*) There is a world-famous newspaper in New York that sees fit to print only the news that is fit to print. That includes expressions of the dark forces of the unconscious apparently. I was reported in *The New York Times* as the first director of the new National Institute on Dying. I think this informs us of a really major problem with which we are trying to contend in our efforts in research, education and service for the older population.

The National Institute on Aging was established for the conduct and support of biomedical, social and behavioral research and training related to the aging process and diseases and other special problems and needs of the aged. I will mention just one of several motivations of Congress which I think has created a flexible law and mandate for us to operate under in such an encompassing field. "The study of the aging process, the one biological condition common to all, has not received research support commensurate with its effects on the lives of every individual."

So, we are not a service institute *per se*, but that does not mean that we do not have a deep and abiding interest in innovative and creative reproducible studies of alternatives of various types of health and service care delivery.

I have felt some regret over the last several days at the fact that we have had such a rich and very important body of papers and not enough time, to my regret, at least, to have intellectual dialogue and interchange among us, and I hope maybe this will be just the beginning. I know I already have fantasies of establishing a traveling medical show in which I have Sir Ferguson Anderson and Professor John Brocklehurst traveling with me and invading Stanford, Harvard, and Johns Hopkins and Washington University, and trying to help acquaint American medical schools and deans with the epidemiological and demographic reality that we can no longer avoid teaching geriatric medicine in the United States.

Now, just a few thoughts on the topic of this conference, meeting the challenges of dependency in the care of the elderly. Our social, economic, health, research and other institutions and processes were not prepared for the demographic revolution, the rising numbers of people and older people with the twentieth century. Thus, a great achievement long sought by humankind has approached a potential tragedy, but as we have learned these last several days, the genuine crunch apparently would come about 2010, 2020, or 2030. So, we have some lead time in mounting effective biomedical, behavioral and social programs that might help us meet this demographic shift.

If we can take, in other words, this human achievement a few steps further and truly enhance the vigor and productivity of older people, extend middle age, we will find that the nature and the length of the dependency about which we have been speaking will change, the length of the dependency, for instance, decreasing. In that sense, basic research in biology and physiology as represented by the intramural and extramural programs of the new National Institute on Aging and similar institutes around the world will be of great, indeed critical, importance.

From one angle, then, we must not be attentive alone to the characterizations of contemporary older people such as we have heard at this conference, but must have in mind a vision of what older people will become, not, of course, only as a result of research, but also as a consequence of more favorable social and economic conditions, health care, housing, social participation, all so vital to the quality of life in the later years. If we could not hope to increase the vigor and productiveness of our population and the quality of life led, it would indeed be a macabre situation to replicate increasing numbers of older people with the same characteristics and characterizations as now, with frailty, multiple diseases, mental impairments, social adversity, and may I say genuine, in my opinion, although not statistically and officially, pauperization with age, the kinds of circumstances that I try to describe in my public policy book, "Why Survive?"

Still another aspect of the dependent elderly is the question of self-responsibility. Again, research is necessary. What I have called self-care behavior and others health behavior relates to the ancient Roman philosopher Seneca's adage, "Man does not die; he kills himself". We must pay much more attention to preventive medicine, which up to now, in the United States, at least, has meant approximately 4 cents of every dollar spent on health. We must be concerned with lifestyles, with social, personal and physical fitness, which means examining specifically and scientifically, dietary, nutrition, physical fitness, exercise, and the like, and to understand better the incentives to smoking, to overeating, to overdrinking, as well as the disincentives which seem to exist against changing from those habits. Physicians who have tended by and large to be privatistic and arcane, practicing the art of medicine as though it were a mystery, must begin to participate actively in health care education, helping people throughout the course of life to more effectively provide self care for themselves. I do think this probably means we have to reach over the professionals and health-care workers directly to the public and educate them, and they in turn, I can tell you, having been a private practitioner, will bring in the articles from the newspapers and magazines and put the pressure on us.

The third and related point concerning the dependent elderly relates specifically to the direct ways in which dependency can be mobilized, and we need specific research to find objectifying techniques as to the measures of dependency and independency. There are those who are responsively dependent, there are those who very much need assistance and help and have a great deal of difficulty asking for it and securing it, and there are those who exploit their dependency and their impairments to gain attention and to gain what they may need for themselves.

The fourth item that I wish to stress briefly is the significance of family lifestyles. Many have emphasized through these several days the great need to study the family more effectively, which does exist for some 75% of older people in these United States. We must bear in mind that 25% who have out-survived their families and for whom we very much need very specific social and medical assistance. But there are those who do have families, and the families also need specific assistance and we need to have research which will better describe the remarkable diversity of family lifestyles: Black, Norwegian, Spanish heritage, Italian American. We have in our pluralistic society the opportunity for an indigenous anthropology which hardly necessitates our traveling abroad. We should begin to look at such things as differential life expectancy among the various radical and ethnic minorities and at the constructive and restitutional aspects within family life that can be so contributory, as well as some of the deleterious elements.

We must look at the immediate situation insofar as older people are concerned in education, research and service. I am quite clear now in my own mind that we must move to a firmly stated, clear geriatric medical education program, including, of course, not only our medical schools but our nursing schools, our social work schools, and our allied health professions. We have got to understand better the changing immuno-competence with age. We must understand drug–drug and drug–age interaction. We must look at sleep. We must look at investigative medical processes of the most fundamental sort. A whole range of time dependent processes require our examination.

I think a natural social experiment has occurred for some time, namely, the absence of geriatric medicine. I suggest this has been deleterious to the health of older people. Nursing homes have not been a source of research, training and service as we would expect and hope, given the fact that there are more than 1.2 million people, more patients than in hospitals, in nursing, personal care, and foster care institutions. But they are outside the mainstream of American medicine, just as, unfortunately, older people are who have been in state mental hospitals, or even in community mental health centers in the United States. No one seems to quite want the older person, and we do not have them in the mainstream of medicine, and therefore we can't teach our medical students because there is not a medical school in the United States that officially, regularly, predictably has its students proceed through a long-term care institution. It just does not exist. How can we begin to learn something about senile dementia, which accounts in such a devastating way for so many of the people in

American nursing homes, clouding the lives of the older people in the later years with the devastation of their personality, of their identity, and their memory? But the opportunities to look at promising immunobiological leads, the chance to develop more specific data concerning diagnosis, effective diagnosis, because we now know that there are many, many types of senility, and that many of these can be reversible, but only, clearly, with effective diagnosis and treatment.

As a physician in research and clinical practice, one of the ironies of Medicare is that it was set up as though older people were younger people. None of the basic elements of prosthetic care, dentures, which mean so much for nutrition and in turn influence intellectual vigor and may even lead to a fall and a broken hip, all of these basic things, outpatient drugs, are not included under Medicare, nor is long-term care. I know that is debatable about the federalization of Medicaid, which for our English visitors is the state federal program, but the humiliation, the humiliation to so many middle class and poor and other families of having to turn, through a means test, for their continuing care in the "dignity" of their later years, of having to become paupers in order to get care, seems to me to necessitate a sensitive reassessment of the Medicare mechanism for long-term care of older people.

It is interesting, and I think the Institute of Medicine has had some studies on the reimbursement of teaching physicians in American hospitals under Medicare. Frankly I am not convinced that much of the teaching reimbursement money is justified in the sense that our teachers in American medical schools have actually used that money in direct teaching of the principles of a body of knowledge, the corpus of knowledge related to geriatric medicine. I think that money should be used for that purpose. It has been used for all sorts of purposes. The Commission on Malpractice has used Medicare trust fund monies, and maybe with some justification, but certainly not directly related to older people.

One important step, certainly, that we must take is creation of a kind of galaxy, a multipurpose type of network of services throughout the country. We can't any longer afford, we just simply can't afford the enormous economic cost that comes about from fragmentation and confusion of services, and research to help clarify those issues is pertinent.

Another aspect related to dependency is the apparently genuine possibility that our courts may decide that it is unconstitutional on the basis solely of age to deny a person their livelihood. Should this happen, are we prepared for it? How much have our economists, our health economists, those who are concerned with employment, how much have they imaginatively considered what the impact of such judgments might be? Yet, from the perspective of a physician and gerontologist, the extent to which the sense of boredom, of mental dysfunction, of extinction of behavior occurs as a consequence of being outside significant roles, meaningful roles, productive roles in our society is quite apparent.

Three more points and I shall stop. One is a great need to develop a science of prosthetics and bioengineering. Dependency at home for the physically disabled by stroke or by severe arthritis could be overcome by many of the — should we call them earthly spin-offs of the NASA program, some of the kinds of techniques for motion and mobility of body, nutrition, and the like.

In Old English, I understand, and Sir Ferguson might correct me on this, they used to refer to the middle-aged period of life as the period of gravity because they recognized how grave middle age certainly is, with its many responsibilities, with its pressures, both from the young and the care of the young and the care of the old; so this transitional group is an important group for us to study and understand to get clear the dimensions of dependency and independency as it exists in this transitional group.

Finally, as life ebbs the opportunities for older people to look back upon their lives and feel that they have interested listeners willing to pay attention to them is of vital importance. It is not enough, I think, to talk popularly, as we do now, about the right to die, or thanatology, or of the profound existential impact of the psychological meaning of death. Life is really the issue, the kind of life that people have led, the kind of life that yet remains, to reconcile oneself with one's neighbor or with a child or with a brother or with oneself. Even our understanding of the dimensions of independence and dependency will be all the better understood simply by our spending a great deal of time listening, truly listening, to older people as they describe their lives, both in the here and now and as they have lived them.

Dr Hamburg Thank you very much, indeed, Bob. It gives us great hope to know that this Institute exists under your leadership. However modest the scale may be at the moment, the quality is certainly going to be very high. Your remarks about the place of the medical problems of the elderly in medical education certainly are well taken. It would be a very interesting proposition to analyze what constitutes a "good patient" in the various teaching services and specialties. It would not by and large include anyone above 65, with the possible exception of people over 65 of very great wealth. One should add that there are other curious gaps in the life cycle. Early adolescence is one, falling between medicine and pediatrics, between adult and child psychiatry, a crucial time from the standpoint of the formation of health-relevant behavior patterns of the kind you were discussing; very much pertinent to the issues of research on health education and possibilities for prevention of disease in the long run; another curious gap in the life cycle clearly not included in the implicit definition of a good patient.

Social Implications: United States and United Kingdom

Social Implications for the United States of America

The Honorable Barber B Conable
Member US House of Representatives

The fact that the Institute of Medicine has chosen to convene a major conference on the "care of the elderly" is a reflection of the growing concern and distress we all share over our collective inability to contend successfully with this sensitive issue. I say sensitive because these people we clinically describe as "dependent elderly" are, after all, our own parents, relatives and neighbors: people who over the course of their lives have given much of the substance and meaning to the values and expectations our civilization has cultivated concerning individual dignity, whose tenacious regard for the common welfare has become part of our heritage, and who must now reconcile those expectations with the relative neglect of their own individuality and welfare in old age. None of us, I suppose, can be wholly objective or impartial on this issue; it is too close to home, and perhaps too painful to confront directly the spectacle of the transformation of our own elders from active, productive and independent individuals into dependents.

As a legislator who is exposed on a daily basis to the economic, emotional and moral problems encountered by our communities in their efforts to develop viable and humane solutions, I tend to seize eagerly on opportunities like this as a source of illumination and guidance. I am hopeful, therefore, that a review of your deliberations will shed some light on the directions we ought to follow. For whatever niche we may occupy in the political spectrum, we all agree, I think, on the compelling need to structure our society somehow so as to assure that those services and resources needed by our aged citizens are available to them in places where they choose to live, under circumstances which preserve their freedom to choose among acceptable alternatives — and without so depleting our resources as to impair our society's capacity to satisfy the multitude of other needs and desires we have. It's a rather tall order; and it will take a good deal of sober thought and careful planning to fill it.

As some of you know, I too have sought to stimulate serious thought on how to address effectively these questions through workable public programs. Some time ago I introduced a legislative proposal designed to provide a comprehensive program for meeting the variety of long-term care needs of the aged (Congressional Record 1975). I did so not in the conviction that my proposal represented the only, or even necessarily the most desirable approach, but rather in the hope that my proposal would generate a critical response leading to the identification of its deficiencies and to the emergence of soundly conceived improvements and alternatives. Regrettably, this has not happened as quickly or to the extent that I anticipated. An analysis of the response indicates some co-sponsorship of my measure but very little evolution of the idea or additional in-put from the many creative minds that make up the Congress. I doubt that my proposal was perfect as presented, and I would like to encourage constructive response rather than passive acceptance. Nevertheless, I am encouraged by the fact that my proposal has helped to focus attention on these issues. Perhaps, also, it may not be presumptuous to assume that the proposal has some merit and may yet be destined to serve as the catalyst for the development of a program that must inevitably emerge from the Congress.

Allow me, therefore, to turn briefly to the proposal I have been identified with, as a way of getting at what I believe are some of the essential elements that will need to be considered in dealing with this issue.

I take it as axiomatic that there are three types of major problems facing us in this area, each of which poses substantial challenges to our present ways of thinking and doing things. First, we have over the years developed a variety of relatively uncoordinated but expensive programs to meet what we have tended to view as isolated, separable problems of the aged. One consequence of this compartmentalization has been that no single agency or community organization assumes responsibility for identifying individual needs or coordinating the provision of services or even becoming sufficiently informed about available resources to refer individuals properly to those services they may need or want. As a result, older people are often left to their own anguished devices and are too often abandoned or lost in the organizational maze, eventually finding their way to the most visible, but not necessarily the most suitable, service — an institution.

Second, in responding to this largely uncoordinated growth of alternative services, we in government have directed our financing to those same highly visible institutions, allowing the other service organizations to compete with one another for clients in a scramble for financial survival. Sadly, this way was the easy way out. Institutions are not only physically visible, they can also be easily counted, grouped, compared, and evaluated on a series of crude scales such as length of stay, qualified staff and physical plant; they can be inspected and reimbursed in a way that makes us comfortable in terms of accountability. But obviously, a consequence of this approach is that we have created incentives for our aged (and their families) to seek out institutional care, even in those cases where institutional care is neither socially desirable nor medically appropriate. And we have just as surely laid a cost burden on them, even when government picks up a good part of the tab, that is really not necessary. Nor can we overlook the limitation this approach has imposed on the aged individual's freedom of choice — too often he is presented with a choice between institutionalization and total abandonment. At the same time this approach offers the rest of us a way to keep the aged and their troublesome demands out of sight.

Third, we have allowed an artificial distinction between health and so-called non-health or social services to grow up and become fixed in our minds and to influence both our funding priorities and organizational arrangements. Thus, health problems are narrowly defined as the onset of acute illness or the intermittent acute flare-up of a chronic ailment; and we dismiss other activities aimed at preserving health status, assuring free movement, or assisting people to accommodate to inevitable changes in their capacity to cope with the environment as less important social services for the provision of which the community need bear little or no responsibility. And in doing this we have inadvertently downgraded the whole idea of the quality of life in old age, so that we need to feel concerned only when someone is critically ill. Thus we foster an image of old age as a time of crisis and pain.

This is to be sure a bleak picture, and not one that can be substantially improved by a casual retouching job here and there. It may help to explain why I have continued to express the hope that my proposal would stimulate the development of broadly conceived improvements and alternatives.

In essence, my approach attempts to address the problems I have outlined through the adoption of a few simple concepts which, admittedly, would entail the implementation of some significant changes. My proposal, for example, would create a system of community long-term care centers to coordinate and direct the provision of all types of appropriate services for the elderly, including such generally neglected services as homemaker, nutrition, outpatient mental health, foster home, and home health services, as well as institutional care. It would require consultation with the individual and his family to assess his or her needs and desires and provide opportunity for the exercise of an informed choice. It would require these long-term care centers to involve and utilize the services of all relevant professional disciplines in the management of its activities and in the provision and evaluation of services to the aged. It would help to assure the continuity of attention and care that is so sadly lacking these days in far too many communities and families. The proposal attempts to put institutional care back into focus as only one among several alternative services the elderly may need. And it attempts to balance the idea of community obligation and individual responsibility, through a financing mechanism that calls for joint financing by the individuals involved and the general community.

The proposal also puts into a more rational perspective the role of the old people themselves; they will participate in the planning and setting of priorities and in the suggestion of appropriate treatment for the elderly in their community under my bill. One of the great concerns of old people is that others who do not understand the problem — like their children — frequently force them to accept the solutions that are most convenient to the children rather than the ones best adapted to preserve some aspect of their independence as individuals. I think they would be reassured by having a peer group of elderly people participating in a significant role in the functioning of the program.

Certainly one must admit that such a system is today only a blueprint. In many of our local communities the range of services is not available; centers of the type I have described do not exist; and established habits of thought relating to long-term care are likely to persist. But it seems to me that nothing less than some such comprehensive approach will be adequate to the need, and that we will very soon have to make a public commitment.

One final point that to me appears crucial to all our deliberations on this issue is this. Some critics may argue that the needs I have emphasized are only materialistic. But the material improvement of human life, if it is genuinely an improvement, directed toward the increase of comfort, convenience and the availability of service for the aged individual is not something to be despised. Such an increase in comfort, convenience and service is also an increase in dignity and in opportunity for meaningful choice; and these matters are too important to our civilization to be disdained.

Reference

Congressional Record, June 25th 1975, **121**, No. 102

Social Policy Implications for the United Kingdom

Sir George Godber
Late Chief Medical Officer,
Department of Health and Social Security,
London

At this Anglo–American occasion we use more or less the same language and that encourages the hope that there might be a consensus amongst us on the most appropriate solutions to our problems. The discussion has already shown how widely different our approaches have been. They have to be different because our political and social organizations are different. The needs of old people may be broadly similar but the assumptions of our two societies about the propriety and method of social intervention by Government, central or local, are not. Therefore, I must begin by some elaboration of the evolution of the British position and the assumptions upon which our future development is likely to proceed in the hope that this will not repeat too much already said — since I had to write this before seeing the other papers. I do not believe that change in health services occurs by revolution. It is an evolutionary process and more continuous than has been implied here. It is guided — it need not be muddling through.

Public provision for the care of old people began under the Poor Law four hundred years ago, when the religious houses were no longer able to continue in this or any other function. The few old people simply shared such care as was available to any other indigent, but it was a legal responsibility of the locality to provide care. That continued for 250 years as a grudgingly met local charge and the care provided was minimal and deliberately so. After the reforms of 140 years ago the attitude was still so grudging, even minatory, that the final resort to it was feared and resisted by the supposed beneficiaries. This outlook changed only slowly through the next hundred years when the need for care of the elderly rapidly expanded as their numbers grew. In 1900 the calculated expectation of life at birth was only 50 years. The cohorts born from 1880 on, in fact, provided far more survivors, but even in 1950 the proportion of the British population over age 65 was only 10.8%; greater than the US figure today, but little more than three quarters the present figure in the UK.

The change in attitude through the second quarter of this century was radical and it coincided with a change in awareness of the constructive possibilities of care for old people — especially sick old people. Few health professionals who really knew the conditions in the former Poor Law Infirmaries now remain, but by the late 1930s when I first knew them, although the attitude was one of far greater concern than in earlier times, the staff were devoted to custodial care and were unaware of the potential for recovery of function. General practice was the main source of care, but National Health Insurance for the work force did not cover dependents in Britain and general practitioner care for many old people was either privately arranged or out-relief provided by a practitioner employed part-time for a district and usually ill-paid.

Change in public and professional attitudes does not happen abruptly. The changes to which we assign dates are legislative and all too often legislation in such matters lags behind public opinion, although legislators are apt to take the credit for progress. I differ sharply from Dr Maddox in his interpretation of events in the late 1960s in Britain. The origins of change were earlier and the expansion, though geometric, was continuous. What becomes defined in statutes, which enable social policy to be stated, is usually no more than national formulation of something already widely supported. The first formulation of need was in a report of 1956, after a survey in 1953–5, and of national policy in a published programme of 1963. For that very reason statutes in Britain are enabling rather than prescriptive in detail. Therefore, our definition of perceived need and its implications for action is hopefully achievable within the legal powers we have. That is a difference we must recognize — you legislate often and in detail; we legislate seldom, in enabling terms, and rely on continuous adjustment by administrative means. Once the guiding principle of universal entitlement and national provision is established, as it was in 1948, method evolves continuously. Sadly the main deficiencies are in understanding and resources. British legislation in the social and health fields was brought together in a group of statutes of which the National Health Service was one, operative from the middle of 1948 and intended to give effect to the Beveridge Report on Social Security published five years earlier. That was the moment of change, not anything that happened in the 1960s. The principle which imbued all that legislation was that society in Britain had a responsibility to ensure the social and health needs were met: so was established a pattern of financial support over a wide range of needs by a central department using funds derived partly from an insurance fund and partly from taxation. Robert Ball described how much the US has done to ensure income but in the UK health services were also mainly supported from taxation and social welfare services from local government agencies using funds about equally derived from central government grants and from local taxation. Subsequent changes have continued this pattern, but with the central responsibility for health becoming more dominant, and a broadening pattern of social welfare better coordinated locally by the changes of 1972–3. All the services consume an increasing share of public expenditure; health expenditure increased between 1953 and 1973 by 141% in real terms, social security by 159% and personal social services by 506%, compared with an increase of 274% in expenditure on education and in general a doubling of public expenditure as a whole. Previous papers have shown how much more could be done if funds were available. Since resources are and will be finite and limited, it is clear that we cannot expect each and all of these desirable activities to grow as those involved in them would wish. We have to think in terms of the best balance between the components to secure the greatest advantage to old people within the total available. Neither health, nor social welfare services nor social security cash benefits can claim automatic priority. David Newell gave some inkling of the difficulties of those choices and Margot Jefferys of the attempts the present government is making to secure agreed choices.

It might seem a logical solution to leave local government to make the choices in spending the resources available to each locality because in the final analysis individual choices are made there. But there are large differences between the wealth of localities from their own tax resources which have to be adjusted by differing grants from central tax funds. Insurance systems such as those of France and Germany bring in money for some purposes in amounts related to the population. France can group the services within a social budget funded largely from social insurances. Britain cannot, under its present system, and does not even have social welfare under the same management as health. Professor Grimley Evans seemed to imply this was mistaken, but I have no doubt that at this juncture it is necessarily so. Social security cash benefits derive partly from insurance (about $\frac{3}{4}$) and partly from central taxation (about $\frac{1}{4}$) and the largest single component comprises retirement or old peoples' pensions which together cost about £4 $\times 10^9$ in 1974–5. If one looks at the present budget for health, personal social services and social security in Britain, health accounts for about one-third, social security for just over three-fifths and the balance goes to personal social services. The forecast of public expenditure to 1979–80 contemplates a reduced total but a slightly increased proportion for health, a greater increase for personal social services and more still for social security payments. This reflects government's belief that the shortfall in provision is most hurtful there.

Somehow the different contributions to the care of old people which these three elements represent have to be brought into the best balance we can devise. Unfortunately, this is one of the points where political considerations can affect decisions which should be made on other grounds. Cash allowances, for instance, may have a strong public and especially electoral appeal and also are the least likely subjects for economy in times of financial stringency. Social forms of service may be more easily understood than technical health requirements, so that the very real need to provide a homely atmosphere in a geriatric unit may take precedence over the provision of active rehabilitation which might allow more to return home. *Vice versa* the provision of a very costly apparatus for radiotherapeutic treatment of cancer may attract outside financial support where a potentially far more fruitful campaign against the cigarette as a cancer producer does not. This only emphasizes the difficulty of providing the best synthesis; however difficult we must still try to do it and I do not think we have said enough about this. No one of us has exclusive access to wisdom, indeed each of us — political, sociological or medical — has his or her own bias. Maybe the elderly know best but which of us asks them. Daphne Krause made this point and it was reiterated in discussion.

The trends in Britain during the last 25 years have been notably different from those in some other countries. In keeping with the increasingly specialized nature of medical and other professional work in hospital, the medical specialty of Geriatrics has been encouraged and has grown from the least recognized to one of the larger non-surgical sub-specialties — almost as large as paediatrics. Professor Brocklehurst stressed this yesterday but I would emphasize that it could only happen fully with medical concurrence, which became general only slowly. The hospital admission rate at later ages has increased but the duration of stay has fallen as more medical and allied effort has been mobilized. Although the use of beds in geriatric wards has been intensified and one bed is used in a year by as many patients as used two in 1949, more than four-fifths of patients aged over 65 are admitted to other wards of General Hospitals. Professor Grimley Evans spoke of the boundaries of geriatric medicine yesterday, but this needs emphasis. Among the older patients admitted are some who stay a very long time so that the average cost of hospital care of geriatric patients is more than twice as great as the average cost of patients with acute illness. Although many of the elderly patients in hospital have the same kinds of mental illness as younger people, others suffer from confused states up to the level of advanced senile dementia so that there are special psychiatric needs of the elderly. The new specialty of psycho-geriatrics has now developed as Tom Arie described and its exponents are finding — as did the geriatricians and psychiatrists earlier — that many of their patients can recover to levels which permit return home. Its functions and its relationships with other specialties, general practice and the social services have been reviewed recently by Colin Godber (1975).

The establishment of out-patient services and day hospitals were natural developments of active geriatric services as they had been in psychiatric services. The number of new out-patients doubled in ten years. Home visits for consultation before admission are used in geriatrics and psycho-geriatrics but I do not think we have emphasized that general practitioners regard their own house calls as essential to home care.

All these developments add up to a smaller amount of hospital time being used in support of the average elderly person than 25 years ago even though that person is older now, but to a far greater concentration of professional efforts in that time. By comparison Sweden, with only a marginally greater proportion of persons aged over 65 in the population, has three times the ratio of beds in hospital for long-term physical illness and a similar advantage — if that is the right word, perhaps one should say burden — in accommodation in old peoples' homes. In Sweden the ratio of psychiatric beds to population is also much larger than in Britain. Here are two countries each with comprehensive health and welfare services available to all without financial deterrent. Britain at any one time accommodates in hospitals or old peoples' homes, including private homes, about 4% of the population aged over 65, whereas Sweden provides through similar means for three times that proportion. Much of the British publicly provided hostel accommodation is of modern construction, whereas most of the hospital accommodation is at best partially modernized.

These contrasting systems pose the fundamental policy question. There is no reason to think British old people need less care than Swedish — except that Sweden has more of the very old. The Swedish population is more widely scattered than the British and home care services are less easily organized. I am a little puzzled by Dr Maddox's figures and would like to check the information. A far higher proportion of Swedish than of British medical manpower is to be found in hospitals, but there is a good public health nurse service. Sweden spends a much larger proportion of the GNP on health than does Britain — perhaps 50% more. But the main reason for the difference has been the deliberate policy over the last thirty years in Britain of keeping and building on a domiciliary support service especially through general practice. The demographic and geographical factors are secondary to this.

Sweden provides the bench mark by which other countries tend to judge their successes in the health field — though it could equally well be Norway or Iceland or even the Netherlands. When we make this kind of comparison we should remember why Sweden's mortality figures are more favourable. It is chronic respiratory disease, malignant disease — especially of the lung — and coronary artery disease which are mainly responsible. British men smoke on average more than twice as many cigarettes as Swedish men. They die early from causes which medical science cannot influence much, but preventive medicine could. There is no reason to believe that the provision of many more hospital beds should be the objective in Britain though there should be some more and much replacement. Since there is no indication that British elderly people seek many more hospital admissions than are now available to them although many suffer delay over elective surgery — there is no valid technical reason to change our policy. We certainly should try to reduce the delay over, for instance, cataract operations or arthroplasties of the hip — respectively 20% and 30% of patients wait over six months. This is not to say there are enough hospital admissions or geriatric beds and many of the existing wards are not good enough. It is to suggest that increases should be modest and the main effort should go into making the hospitals better — especially in amenities and nursing and rehabilitation facilities. We could use the numbers we have much better than we do now. A recent consultative document published for England by the DHSS appears to have fallen into an old error of setting too much store on increasing long-stay beds. The same attitude surrounded mental illness provision 25 years ago. The over 65s need the services of the other specialties at least four times as often as they need geriatrics.

In our concern for the well-being of old people in hospital, however, we must not make the mistake of concentrating only on conditions for which patients enter geriatric wards or their equivalent. Only one-sixth of patients over 65 admitted to general hospitals in England and Wales enter such wards; even in the over 75 age group just over one-quarter enter such wards. One-quarter of the patients admitted to all wards other than obstetric and psychiatric are aged over 65. The hospital contribution to the care of old people is, therefore, mainly through such services as are also used by young people. If choices must be made because of overall shortage most patients will benefit from good general hospital services. It is the old question — three-quarters of the over 65s are treated in one-half of the total beds used by them. It is a regrettable aspect of this that "acute" specialists consult their geriatric and psycho-geriatric colleagues too seldom and too late, from sheer ignorance of social factors in the illness of old people. This sort of statistical exercise is endlessly wearisome, but it must be borne a little, because so many wrong conclusions are reached on the basis of superficial judgements about areas of greatest needs.

Nevertheless high technology in hospitals does compete for the limited funds available with simpler forms of care which help many more people. The technology is likely to be highly expensive in proportion to the actual benefit conferred on a few individuals. It must be conserved and used on a regional scale for the real benefit of patients and never for the greater glory of their professional attendants. I commend to you a recent letter from Dr I R Lawson in the *Lancet* (Lawson 1976). He describes a "low income elderly" patient in the United States who went through $6000 worth of in-patient hospital care to emerge with a recommendation for a gluten-free diet but still without attention to the broken denture and some other disabilities for which he really needed help he had not received. It was difficult to get him meals on wheels at $10 a week, but says Dr Lawson "I can get him an endoscopy or a hospital work-up any time". We can do the ordinary things for the majority of the patients all the time. Our highest priority should be to do them better, with less delay and with greater consideration. That is what hospitals are for. It is especially what geriatric medicine is for and maybe the nurses and the general practitioners know that even better than the physicians. I must say that I greatly regret the absence of a general practitioner and both a hospital and a home nurse from the British team. Not all geriatric units make the best of what they have and we need to foster the best as demonstration units — a point well taken by Sir Keith Joseph when he was Secretary of State for Social Services. But the geriatric units should be in the general hospital with the other specialties notwithstanding their links with many beds in outlying units for long-term care.

In the British context the solution chosen remains the use of hospital facilities only where this is necessary and then intensively with the object of restoring the patient to the best level of function he can reach and in a residential situation usually of his own home — perhaps in purpose-built housing, failing that, in a residential group home and only in a hospital ward as a last resort. That this has long been recognized is reflected in the five-fold increase in expenditure on personal social services in the last twenty years, though this is still far from sufficient. The forecast allows for double the rate of increase in this area by 1979–80 as compared with the increase in strictly health expenditure, but of course, they are inter-linked.

Is there any reason to change this policy, which is indeed in line with the policy toward hospital accommodation for other age groups? If this discussion leads us to endorsement of the present policy — as I think it must — the implications for future social policy are clear. Hospital facilities and staffing must be planned to this end. Residential accommodation other than private houses must be planned, distributed and staffed in a way best suited to carrying out the larger share of long-stay support which will fall to them. Support for those able, despite handicap or frailty, to live independently or with their families, in special housing, or with assistance by social welfare staff, meals on wheels or some kind of discreet surveillance and cash allowances must be available. Good neighbourliness and family support already provide far more than the organized services and at an earlier stage, but not for everyone, and there is room for more voluntary intervention here, as several speakers have emphasized. Health care in Britain is part of the public services and the most important component in it is general practice in that broader sense which includes home nursing. There are other reasons why one would hope that the practice of making house calls will not be reduced in Britain as it has in the US, but in the care of old people it is crucial. Moreover, the emergence of the doctor/nurse/health visitor group in British general practice is peculiarly well fitted to the needs of the elderly — especially if it is used as described by Law and Chalmers (1976) in a recent study of people aged 75 years old and over.

The panel is better equipped than I am to discuss these different aspects and I will only attempt to suggest directions of change in each. The order in which I have introduced them is in inverse proportion to their social contributions to the total pattern of care.

Obviously the first requirement for the seven-and-a-half millions aged over 65 is that they should have sufficient funds for their support, be acceptably housed, warmed and fed and, as Dr Butler emphasizes, occupied usefully. The Social Security cash support includes both basic retirement, old people's or widow's pensions and supplementary pensions for those with demonstrable need. So long as the old person is mobile and mentally competent this is meant to be sufficient to meet the rent, food and the other ordinary expenses of living. But everything depends on the social competence of the individual or couple and that may diminish with age or abruptly on the death of one spouse. There are arrangements to pay constant attendance allowances to help the family cope, but there are also many ways in which support — especially voluntary support — can move in unobtrusively if family support is insufficient, and we must not let the burden on families overwhelm them. For that there must be awareness, for the individual may not relish intervention which he or she thinks signals a decline not yet accepted. Having lived most of my life in two small villages, I know how much easier that setting is, but four-fifths of the British population are not villagers. We have much to learn from the way in which health aides of various non-professional kinds work in countries such as the USSR and China. But formal registration and intrusive surveillance are not wanted.

Once need is recognized there is a wide range of direct support — meals on wheels, domestic help in the home, home nursing. Half-a-million old people receive each of these reliefs in a year and even if this may be less than a million separate individuals it is still a far larger proportion of the old than any other service except general practice touches. That it is insufficient is well shown by the occurrence of deaths from hypothermia every winter. It should be a major concern to improve our knowledge of, and support for sound nutrition and adequate warmth for the old. Over a million old people are given chiropody treatment in a year. There is a nice balance to be struck between support for the individual's own actions through cash allowances related to need and actual provision of meals or space heating. A recent study has shown that in winter body temperatures of a sample of old people living at home were on average slightly lower than those of a similar group living in hostels. Professor Exton-Smith brought out this and much else in his paper. An earlier follow-up study of a group of women in their eighties living alone revealed that physical and mental state of those on a good diet was better maintained over a seven-year period than in those on a poor diet. Which was cause and which effect none could say; but for all the potential benefits in the remote future from our concern with abstruse biochemistry and rat encephalography, the work in California, which was not mentioned, on the benefits of a better life-style in middle age, seems far more important (Belloc 1973).

There are many ways of supporting those living at home, up to group homes with warden surveillance. Eventually hostel-type accommodation becomes necessary with all its social problems. There are more than twice as many elderly hostel residents as there are patients in wards for the chronic sick, but rather fewer than in all hospital beds on a particular day. There is a shortage of places even though we do not aspire to the Swedish level of provision; we probably need to modify our policy of concentration as the DHSS consultative document proposes. That need will become greater as the numbers aged over 75 increase — perhaps by one-third in the next 25 years. The most difficult area may well be that of liaison between hospital and hostel — a matter of administrative coordination which should be easy, but is too often as cranky as the human race can be.

Very little is known about changes in the frequency or severity of frailty at later ages. Some psychiatrists believe that senile dementia is now arising at later ages than formerly. Margot Jefferys mentioned the progressive decline in psychiatric admissions of old people. Certainly blindness is certified less frequently than the age of the population would have suggested on earlier experience and Professor Ferguson Anderson quoted work listing a dozen other conditions which now occur later. The average age of patients in long-stay wards has risen steadily and we have a substantially higher proportion of old people living at home now than in 1948. This may be due to better care at an earlier stage than before the NHS, to better supporting services or to later onset or slower progression of degenerative disease. Obviously the last is the explanation we would hope to justify, but it is not supported by the continuous increase in the proportion of men aged 64 who have already been certified unfit to work for a year or more; that is now one-eighth. Any effective prevention of degenerative disease should have the highest priority — but most of the contribution would come from changed life-style — smoking, abuse of alcohol, physical inactivity, overweight, failure to use fluoridated water. Bjork has shown that Swedish men gain their greatest advantage in longevity over British or American men from the fact that the increase in myocardial infarction with age occurs five or six years later in Swedish men. There is great scope for prevention that could help young adults in their later lives. Help for the old now can only come from earlier service to limit disability.

This brings me finally to the factor in care of old people within the NHS which I deem by far the most important — better use of general practice in its widest sense. By general practice I mean a practice of doctors with nurses and closely linked with the social services. The geriatric, psychiatric and psycho-geriatric services can only work effectively if supporting and supported by general practice. They are central, as the hospital is central, but they are the support and not the main service. It follows that those entering general practice must be properly trained in this most important part of the work: indeed all physicians should know it. That means that pre-qualification and vocational training in medicine must include sufficient exposure to the community and institutional components of this work and an appreciation of the still greater social service component. Moreover, the rate of progress in medicine — especially in therapeutics — is unlikely to diminish, and that makes continuity of education for all physicians essential — especially for general practitioners who need to know most. All the health professions must share in this.

My orientation is toward the health side of the provision we make for the elderly, but it is, if anything, the less important component. The health services are part of the wider field of social services, but too often they operate as if they were not only separate, but over-riding in importance. Even within health institutions for long-stay care the social component is of great importance and too often neglected. In both our countries the great majority of members of the present generation will grow old and commonly infirm before they die. Support in that infirmity and even its postponement is more social than medical. Housing, domestic help, nutrition, warmth, and even continuing human relationships may be far more important to active survival than all our medical technology. The social view may well emphasize activity even at risk of final breakdown rather than technological effort to postpone death. We all of us need a little humility among ourselves and most of all before our clients or patients — perhaps the administrators and planners most of all.

As you all know the local administration of health services in Britain is in the hands of appointed authorities and centrally financed; whereas the personal social services are administered by elected local councils and partly financed by them. It is often said that this is a wrong and harmful division. As of the present, this is not true. The advantages to my mind, heavily outweigh the disadvantages on both sides. There are disadvantages and we may one day reach a point when local government evolves a further stage and the two can combine. But I believe a regional and district level would be necessary for that. The present compromise must continue at least well into the 1980s, and, I suspect, longer than that.

This talk has not pulled things together for you, but I hope it has given something for the panel members to bite on. One of them, Michael Green, has published a far better synthesis (Green 1975). The presentation I have chosen is historical because I am convinced that that perspective of our further evolution is essential. There are no slick solutions; we must build as we can on the foundations of what we have.

References

Belloc, N. B. (1973). *Preventive Medicine* **2**, 67–81

Godber, G. (1975). *Journal of the Royal College of Physicians* **10**, 101–112

Green, M. (1975). "Specialised Futures: Essays in honour of Sir George Godber, GCB." OUP: *Nuffield Provincial Hospitals Trust* pp 99–153

Law, R. and Chalmers, C. (1976). *British Medical Journal* **1**, 565–568

Lawson, I. R. (1976). *Lancet* **i**, 481–482

Panel Commentary

Michael Green

Royal Free Hospital, London

The message we must take from this conference is a compelling need to inform and instruct and demand from politicians and health and social service administrators. One memory I will take back. I turned on my television and a commentator said: "Have you a confused elderly relative? He may be remediable". We do not have that in Britain. We have hardly any media involvement in instruction and education about old age.

We are often reminded that self-interest for the future should persuade us and politicians to improve services for the elderly. Physical disability and dementia are no respecters of persons, but are we prepared to admit our mothers to geriatric wards and nursing homes? I have seen some fairly opulent nursing homes here, but in general the difficulties in staffing, in fabric, in food of many of these institutions would certainly outweigh the benefits of a multidisciplinary team.

The problems of institutions fostering excessive dependency have been mentioned, and I would suggest that so-called homes are not homes, however good their accoutrements, and admission to them should largely be restricted to those who really do need physical and mental support, and the admission should be only after very careful assessment aimed at treating any remediable problems so as to preclude admission.

At present I suspect that we are not only admitting or forcing some old people into these "homes" unnecessarily, but are missing some disabled, dependent, depressed people who need help and might reluctantly leave their own homes and move into sheltered accommodation or even a residential home. The non-white group in the US has been mentioned, and I wonder whether this is a group where many of these lost souls could be found, poorer than average, rejected by doctors for acute and preventive care, and with diminishing family ties.

As well as talking about dependency, I want to make a point that we should be talking about a national health service rather than a national illness service. Although we have talked about dependency, we really have to have preventive measures and measures for the health as well as the national illness service aimed at maintenance of even limited independence. In the preventive area I will just mention screening in the elderly. You all know the principles of screening — that you must look for easy things — eyes, ears, teeth and feet are very easy things to look for, but you cannot do this by telephone. You cannot see the breakfast on the spectacles unless you look at the person wearing them.

Of course, we are dealing with a range of problems from the purely medical, physical, mental, through medical-social, malnutrition, poverty, locomotor disability, housing, heating, to purely social and philosophical. We have recently described a Diogenes syndrome where people refused help. They wanted to opt out of society.

An important point about geriatric practice in the UK is the visiting at home. Even General Practitioners do it, reluctantly. Our department does some 250 home visits a year to offer specialist advice to General Practitioners, and sometimes this visit does not just give you an idea of how the person lives. It stops them from coming to hospital and this is an important cost point. It really may prevent unnecessary admission.

In our hospital department patients have almost twice the number of things wrong with them that Professor Williamson found in his community studies. We use a problem-orientated system to record what is going on, not only to allow me to do a ward round without anybody else there, but to help everybody cope with all the problems of handling information about old people. In the States, of course, Professor Weed's system has rather been diverted into checking on the reimbursement system. Perhaps that is unfair. When I look in my colleagues' wards and other hospital wards, I find people who did not need to come into hospital and yet my colleagues complain about the number of old people in their wards. This is another point about admission and assessment and diagnosis beforehand.

Hospital is a very expensive resource. My department costs the equivalent of $100 000 a week to run. That is a lot of money and we are not really very businesslike about it. We need to monitor and challenge the cost-effectiveness of caring for people in hospital, not only in terms of money, but in terms of resources. In the end, it is going to be whether you can get incontinence nurses for night as well as whether you are able to pay them. We are looking at various experiments of how people look after themselves in long-stay wards, how sheltered housing should exist, perhaps getting six flats in an existing block converted when they become vacant rather than hopelessly expecting a big, purpose-built block to be produced from somewhere.

We stressfully manipulated the environment in one experiment and took incontinent people out to a shopping centre. They managed to be continent for three hours and were less confused. It was just a new thing to try.

There is an important point I want to make. We go on about age, but old people are individuals. In practice I forget about the ages of my patients. I know where they live and what is wrong with them, but I cannot remember whether they are 93 or 92. But on the other hand, the paradox is that we do need to know about old people because advancing chronological age does have very serious problems in terms of mental deterioration, for instance. In some of our hypothermia work, where we thought there were various factors connected with cold injury, it is probable that many of these are in fact a function of old age: the poverty, the isolation, the medical problems. In fact, the common link is the age of the person, the chronological age.

Various facts that we should not accept at face value — we mention sleeping. There are different EEG patterns. We have found, in fact, that people sleep in the daytime if they are old. That has got implications for the staff and the people in homes and hospitals. About 50% of elderly people get up at night to go to the lavatory and that, too, may affect the EEG, but it is an important practical point.

I am not going to refer to much literature, because there is a vast amount, but I want to refer to three things which might be relevant to people going away from this conference. One is the Age Concern booklets, the manifesto on the place of the retired and the elderly; Professor Brocklehurst's book, "Geriatric Care in Advanced Societies", which covers a lot of the ground we should be thinking about here; and Nicholas Bosanquet's short pamphlet on "A New Deal for the Elderly". These have got some of the facts, some of the discussions about the elderly, and about policies.

I want to make a very crucial point. I think one of the main needs that has been expressed here, and I have an absolute obsession with it, is the need to relate training and education of students, medical students, qualified doctors and, for the want of a better word, other "careers" to the real needs of their patients and not just continue in the same old rut.

I think we need to continue to expand in the UK, and the US needs to start — I am being rude — training in medicine, nursing, sociology in old age, in and out of hospital. A cadre of specialized geriatricians should continue to have their own little empires, but also somehow continue to be involved with old people in other departments. There are 60 people with strokes in my hospital, 30 in my beds and 30 in other wards. That is a particular group we should be concentrating on in general policy planning, in the choice of drugs and so on.

I would like to summarize. There are different ways of compartmentalizing things. The dependent elderly can only, to my mind, live and die in three compartments — their own domicile with or without friends or relatives or support; in some specialist accommodation — sheltered housing, residential homes, whatever you call them; in hospitals. These are three compartments that we need to review to identify our priorities to see what sort of style we want to make each compartment and how people move between them.

Another way of dividing and marshalling our thoughts about elderly people is under four heads. First, service needs. We should use people in their 50s, 60s and 70s to care, to help, to contribute to the 70s, 80s and 90s. Second, education we have mentioned. Third, politics and politicians and the elderly themselves. Why do the elderly in our country not have a Party, have more political power, have a Minister, have the sort of strength they have in some other countries? I do not know; perhaps David Hobman will mention that. We should also mention research, some of it mundane, some of it exhaustive. A recent survey showed that old people benefit from having pets. When they had budgies and they died, they replaced the budgies. When they had begonias and they died, they did not, so they got depressed. That was one sort of research at a good, practical level.

Finally, I would like just to return to education. I am a young man, perhaps, but geriatrics is exciting. Care of the elderly is exciting. It is not just a matter of worry and sadness and depression with the problems we have. I am looking for one of the lapel badges people are going around with saying "I am getting better with age". I think I feel like that.

David Hobman

Age Concern, London

The Washington Post carries a story today about the apparent failure of 75% of 7000 hospitals to put into effect a patients' "Bill of Rights" recommended by the American Hospitals Association three years ago.

I do not know the essence of the Charter, and, of course, terms such as patients' or pensioners' rights can be very emotive in relation to current debates about student power, the power of labour, and of other forces which work within and without the traditional mechanisms of decision-making in contemporary society.

Some of these groups, which may well represent the consumers of the health and social services, in the context of this conference, often function without the benefit of the advice of administrators, professionals and researchers; but many of them do not need to study the results of an in-depth study on deprivation to know that their money will run out before the end of each week or that there is no adequate home in which they can find a degree of comfort and personal fulfilment.

Their inability to relate may not require the services of a psychotherapist, but as Ferguson Anderson suggested an extra twelve inches of hand-rail. John Brocklehurst referred metaphorically, if not literally, to the pleasures of good brandy and a cigar: by implication, to the importance of living a little dangerously which gives a continued sense of meaning and purpose to life; in spite of the health educators' serious and responsible advice about many of the hazards from which we must be protected.

Perhaps it was the consumer's perception of the many good things on offer which has been the only missing element in this otherwise stimulating and full agenda.

It may well be argued that this is not the time or the place for the consumer's view to be aired and that there are adequate opportunities for consumer inputs to be made whether they are spontaneous or now part of the whole process of consultation. For example, in England through the recently established Community Health Councils which provide one interesting model.

Sometimes the process of consultation is more symbolic than real: when conversations with consumer representatives take place after plans have been formulated or even finalised, although there is increasing evidence of their influence: but in the final analysis, judgements and decisions about services still largely reflect the views of relatively small élitist groups whose social economic and cultural values may differ widely from those on whose behalf they administer. Once it was the Church and the long tradition of middle-class philanthropy; at best caring and compassionate; at worst, judgemental and patronizing. Then came the social activists, at best looking for the new millenium and an egalitarian society; at worst, harsh, cruel and destructive. And now, the professionals; at best skilled and sensitive; at worst management obsessed, system orientated, sunk in a slough of cost-benefit analysis.

What each successive approach seems to have failed to acknowledge is the fact that someone who has managed to survive 60, 70 or 80 years has also assumed some skills in an albeit random, untidy, unrecorded process, based on the accumulation of experience, who would find greater satisfaction in continuing to function as an independent agent; for whom the capacity to shuffle round to the shop at the corner, to fumble at the stove and to produce a not very nutritious plateful of food; perhaps even to continue to play the role of host may represent better medicine than some of the more clinical alternatives. The argument is perhaps analogous to the debate about the degree to which the benefits of pet-owning, in terms of good psychotherapy, outweigh the hazards of parasitology.

Sir Ferguson Anderson, describing the physician's role, rightly stressed the importance of identifying the patient's social circumstances. Elaine Brody referred to the inter-dependence of the agency and the environment. Put crudely this means that skilled diagnosis, prognosis and treatment are not merely dependent upon technology, drugs, and rehabilitation programmes. They cannot be administered in a vacuum. They have to be related to the conditions in which people live, or to which they must return.

The prescription of a balanced diet is useless unless it is related to the capacity to pay for special food; to shop for it; to be able to purchase it in suitable quantities and store it, as well as the ability to cook it.

Recognition of the need for sustained social relationships for the elderly isolate is of little use if life on the first or the thirty-first floor is the extent of the horizon for someone who is dependent upon fast disappearing or inconveniently designed public transport.

The need for sustained warmth may be recognized in relation to the prevention of hypothermia; but there are no cures for those who live in damp or uninsulated rooms and, as Margot Jefferys and others said, it is the elderly who are most likely to live in substandard accommodation.

The physician must, therefore, be conscious of the wide range of services, the effectiveness of community-based agencies and the contribution of other professional skills involved in the problem-solving process as well as in the prevention of breakdown. This is well understood by the most experienced geriatricians; but it has not, perhaps, been sufficiently acknowledged at this conference, which has lacked contributions from a number of critical areas including the personal social services, nursing, education, architecture, planning, marketing and the churches as well as other disciplines; many of the multiple disabilities associated with aging may demand multi-professional solutions.

It is true that references have been made to the need for a multidisciplinary approach and to the role of the doctor as a teacher in community medicine and health education; but less has been said about the extra-curricular skills the doctor needs to draw upon and about his role as a social advocate because, in the final analysis, it is political judgements which ultimately determine the allocation of available resources, rather than the application of management theories when making decisions about their amounts, priorities and the way they are to be distributed. This point was recently made by a senior British civil servant in relation to the personal social services, but it applies equally well to health.

The argument here, therefore, is not just for an increase of time in the medical schools for the teaching of geriatric medicine or for the schools of social work to accept that human growth and development do not finish at the threshold of adulthood, but to see doctors involved in the poverty lobby; influencing schools of architecture to put people before aesthetics or in helping the clergy to accept that they might be better deployed in counselling the living to assist the dying and in breaking the conspiracy of silence which has come to surround death in a pluralist secular society.

The basis that death is the point of departure and the growing recognition that social policies will increasingly need to concentrate on the very old "at risk" group could well suggest that a more dynamic policy for aging might be to work backwards from the end, from the final moment until the point at which service is needed, rather than in taking the arbitrary chronological date at which services for the elderly begin: this is both irrelevant and psychologically damaging. The phased introduction of services at a considered pace, which recipients could absorb without an overwhelming feeling of social incompetence, should be offered at a point in time at which some, at least, of the options remain open and a reasonable degree of choice can still be exercised.

Here I want to go back to two early contributions. Firstly to Margot Jefferys, who concluded her analysis of the needs of others by describing her own in retirement as far as she was now able to anticipate them. She implied that she did not relish the geriatric label which society would hang around her neck when she reached an arbitrary birthday. She wants to continue to be seen as a creative personality with intrinsic qualities; but in a work-ethic society, as things stand at the moment she is likely to be devalued because she will no longer be part of the wealth-producing process. Margot Jefferys did not say so, but I believe she would also resent the sentimentality associated with old age so closely identified with the silver threads/autumn leaves ethos based on the notion of low expectations, limited social functioning and a passive acceptance of whatever crumbs may fall from the working man's table.

Indeed, one of the the problems facing the current generation of elderly retired people is not merely the "mis-match" of too much or too little, as George Maddox described the position; but their ready acceptance of standards of service and a life-style which those who are younger, more sophisticated, manipulative and better educated, would not tolerate.

In a manifesto of the place of the retired and elderly published in the United Kingdom in 1975 by Age Concern, it was suggested that the most powerful motivating force for social change is enlightened self-interest — the point in time at which providers of services begin to perceive themselves as consumers. This has always been true in any reforming movement. It had a profound influence on the child and maternal welfare services. Now we must hope the same thing will happen with the elderly, stimulated by changing attitudes within society; by the same process within the caring professions and, most important, when those increasingly significant organizations of the retired which reflect a much more potent force in the United States than in Britain begin to make their presence felt in social policy making and planning.

Margot Jefferys and Nelson Cruikshank in the panel commentary yesterday both made reference to the vital element of occupation amongst the elderly in relation to health.

For some people continued employment after the statutory retirement date may be economically necessary; but for many more it can provide a stimulus and a continued role in the community. The majority of retired people who wish to work are not a threat in terms of increasing unemployment amongst the young; but although the Trade Unions have played a valuable and positive role in urging higher state pensions, in neither the UK nor the US do the Unions appear to have been active in the debate about the need to change the legislation which reduces pension entitlements in relation to earnings during the first five years of retirement and which acts as a powerful disincentive.

But there are many variations on the employment front, ranging from increasing voluntary service amongst the young retired to mutual-aid, barter and co-operative schemes in which they can pool their skills for their own benefit as well as for those of their wider community. There are a number of interesting innovative schemes in this field, including one which uses the exchange of stamps for time and service given, rather than cash.

It was inevitable that any conference discussing the health or personal services should be concerned with the amount of financial resources available as well as the basis of their allocation. In this connection there is perhaps one important point to make about the relative merits of community care over institutionalism. Whilst there can be no doubt that policies should reflect a philosophy of extended independence in terms of its social desirability, it is arguable whether it would be less costly than institutionalized care if the full range of domiciliary services were readily available at a sustained level. Arguments about community care should not, therefore, simply be based on crude cost-effective yardsticks; but on assessments which relate to the quality of the life-style of those to whom they are directed. By the same token, voluntary service should not be seen as a cheap alternative to under-manned public services but as a crucial element in community enterprise in recognition of the fact that the recruitment, deployment and support of volunteers is itself a skilled and demanding task.

Finally, the title of this conference, "the challenge of dependency", might perhaps more appropriately have been stated in terms of a better understanding of interdependency. Dependency as such is not itself necessarily negative or unacceptable. It is only when the terms on which service is offered are unacceptable, or the needs of those who provide it take precedence over those who receive it, that it may become intolerable. Dependency on those in whom one has trust, or holds in affection, with whom exchanges are reciprocal, are important at all stages of life; but in none more than in old age, as an elderly lady illustrated when complaining about the inconvenience of the need to be at home on Thursday afternoons because she did not know what her well-meaning voluntary visitor would do if she were out! This comment seems to epitomise the underlying nature of the mutuality of relationships at a personal and professional level which need to be acknowledged in both policy and practice.

Melvin A Glasser

Director, Social Security Department,
International Union UAW,
Member Governing Council, Institute of Medicine

New Social Mechanism

In proposing a new initiative for the organization and delivery of services to the elderly, Congressman Conable has focused on a major problem and defined a most constructive approach to its solution. As older people have increased in numbers, and their unmet needs have become more apparent, there has been almost universal agreement that too many of them have been placed in institutions where they often receive inferior care, for excessive lengths of time, and at unnecessarily great costs to themselves and society.

There are numerous demonstrations in the United States, and more extensive models in Great Britain, which illustrate that a system of community centers capable of providing a wide range of support services is a desirable and a viable alternative to the present rush to "warehouse" the impaired older person. But our society has not yet created the social institution to achieve this objective. By proposing to establish such a social mechanism, Mr Conable would make possible not only the integration of services around people, but the creation of needed new services to fill gaps as identified in individual community situations. This new social institution would also reduce the pressure on welfare programs and upon health programs to add to their functions services which may be neither feasible nor appropriate because their own mandates are too limited.

The community center, or as some have called it, the "personal care organization" concept, to be successful, will require the back-up of institutions, many of which would be of a different character from those which predominate in our country today. These include what Tobin has described as the long-term care institution for those aged persons who must have custodial care (primarily women in their late eighties and nineties), and terminal care centers or hospices, for persons who are in the final phase of life (Tobin 1975). And of course unlike our present situation it will be essential that there be strong linkages among these alternative care mechanisms, as well as with established hospitals, skilled nursing homes, recreational centers and the like to provide the continuity of care largely absent in our current programs.

This Conference has illustrated dramatically how very little the United States has to offer in effective programs to care for the elderly compared to what we could and should have, or compared to what is available in the United Kingdom and a number of other European countries. This perhaps is the over-riding social policy implication of these sessions.

Congressman Conable's proposal is a major move in the direction of closing the gap. It has an added advantage in that it makes possible continuing funding from a combination of public and private sources. In addition to the usual sources, I see in such a program the possibility of substantial support from unions and industry. Once these service systems are sufficiently institutionalized, it should be possible to write into management-labor contracts and employee benefit programs provisions to fund integrated care for retirees, at their choice, as alternatives to separate, categorical cash payment pensions and health insurance premium benefits.

Health Care

As the papers presented at this Conference richly illustrate, there is need for major changes in the way the health problems of the elderly are understood, how the services are provided, under what conditions and by whom. Older people, in our traditional fee-for-service, solo practice medical care system, all too frequently obtain too little care too late. They spend too much time in hospitals where they don't belong and too little time seeing health professionals outside of hospitals. Their problems are complex, they sometimes are confused and not well organized, and many learn to their sorrow, that they are not particularly welcome in busy private practices—even if they have the funds to pay for needed services. And the element of caring, of human understanding, is all too often absent in a system which puts a cash premium on efficiency and productivity.

Preventive medicine and rehabilitation are today recognized as essential components of health care for the elderly, but by and large they are able to avail themselves of these services to an even lesser extent than younger Americans.

The US today operates public and private programs designed to meet the personal health services needs of the elderly. Medicare and Medicaid have proved invaluable. But they have also demonstrated that a system that only pays for services and does not deal with the organization and delivery of those services, and which in major ways is not able to control costs or protect quality of care leaves a great deal to be desired, from both the point of view of the recipient and the taxpayers who pay for the programs.

It is realistic to expect that the experience of the US with Medicare and Medicaid will lead in the not too distant future to the extension of national health insurance to the entire population. If the lessons of Medicare and Medicaid are understood, and the special interests of those who have profited so richly from these programs can be overcome—and I believe they can—the extension of national health insurance to the total population will encompass payment mechanisms related to reorganized delivery programs. We need to see not only that providers are compensated; accessible services of good quality, at reasonable costs must also be assured.

A second social policy implication therefore is that our experience with national payments for personal health services has demonstrated that the leverage of the payment mechanism is required to bring about needed system changes in the provision of health services to the aged, and indeed to all Americans.

Income

In his lucid and encyclopedic opening address, Robert Ball commented that the US policy for the elderly is primarily an income policy. We were among the last industrial nations to develop a Social Security mechanism, but we now have it as a means of providing adequate income to those whom Walter Reuther used to describe as "too old to work and too young to die."

It seems to me our value system has changed from the mid-1930s when the program was initiated. Ball points out that the percentage of the elderly below the government defined "rock bottom low income level in 1974 was only 16%". This, together with the recently added cost of living increases in Social Security, is considered by many to be a satisfactory response to meeting the income needs of the elderly. Those who examine that "rock bottom level" recognize it's a hard bed. Retirees feel, as do the rest of us, they should be able to lead satisfying lives. Further, as the standard of living improves, even with their cost of living increase, the gap between them and the generations following widens.

A continuing public policy issue therefore will be the inadequacy of Social Security benefits, particularly for those already retired or who will be retiring in the next decade. As a nation we may well need to follow the other industrial countries of the world by introducing general revenue contributions to Social Security financing, so that larger benefits can be paid.

An income policy in retirement is further complicated by the accelerated movement in the United States toward early retirement. Ball reports that over half the Social Security retirements in the US are of persons under 65. In private industry and in public employment retirements in the 50–60 age brackets are increasing rapidly. In recent years, the movement has spread to blue collar workers. In the automobile industry for example, a worker may retire with full pension benefits after 30 years of service, regardless of age. He may not take another full-time job, but he is assured a level income for life, first in private pension payments, then in his older years through a combination of his private pension and Social Security payments.

In the first years of this new program an astonishing third of eligible workers under the age of fifty elected to retire, and essentially leave the workforce. Nearly 40% of those eligible between the ages of 50 and 55 also followed this pattern.

Our increased technology is enabling fewer workers to produce larger quantities of goods. It does not appear likely that the service industries will be able to provide nearly enough jobs to keep unemployment at an acceptable level. Hence the pressure to create job opportunities through early retirements is likely to increase.

There are many who believe that meaningful, productive employment, perhaps at less than full time, should be provided for retirees who wish it. The experience of the US post-World War II economy does not give much support to the view that such an objective is achievable in the forseeable future — certainly not while large numbers of teenage first workers, ethnic minorities and women have been unable to find adequate and continuing attachment to the workforce.

And why shouldn't a worker be encouraged to live a life of decency and dignity in retirement without continuing to be evaluated by the Protestant work ethic? The thesis that jobs are required to support satisfying lives for those who have worked steadily for 30 or 40 years is questionable — and particularly so for those who have bucked the production lines or sweated in the steel mills for most of their adult lives.

Studies of auto workers who elected to take early retirement well before reaching the mandatory age 65 have shown that most have been well satisfied with their decision. They report they are living good lives without attachment to the workforce (Barfield and Morgan 1969; Barfield 1970).

Competitive Demands

The unsatisfactory and inappropriate nature of much of the housing of the elderly, the scanty production of new housing suited to their needs and pocketbooks, the very real threat to life and security that most older people must live with because of widespread crime in our cities, the inadequacy of public transportation which in special ways further isolates older people, separately and together are other major causes of dependency in the elderly in the United States. In viewing the needs and the demands, they often appear to compete with each other and with the needs and priorities of the society as a whole.

For the first time we have a national institute to help us add to knowledge and look in depth at trends in the field. But we have no mechanism for effectively determining priorities in programs for the aged, for balancing needs versus opportunities, and translating new information into activities of substance. We are not short of goals in programs for the elderly. Many of them were enunciated at the 1971 White House Conference on Aging. The theme of that Conference was "Toward a National Policy on Aging." How far we have progressed since then is questionable.

There is potential for such policy setting mechanisms in the Senate Committee on Aging and in the Federal Council on the Aging. The power base of both groups has not until now mobilized enough strength to enable them to achieve independent leadership roles.

Today, however, there are more retirees than ever before. They are better organized, younger, and better educated than their predecessors. We in the US can expect that the years immediately ahead will witness a growing political force pressing for the social and organizational changes delineated in this Conference.

References

Barfield, R. (1970). "The Auto Worker and Retirement: a Second Look." Survey Research Center, University of Michigan, Ann Arbor

Barfield, R. and Morgan, J. (1969). "Early Retirement: the Decision and the Experience." Survey Research Center, University of Michigan, Ann Arbor

Tobin, S. S. (1975). *Gerontologist*, **15**, p 32

Anne R Somers

*Departments of Community Medicine and Family Practice,
College of Medicine and Dentistry of New Jersey-Rutgers Medical School,
New Jersey 08854*

I join enthusiastically with my colleagues in congratulating the three sponsoring organizations for this conference. It could not be more timely. And it was a very good conference.

But conferences like this tend to be misleading. After two and a half days of talking among ourselves, of listening to congenial thoughts and ideas, we could go away thinking we had made real progress toward crystallization of a national policy on care of the dependent elderly.

I cannot presume to speak for the British. There is no doubt that they are well ahead of us in this respect. But, as for the US, I think we are still very, very far from any real consensus, or even a bare majority agreement on most of the issues raised here today. Indeed, I think we have just begun to define the issues — let alone the solutions.

I do not think this stems from stupidity, venality, or lack of compassion. I agree with Bob Ball's opening statement that we, in this country, have given a great deal of thought, especially during the past two decades, to this subject and we've also made substantial progress both with respect to income maintenance and medical care. It is worth noting that the Federal Government is now spending over $\$100 \times 10^9$ a year for income security benefits for the elderly and for the share of Medicare, Medicaid, and other in-kind benefits going to the elderly.

Parenthetically, I would like to take this opportunity to pay special tribute to Bob Ball, as Social Security Commissioner for many creative years, and to Arthur Hess, as first Director of the Bureau of Health Insurance and a principal architect of Medicare. Whatever shortcomings some of us may now find in these two programs, we need only ask ourselves what the world of the elderly would be like without them, to appreciate how important they have been in the evolution of US policy for the elderly.

Nearly five years ago, I wrote:

> Probably the most difficult, the most intractable of all health care issues facing the American people is the long-term care of the aged and the disabled (Somers 1972).

I have not changed my mind — which is perhaps one reason that I, like many others — physicians, health insurance executives, public officials and others — have been, consciously or unconsciously, somewhat reluctant to become involved in this area.

But really there is no choice. This is an issue that cannot be run away from. It may, indeed, be *the* domestic issue of the late twentieth century.

What is involved is a reconciliation of a number of competing values, each of which is cherished by large numbers of Americans and none of which can be ignored by Congressmen, at least those who care to be re-elected in this democracy. These include: (1) a vigorous economy growing fast enough to provide jobs and good take-home pay for all Americans who want to work; (2) an elaborate and expensive system of health, education, and welfare benefits, including lifetime retirement pensions of two-thirds to three-fourths of final pay and all essential health and social services; (3) a military establishment guaranteed to make us "Number One" in the world and (4) to do all of this without harming the environment or exhausting our resources.

Whether our resources are finite or not in the long run is perhaps debatable. Here, in the halls of the National Academy of Sciences, men and women are pitting their brains against time in the hope that science and technology can save us from the inevitable results of finite resources. There can be no question, however, that resources are limited at any given time. Thus it is highly unlikely that we will succeed in all four of these areas simultaneously to the extent that would satisfy the advocates of each.

This is *not* a call for retreat or defeatism. It *is* a plea for realism in facing up to the inherent difficulties of the task that I believe we are committing ourselves to at this conference. It is also a caution that we are not likely to achieve our goals, no matter how reasonably and realistically defined, without a great deal of effort and considerable travail. We will need all the allies we can muster.

In this connection, I urge a strong follow-up to this conference — perhaps in the form of a "working party" or committee to continue formal dialogue between our two countries on some of the problems involved in gerontology and geriatrics. This is not the appropriate place to discuss the precise form of this cooperative effort or the precise agenda. But I'm sure I speak for all the Americans present in expressing our gratitude to our British guests for their contribution and our desire for a new type of "Atlantic Alliance" in this difficult and portentous undertaking.

What might be the outlines of a viable US health policy for the dependent elderly? After all the words of wisdom you have heard in the past two days, I assure you that you will not be subjected to another speech from me on this subject. Time alone precludes anything but the barest outline. Moreover, the formulation of viable policies in this incredibly complex area will require a great deal more study, thought, public and Congressional debate.

Still, we are not entirely in the dark as the near unanimity expressed in this conference on numerous points has indicated. Let me summarize several of the major ingredients of such a policy. For the most part these are points that have already been made by others, although you will recognize that I have added a few special concerns of my own.

There are ten on my list. They are as heterogeneous and multidimensional as the problems themselves. Also, needless to say, there are many additional elements which should be included if time permitted.

1. We must find some way of providing productive employment to a substantial portion of those over 65. This is essential not only for fiscal reasons (on this score, I remind you of just one relevant statistic: the woman who retires at 65 faces an average remaining life expectancy of over 17 years!) but to maintain the independence and self-respect of the elderly themselves and to permit them to exercise maximum control over their own lives and the institutions that seek to serve them.

How should we do this? I don't know for sure. There are many possibilities: should we postpone the conventional retirement age to 68? to 70? Should we, and could we, outlaw compulsory retirement? Should we start to think in terms of "phased" retirement? Should we leave the present retirement system pretty much as it is and concentrate, instead, on developing new part-time jobs for the healthy retired? If so, should they be in the regular job market or confined to some form of "sheltered" employment? Should we concentrate on the development of voluntary activities, including programs in which the "young old" would take care of the "old old"? Is there a place for a new form of "barter economy", under which the elderly might exchange useful services among themselves or with other segments of society totally outside the money economy?

These are extremely complex issues which must be very carefully studied for all the possible side effects. Clearly, anything effective in this respect can only be accomplished politically in a context of relatively full employment.

2. We must find some way to improve amenities in our cities, where so many of the dependent elderly live. This involves, at the very minimum, vastly improved housing, better public transportation, and effective crime control.

3. We must abolish all remnants of racial discrimination which has contributed so much to the current backlog of poverty, dependence, and ill health among our elderly.

4. We must find some way to minimize the environmental, behavioral, and lifestyle threats to health that now take such a heavy toll of the elderly in the United States. I am not suggesting prohibition of smoking, alcohol, juicy steaks, eggs, and other actual or potential

threats to health. I am not suggesting that we put the entire plastics industry, the paint industry, or the rubber tire industry out of business.

I am suggesting that we mount a large scale and serious national consumer health education effort, utilizing the same techniques of mass persuasion that are now used to seduce the public into health-threatening activities. I am also urging a wide-scale review and, where necessary, modification of national policies that are contrary to the health interests of the public. Among the first that come to mind are the federal tobacco subsidies and support of school lunch programs keyed to interests other than the health of the children.

I am also suggesting renewed attack on occupational illness and disability, including industrial cancer. I want to particularly take exception to President Ford's remark a few months ago, "OSHA (Occupational Safety and Health Administration) should be thrown into the ocean."

5. We must make "long-term care" a respectable and respected aspect of comprehensive health care — in terms of professional interests, public understanding, and third-party reimbursement.

Should this be done by adding "long-term care" to the familiar triad — "primary, secondary, and tertiary" thus providing a quartet "primary, secondary, tertiary, and long-term?" Or, should long-term care be subsumed under the general heading of "primary care"?

I am not sure. Arguments could be made for and against each view. But of this I am sure: long-term care has to be brought into the mainstream of health care, one way or another, and not isolated as it typically is now, even under the broadest national health insurance proposals.

6. Long-term care and geriatric care must be made essential parts of the education of the health professions, especially physicians and nurses. This is necessary not only to assure the quality of such care as it is provided to individual patients, but to provide the sense of professional excitement and leadership necessary to attract the health-care teams, funds, and other resources.

Does this mean, for medicine, that we should develop a specialty of geriatrics, as there is in Britain today? I am inclined to think so, largely on the basis of the impressive record of the British geriatricians and the creative leadership that this relatively small group has been able to give to general medicine throughout that country.

However, the structure and traditions of medical practice in the US may be sufficiently different from those in the UK to justify a different approach. This is an issue that needs to be vigorously and promptly debated, both by the health professions and our public representatives. Among other things, there are important implications for federal support of medical education and reimbursement policies with respect to hospital house staff.

7. Public and private investment in health-care resources for the next five years should be heavily concentrated on long-term care facilities and programs rather than acute care.

There are two sides to this coin. On the one hand, we probably need a federally-supported loan program for construction or expansion of the needed spectrum of long-term care facilities, including minimum care homes, "sheltered homes", and something like the "community long-term care centers" contemplated in the Conable–Heinz bills (e.g., H.R. 10908). In my view, the latter should frequently be physically located in community hospitals, although with clear consumer control.

On the other hand, we will probably have to balance additional expenditures in these areas by a moratorium on all new acute-care beds and equipment. The only exceptions for the latter should be for replacement or certain new developments whose major contribution to life or health is documented by clinical trials.

8. The potential of the new national health planning and resource development program and PSROs should be fully utilized to assure that all new long-term care construction and programs be developed in accordance with a balanced continuum of comprehensive care, including personal social services, and with effective provision for assessment, placement, quality and utilization review.

In this connection, it is encouraging to note that the Rochester, New York, PSRO already has a functioning long-term care committee, carrying out both utilization and quality review.

9. Pending the advent of national health insurance — and I agree completely with Bob Ball that this is still probably a number of years away — Medicare should be extended to cover long-term care including home care and related essential personal social services, for all its beneficiaries. The necessity for objective assessment, placement, utilization and quality review was noted in point 8.

I came to this conclusion long before reading the Conable–Heinz bills. However, I am now prepared to accept the list of benefits spelled out in H.R. 10908 as a good starting point for Congressional and public debate and discussion.

It is particularly important that we act now, before the present exclusively medical model is written into legislative concrete in NHI legislation, to make sure that the social services are included. To those who say that abuse would be uncontrollable and costs prohibitive, I urge them to study the British record. With full coverage of essential social services, the combined cost of their health and social services is dramatically less than ours, whether measured on a per capita basis or in relation to gross national product. Certainly there can be abuse of any benefit. But I am convinced that the potential for abuse is far less than under our present Medicare/Medicaid system with its overemphasis on medical care and acute care.

I am also prepared to go along, for the moment, with Congressmen Heinz and Conable in their proposal to tie the new long-term care benefits into Part B of Medicare, with some adjustment in financing. This may not be the best possible way, but it is a good taking-off point to start discussing the whole question of financing and administration of long-term benefits.

These new benefits will, of course, result in additional costs. As a result, we may have to accept some limits on acute care expenditures as a trade-off. Among the most equitable limits that come to mind and which have already been widely discussed are: (a) negotiated prospective rates for hospitals and other institutions; (b) negotiated fee schedules for practitioners; and (c) a requirement that physicians and other practitioners should choose between participating or non-participating status for their Part B patients.

10. We must expand support for research, demonstration, development, and evaluation in this whole area. I refer not only to research in the biomedical, environmental, and behavioral aspects of aging, but in the clinical, socioeconomic, and political problems of delivering care to the elderly.

Demonstration projects should be funded and set up not to discredit or postpone new programs, but to assess objectively, to improve and facilitate them.

Evaluation cannot continue to be based on the current double-standard which always gives the benefit of the doubt to acute care and curative medicine and always demands irrefutable proof from long-term care and preventive medicine. Given the application of a single objective cost-benefit standard, I have no doubt that long-term care and preventive medicine will come out very well in such tests.

Reference

Somers, A. R. (1972). *Annals American Academy of Political and Social Science* **399**, 173

Harriet Miller

American Association of Retired Persons,
National Retired Teachers' Association

I am pleased to have the opportunity to comment on how our conference discussions may be translated into significant improvements in the lives of older people. As always, it is gratifying to meet with the people who are actively concerned with bettering the care that is afforded to our older people. It has been repeatedly heard here at this conference that present approaches to the care of the elderly, particularly in the United States, are in urgent need of improvement.

In reviewing the presentations of the earlier speakers, I have pinpointed five major processes which I believe must occur in order for the care of the elderly to reach an optimum of service, availability, proficiency and, above all, humanity. Briefly these five processes are: one, a change in professional and lay attitudes regarding the nature of dependency and the range of older people's needs: two, major improvements in and integration of existing health care and social service systems; three, the provision of wide-ranging alternatives to the present limited care options; four, an acceptance of the responsibility for adequate care to the elderly on the part of the younger population; and five, most importantly, an unrelenting commitment to retaining and protecting the individuality, independence and dignity of older people in need of care. This is a big order but not impossible.

The first process I mentioned, changing attitudes towards dependency and the needs of the elderly, may be the most difficult. As social scientists long ago discovered, changing attitudes is no simple matter. Nonetheless, no matter how difficult the task may be, the adoption of attitudes free of stereotypes and blanket solutions is a necessary component in achieving the desired quality of care. As Elaine Brody has pointed out, varying levels of dependency in old age should be viewed as part of the life process, just as much a part of that process as the expected and well provided for dependencies of childhood. The dependencies of old age, of course, are not like the dependencies of childhood. In childhood the dependencies are temporary stages preceding increasing independence, while in old age dependencies are often the sign of continuing or increasing dependency.

Yet it must be underscored that these dependencies of old age do not equally affect everyone that is old. The associations I serve maintain and promote the view that older people are active and want to remain as active as possible for as long as possible. Not all older people are dependent. Some are more dependent than others. National recognition that dependencies come in varying degrees is a necessary precursor to broadening the levels and kinds of care available to the elderly.

Just as dependency should be viewed as part of the life process which manifests itself in a number of ways and on differing levels, dependency must also be recognized as the result of both medical and social needs. It must be recognized that some factors which determine dependency, such as housing deficiency and high crime neighborhoods, do not arise from older persons' infirmities but are related contributory problems.

For too long care of the elderly has been regarded as primarily a medical problem. The negative effects of this adherence to a strictly medical care model have been well-documented at this conference. As Sir George Godber has said, support in old age and the postponement of dependency may be more social than medical. Only recently have our countries begun to recognize this view that housing, domestic help, nutrition, warmth, and even continuing human relationships may be far more important to active survival than all our medical technology. The need for addressing the social problems of old age as well as the medical concerns still escapes the attention of most of today's health care providers.

The emphasis remains on medical routines, the treatment of older people solely as patients, the crisis and cure orientation, as Dr Brody aptly described. This approach has little regard for ongoing social needs. Our attitudes toward dependency are in need of revision, as is our definition of health. Daphne Krause outlined this broader concept of health. Health, she said, is not just medical well-being, but also our environmental, nutritional and emotional well-being, and really anything that goes into making up the quality of our lives.

It is within this encompassing view of health that we need to redesign existing health care programs as well as to build comprehensive new services. The need to improve existing elderly care institutions has been dramatically demonstrated in a number of state and federal investigations, but one 80-year old woman's attitude toward today's institutions says it better than all the investigation reports. At a recent conference, a young man of 18 asked this outspoken lady if she were afraid of dying. She replied, "I'm not afraid of dying, but I am afraid I will have to go to a nursing home before I die. That thought is the only thing that keeps me from being really happy in my old age".

To this woman there was a greater fear than death: living in a nursing home, an institution designed to provide comprehensive care to the elderly. The case for improving existing elderly care facilities needs no other testimony than the overwhelming number of older people who say they would prefer to commit suicide rather than live in a nursing home.

Present elderly care institutions are fertile ground for long-winded criticism, but I believe, as Robert Ball has said, that it behooves us not to attack the institutions or abandon them, but to improve them. Institutions should not and cannot be the answer to all problems of dependency. However, a certain small percentage of older people will need the total care of institutions at some time in their lives.

Because this need will not diminish, we need to concentrate efforts to upgrade these institutions while simultaneously developing comprehensive alternatives to institutionalization of those not requiring a level of total care. We cannot afford to abandon one approach in favor of the other.

Both the alternatives to institutionalization and the institutions themselves should share a common goal, to encourage independence to the maximum extent possible for as long as possible. In the United States the independence of older people is too often drained away due to a scarcity of enabling services or an over-abundant institutional package of care. The over-use of total care facilities because lesser levels of care are not available is one of the most tragic, not to mention costly, examples of America's all-or-none approach to elderly care.

Clinging to a medical model of elderly health care has only deepened America's phenomenon of total care or total absence of care. Medicare and Medicaid as they are today cannot supply all the elderly care needs. They are medical programs whose services are prescribed by physicians. As has been repeatedly proven, medical needs are only one small aspect of the services required to keep elderly independence at its highest possible level.

Furthermore, as George Maddox has noted, when provisions are made for some level of community and home help care, complex legislative and administrative regulations often rely again on the long-established medical model requiring medical certification and the use of skilled professionals. The net result, of course, has been a paucity of home health services and a disproportionate reliance on existing medical approaches. What is needed is a comprehensive and integrated social and medical approach to the care of the elderly.

I think Congressman Conable's long-term care act is certainly in the right direction, and our associations support this approach. At least one area of the United States already has a comprehensive full service center, and you had the description of Daphne Krause about that program, which I think is excellent. Let me just mention one thing George Maddox said. He referred to the issue of cost effectiveness as being a diversion from the issue to be addressed, the development of a comprehensive, systematic coordination of services available to the elderly population. He has said that the quality of care and the costs should be discussed together, and I would add to that discussion a consideration of the older person's preference regarding the kind and amount of care he or she desires. A theoretically cost effective system of care which is rejected by those it is intended to serve will be neither useful nor economical.

I think we must not be tempted to mold individuals into existing systems or programs. We must strive to design the programs to allow consumers to determine what is most appropriate for their needs. If there is anything outstandingly wrong with health care today apart from its cost, it is the impersonalization. We must build the human element into our health care programs and abandon the present "we know what's best for you" attitude. The results of the doing-for and doing-to approach to elderly health care have been extensively documented, and I think it is the recognition of these results that makes many an older person prefer sudden death to being found in any kind of an institution.

As a person grows older he or she does not owe it to society to sacrifice the rights to independence and freedom of choice. Our health care systems must acknowledge and protect these rights. Our most elaborate, well-coordinated care delivery system will be meaningless without an accompanying respect for the older person as an individual with rights of independence and choice. Older people want to remain active and independent, alert and free to make their own decisions. I think this is what people want for their lives in general, and appropriately they expect assistance in reaching and maintaining these goals from the health care systems available to them.

Discussion

Ms Gloriana Arceneau (*American Nurses Association*) I wanted to express disappointment that the nursing component of care of the elderly did not have formal input into the conference. Nursing traditionally has been in charge of the care of the elderly, particularly in nursing homes and in health care services, and this has been done under the nursing services. Nurses do not see the care of the elderly as basically sick care. We are concerned with maximizing the potential of the elderly individual and maintaining that potential. I would like to comment that I do not think this conference has had the nurses' opinions voiced sufficiently explicitly and would hope that in a future conference of this type more active participation by nurses could be included.

Dr Martin Loeb (*Institute on Aging, University of Wisconsin*) One very brief suggestion that might start something for the United States, while Bill Oriol and Bob Butler are here. I just figured out that if, through the National Institute on Aging, two medical schools in each of the 10 federal regions were provided with $100 000 a year to start a geriatric training program, and they were guaranteed for seven years, we would be well on our way. The one thing that convinces medical schools about what to do is to bait them, and this would do it sufficiently and would cost only a little over $2 000 000 a year, which would be a small addition to the NIA budget. I think that we will never get geriatrics going in this country until we start somewhere, and it seems to me we ought to start there right away.

Dr P R Greenfield (*Department of Health and Social Security, London*) The session on research dealt in some detail with basic gerontology, but I regret the omission of any reference to research into the provision of services for the elderly. A number of speakers have noted that the elderly are rarely involved in decisions about themselves, and Dr Maddox mentioned our ignorance of the cost of home care and the fact that, for some 12% of elderly people, forms of care were interchangeable.

I would like to say that the Department of Health and Social Security is very conscious of these factors, and some 12 months ago launched a major research project to determine the needs of old people as perceived by themselves. Within the last two weeks we have set up another research project concerned with alternative patterns of care for the elderly, in which particular objectives will be to attempt to determine the true cost of home care, and to determine the point at which, with increasing dependency, the cost of home care exceeds institutional care. We are also looking at the support needs of families who are looking after elderly relatives in their homes, though no formal research initiatives have yet been taken.

Mr William Oriol (*Staff Director, US Senate Special Committee on Aging*) Very briefly, I do not like to speak towards the end of a conference about the possibility of another conference, but last Thursday, Senator Church, Chairman of the Senate Committee on Aging, introduced a resolution calling for a midway conference on aging, meaning midway between two White House conferences on aging; not to be a miniature version of what happened in 1971, but to focus on a manageable theme. He has chosen the theme of "Toward Longer Independent Living in Aging" which, as we know from this conference, can cover a multitude of subjects. He has built into the resolution certain actions which would make it more than just a conference, but a culmination. I just want to add the note that with the exception of Daphne Krause's presentation, we were talking as if we were at the beginning of things in providing comprehensive options for the care of older people. But I merely want to point out the urgency of the situation by saying that there are many, many things happening in a very uncoordinated fashion in providing the kind of care we were talking about.

At this very moment, in about 450 area agencies on aging under the Older American Act, people are attempting to cope with or to develop some of the programs we are talking about here. We are spending greater amounts of money by the minute, and that is why what was discussed at this conference is so urgent.

Sir Gordon Wolstenholme Now, I am extremely sorry but I have to close this conference. I thank all the speakers, both those who prepared full papers and those who took part in the panel discussions. I want to thank particularly our hosts, the Institute of Medicine, and in doing that, not only its President, Dr Hamburg, but all the people in the background — engineers, secretaries and everybody else — without whose co-operation so smoothly run a conference would never have been possible.

We are deeply appreciative, Dr Hamburg. We ask you to convey to every member of the Institute our very, very great gratitude and our very best wishes for the future work of the Institute.

Appendix

Conference Attenders

ABRAMS, Mrs W. June, M.S.W., State of Delaware, Division on Aging, 2413 Lancaster Avenue, Wilmington, Delaware 19805

ACLAND, Sarah, M.D., Consultation-Liaison Psychiatry Program, Department of Psychiatry and Behavioral Sciences, University of Louisville Health Sciences Center, P.O. Box 1055, Louisville, Kentucky 40201

ADAMOVICH, George, Minneapolis Age and Opportunity Center, 1801 Nicollet Avenue South, Minneapolis, Minnesota 55403

ADAMS, Mrs Carolyn, R.N., Lutheran Hospital of Maryland, Inc., 730 Ashburton Street, Baltimore, Maryland 21216

ANDRES, Reubin, M.D., Gerontology Research Center, NIA, Baltimore City Hospitals, Baltimore, Maryland 21224

ANWAR, Dr Masud, Consultant Physician in Geriatric Medicine, The General Hospital, Hartlepool, Cleveland, England

ARCENEAU, Gloriana, R.N., American Nurses' Association, 1030 — 15th Street, N.W., Washington, D.C. 20005

ARNOLD, Margaret, National Retired Teachers Association/American Association of Retired Persons, 1909 K Street, N.W., Washington, DC 20049

BAUSMAN, Jane, Yonkers Office for the Aging, 87 Nepperhan Avenue, Yonkers, New York 10701

BEALL, George Thomas, International Center for Social Gerontology, 425 13th Street, N.W., Suite 350, Washington, DC 20004

BEARN, Alexander G., M.D., New York Hospital-Cornell Medical Center, 525 East 68th Street, New York, New York 10021

BENNETT, Robin I., M.D., 850 N. Orange Grove, Suite 1, Pasadena, California 91103

BESDINE, Richard W., M.D., Hebrew Rehabilitation Center for the Aged, 1200 Centre Street, Roslindale, Massachusetts 02131

BEVERLEY, E. Virginia, Senior Editor, *Geriatrics* Magazine, 4015 West 65th Street, Minneapolis, Minnesota 55435

BICKNELL, William J., M.D., Harvard School of Public Health, 677 Huntington Avenue, Boston, Massachusetts 02115

BLUMENTHAL, Monica D., M.D., Ph.D., Department of Psychiatry, University of Michigan Medical Center, Ann Arbor, Michigan 48109

BOREN, Nona, The George Washington University School of Medicine and Health Sciences, 2300 Eye Street, N.W., Washington, DC 20037

BREEN, Faith Lee, American Enterprise Institute, 1150 — 17th Street, N.W., Washington, DC 20036

BRIGHAM, Mrs Elizabeth N., George Washington University School of Sociology, 4005 N. 22nd Street, Arlington, Virginia 22207

BROCK, Ann, 6000 Springhill Drive, Greenbelt, Maryland 20770

BROTMAN, Herman B., Consultant, House Select Committee on Aging, 3108 Holmes Run Road, Falls Church, Virginia 22042

BROWN, Mrs Anna V., Executive Director of the Mayor's Commission on Aging, City Hall, 601 Lakeside Drive, Cleveland, Ohio 44114

BROWN, Robert Guy, The George Washington University, Department of Sociology, Washington, DC 20052

BURKE, Steven, Greenville Hospital System, 701 Grove Road, Greenville, South Carolina 29602

BUTLER, Robert N., M.D., Director, National Institute on Aging, Building 31, Room 4B-59, Bethesda, Maryland 20014

CALKINS, Evan, M.D., SUNY-Buffalo, E.J. Meyer Memorial Hospital, Buffalo, New York 14215

CARBONI, David K., University of Connecticut Medical School, Department of Community Medicine, Farmington, Connecticut 06032

CASGRANDE, Ann, Mt Sinai Hospital-Smith Towers Clinic, 500 Blue Hills Avenue, Hartford, Connecticut 06112

CHRISTMAS, The Reverend Clyde J. III, Lutheran Social Services, 715 Falconer Street, Jamestown, New York 14701

CLARK, Cary, Association of Univeristy Programs in Health Administration, 1755 Massachusetts Avenue, Suite 312, Washington, DC 20036

CLARK, Malcolm, Minneapolis Age and Opportunity Center, 1801 Nicollet Avenue South, Minneapolis, Minnesota 55403

CLARKE, Elsie B., Office of Services to the Aged of DC 1329 E Street, N.W., Suite 1031, Washington, DC 20004

COBURN, Herbert, Executive Secretary, Social Problems Research Review Committee, National Institute of Mental Health, 5600 Fishers Lane, Rockville, Maryland 20852

COHEN, Gene D., M.D., Chief, Center for Studies of the Mental Health of the Aging, Parklawn Building, Rm. 18–97, 5600 Fishers Lane, Rockville, Maryland 20852

CROMER, Janice, National Retired Teachers Association/American Association of Retired Persons, 1909 K Street, N.W., Washington, DC 20049

CYR, Michelle, Triage Project, 269 N. Washington Street, Plainville, Connecticut 06062

DANIEL, Gerard L., M.D., RHODIA, Inc., 600 Madison Avenue, New York, New York 10022

DAVIS, Clarice, 104 Twin Willow Court, Owings Mills, Maryland 21117

DECOTIS, Tony, Georgetown Medical School, Washington, DC

DEIRANIEH, Mrs Mary Jane, National Retired Teachers Association/American Association of Retired Persons, 1909 K Street, N.W., Washington, DC 20049

DELEON, Jean, D.C. Village, 1600 S. Eads Street, Apt. 215-N, Arlington, Virginia 22202

DELEON, Patrick, Legislative Assistant to Senator Inouye, 442 Rayburn Senate Office Building, Washington, DC 20510

DONAHUE, Wilma T., Director, International Center for Social Gerontology, 425 — 13th Street, N.W., Suite 350, Washington, DC 20004

ELWOOD, Thomas, National Retired Teachers Association/American Association of Retired Persons, 1909 K Street, N.W., Washington, DC 20049

FELDER, Miriam R., Homemaker Health Aide Service of the NCA, Inc., 1825 Connecticut Avenue, N.W., Room 100, Washington, DC 20009

FELDMAN, Leonard, Johns Hopkins University, 621 N. Castle Street, Baltimore, Maryland 21205

FELTIN, Marie, M.D., East Boston Neighborhood Health Center, 527B Franklin Street, Cambridge, Massachusetts

FERGUSON, Leon, Stoddard Baptist Home, 1818 Newton Street, N.W., Washington, DC 20010

FERNANDES, Marge, Jewish Institute for Geriatric Care, 608 Hicksville Road, Massapequa, New York 11758

FERRIS, Dr Frederick J., National Retired Teachers Association/American Association of Retired Persons, 1909 K Street, N.W., Washington, DC 20049

FIELDS, Clavin, Director, Institute of Gerontology, Federal City College, 425 Second Street, N.W., Washington, DC 20001

FISHER, R. H., M.D., Sunnybrook Medical Centre, Rm. G321A, K-Wing, 2075 Bayview Avenue, Toronto, Ontario M4N 3M5 Canada

FOLKEMER, Donna, Office on Aging, 301 W. Preston Street, Baltimore, Maryland 21201

FRISCH, Robert A., M.D., 425 E. Wisconsin Avenue, Milwaukee, Wisconsin 53202

GERMAN, Pearl S., Sc.D., The Johns Hopkins Medical Institute Health Services R&D Center, 624 N. Broadway, Baltimore, Maryland 21205

GERTMAN, Jessie S., M.S.W., National Institute on Aging, Building 31, NIH, Bethesda, Maryland 20014

GIBBS, Doris M., Federal City College, 1220 — 12th Street, N.W., 501, Washington, DC 20005

GILROY, Patricia A., Homemaker Health Aide Service of the NCA, Inc., 1825 Connecticut Avenue, N.W., Washington, DC 20009

GLOVER, B. H., M.D., University of Wisconsin Medical School, 4th Floor WARF Building, 610 Walnut Street, Madison, Wisconsin 53706

GOLDKUHLE, Ute, George Mason University School of Nursing, 11219 South Shore, Reston, Virginia 22090

GONIK, Aleksander, American Joint Distribution Committee, 75 Rue de Lyon, 1211 Geneva 13, Switzerland

GOODMAN, Grace, Association of University Programs in Health Administration, 1755 Massachusetts Avenue, Suite 312, Washington, DC 20036

GOSS, Kenneth G., M.D., Department of Family Practice, College of Medicine, Medical University of South Carolina, 80 Barre Street, Charleston, South Carolina 29401

GREEN, Bernadette L., Area A Outreach to the Elderly, 5671 Western Avenue, N.W., Washington, DC 20015

GREEN, Dr Daniel B., Virginia Commonwealth University, MCV Station Box 637, Richmond, Virginia 23298

GREENFIELD, Peter R., Senior Medical Officer, Department of Health and Social Security, Alexander Fleming House, Elephant and Castle, London SE1 6BY, England

GUSTAFSON, Nancy, Hebrew Home for the Aged, 615 Tower Avenue, Hartford, Connecticut 06112

GURLAND, Barry, M.D., Department of Geriatrics Research, Columbia University, 722 W. 168th Street, New York, New York 10032

HALL, William, M.D., Lutheran Hospital of Maryland 730 Ashburton Street, Baltimore, Maryland 21216

HARPER, Mary S., Ph.D., R.N., Special Assistant, Center for Studies of Mental Health of the Aging, National Institute of Mental Health, 5600 Fishers Lane, Rockville, Maryland 20852

HASAN, Dr A. M., Consultant Physician, Geriatric Unit, South Shields General Hospital, South Shields, England

HELLER, Muriel, Jewish Institute for Geriatric Care, 31-03 88th Street, Jackson Heights, New York 11369

HELLER, Sheila J., Triage Inc., 269 N. Washington Street, Plainville, Connecticut 06052

HELM, Jocelyn, Director, Princeton Senior Resource Center, and Princeton Commission on Aging, 207 Mt. Lucas Road, Princeton, New Jersey 08540

HEMPHIL, Alex, School of Medicine, Howard University, 520 W Street, N.W., Washington, DC 20059

HENDERSON, Kathryn S., Executive Director, American Geriatrics Society, 10 Columbus Circle, New York, New York 10019

HERSH, Alice S., Assistant to the Director, Health Staff Seminar, Suite 305, 1901 Pennsylvania Avenue, N.W., Washington, DC 20006

HESS, Arthur E., Commission on Public General Hospitals, Suite 1016, 10001 Connnecticut Avenue, N.W., Washington, DC 20036

HEWITT, Richard, Executive Director, Royal Society of Medicine, 1 Wimpole Street, London W1M 8AE, England

HILDEBRANDT, Eugenie, 2105 Colts Neck Court, Reston, Virginia 22091

HILL, John, Minneapolis Age and Opportunity Center, 1801 Nicollet Avenue South, Minneapolis, Minnesota 55403

HOLT, Helen, Assistant to the Secretary for Programs for the Elderly and the Handicapped, Department of Housing and Urban Development, 451 — 7th Street, S.W., Washington, DC DC 20410

HORTON, Jacqueline A., Johns Hopkins University School of Hygiene and

Public Health, 1620 Winding Way Lane, Silver Spring, Maryland 20902

HUDSON, Paul, Johns Hopkins University, 525 N. Washington Street, Baltimore, Maryland 21205

IRVINE, Patrick, M.D., St Paul-Ramsey Hospital, 640 Jackson Street, St. Paul, Minnesota 55101

JACKSON, Nell, US Office of Education, Community Service and Continuing Education, 7th and D Streets, S.W., Washington, DC 20202

JENKINS, Mary, R.N., Lutheran Hospital of Maryland, Inc., 730 Ashburton Street, Baltimore, Maryland 21216

KAMEL, Wadie W., M.D., 816 Heritage Drive, Addison, Illinois 60101

KAYAN, Dr Sabih, Ciba-Geigy Corporation, 556 Morris Avenue, Summit, New Jersey 07906

KELLY, Ann Agnus, 813 South Veitch Street, Arlington, Virginia 22204

KELLY, Ann M., Baltimore County Department of Health, 105 W. Chesapeake Avenue, Towson, Maryland 21204

KELLY, Margaret, Social Integration and Welfare Section, Social Development Division, United Nations, New York 10027

KERRIGAN, William, National Retired Teachers Association/American Association of Retired Persons, 1909 K Street, N.W., Washington, DC 20049

KLAFTER, Frances, Gray Panthers, 1734 P Street, N.W., Washington, DC 20036

KNOX, Julian J., Secretary of Islington Community Health Council, London, and Senior Research Associate, School of Family Psychiatry and Community Mental Health, Tavistock Institute, London, England

KOVAR, Mary Grace, National Center for Health Statistics, Room 8A-55, 5600 Fishers Lane, Rockville, Maryland 20852

KOVNAT, Maurice, M.D., 1024 W. 47th Court, Miami Beach, Florida 33140

KUNZ, Jeffrey, University of Wisconsin Medical School, 6010 Old Saulk Road, Madison, Wisconsin 53705

LAMPERT, Judy, Minneapolis Age and Opportunity Center, 1801 Nicolett Avenue South, Minneapolis, Minnesota 55403

LANE, Larry, National Retired Teachers Association/American Association of Retired Persons, 1909 K Street, N.W., Washington, DC 20049

LANOY, Anne-Marie, M.D., Consultant, Centre de Psycho-Geriatrie, rue de Naut, 8 Geneva, Switzerland

LAUGHLIN, Thomas, Associate Commissioner, Medical Services Administration, Social and Rehabilitation Services, 330 Independence Avenue, S.W. Washington, DC 20201

LAURICE, Sr. M., OSF, Catholic Hospital Association, 1438 South Grand Boulevard, St. Louis, Missouri 63104

LEVESTON, Alice P., Triage, Inc., 269 N. Washington Street, Plainville, Connecticut 06062

LEVY, Morris B., Bureau of Health Insurance, Social Security Administration, Room 1-Q-4, East Building, Security Boulevard, Baltimore, Maryland 21235

LEWIS, Irene, Department of Family Care Nursing, University of California, 432 Lanyard Street, Redwood City, California 94065

LIDOFF, Lorraine, National Council on the Aging, 1828 L Street, N.W., Washington, DC 20036

LIPSKY, Hannah K., Mt Sinai Hospital Medical Center, 100 Street and Madison Avenue, New York, New York 10029

LOEB, Martin B., Faye McBeath Institute on Aging, University of Wisconsin, 425 Henry Mall, Madison, Wisconsin 53706

LUBITZ, James, Social Security Administration, Room 940, 1875 Connecticut Avenue, N.W., Washington, DC 20009

LUSTMAN, Claire, Veterans Administration, 2001 N. Adams Street, Apt. 1002, Arlington, Virginia 22201

MADISON, Ann, School of Nursing, University of Maryland, 655 West Lombard Street, Baltimore, Maryland 21201

MAHON, Melvin, School of Medicine,

Howard University, 520 W Street, N.W., Washington, DC 20059

MAHONEY, Florence, 3600 Prospect Street, N.W., Washington, DC 20007

MARSHALL, Mary A., Virginia General Assembly, 2256 N. Wakefield Street, Arlington, Virginia 22207

MARTIN, John, National Retired Teachers Association/American Association of Retired Persons, 1909 K Street, N.W., Washington, DC 20049

MARTIN, Martha, 2829 Connecticut Avenue, N.W., 409, Washington, DC 20008

MAY, John, Executive Secretary, W.R. Hewlitt Foundation, 1801 Page Mill Road, Palo Alto, California 94304

MCCALLY, Michael, M.D., Ph.D., The George Washington University School of Medicine and Health Sciences, 2300 Eye Street, N.W., Washington DC 20037

MCGLONE, Frank B., M.D., Medical Care and Research Foundation, 1565 Clarkson Street, Denver, Colorado 80218

MEEK, Peter G., 210 Fairmount Road, Ridgewood, New Jersey 07450

MELTZER, Judith, University of California Health Policy Program, c/o Lewin and Associates, 470 L'Enfant Plaza, Suite 4100, Washington, DC 20024

MILLER, Judith K., Director, Health Staff Seminar, 1901 Pennsylvania Avenue, N.W., Suite 305, Washington, DC 20006

MORAVEC, Jule, M.D., Veterans Administration, 6151 Loch Raven Drive, McLean, Virginia 22101

MURPHY, Mary Brugger, National Association of Counties, 1735 New York Avenue, N.W., Washington, DC 20006

NADON, Dr G. W., Sunnybrook Medical Centre, 2075 Bayview Avenue, K-Wing, Room G321C, Toronto, Ontario M4N 3M5, Canada

NASH, Bernard, President, International Federation on Aging, 1345 Connecticut Avenue, N.W., Suite 619, Washington, DC 20036

NIEMEYER, Mary, 2829 Connecticut Avenue, N.W., 409, Washington, DC 20008

O'BRIEN, Judith A., Director, Special Projects, American Pharmaceutical Association, 2215 Constitution Avenue, N.W., Washington, DC 20037

OLUMBA, Agnes, Howard University School of Nursing, 1401 Sheridan Street, N.W., Washington, DC 20011

ONYEMELUKWE, Obidima I.O., National Center on Black Aged, Inc., 1730 M Street, N.W., Washington, DC

ORAHOVATS, Peter D., M.D., Vice President/Scientific Director, Bristol-Myers Company, 345 Park Avenue, New York, New York 07024

ORIOL, William, Staff Director, US Senate Special Committee on Aging, G-225, Dirksen Senate Office Building, Washington, DC 20510

PADULA, Helen, Consultant, Long-Term Care, State of Maryland Office on Aging, 301 W. Preston Street, Baltimore, Maryland 21201

PAUL, Jeanne, National Retired Teachers Association/American Association of Retired Persons, 1909 K Street, N.W., Washington, DC 20049

PORTE, Phillip, Health Staff Seminar, 1901 Pennsylvania Avenue, N.W., Suite 305, Washington, DC 20006

POWER, Mary F., National Retired Teachers Association/American Association of Retired Persons, 1909 K Street, N.W., Washington, DC 20049

READ, Dr William A., University of Washington, D-670 H.S.B.—SM-54, Seattle, Washington 98195

REID, Sharland, Howard University School of Social Work, 14229 Woodwell Terrace, Silver Spring, Maryland 20906

RENNER, Jayne, Ethel Percy Andrus Gerontology Center, University of Southern California, University Park, Los Angeles, California 90007

RETTIG, Paul C., Professional Assistant, US House Committee on Ways and Means, 412 Congressional Annex, Washington, DC 20515

RICE, Dorothy P., Director, National

Center for Health Statistics, 5600 Fishers Lane, Rockville, Maryland 20852

RIDDICK, Vera, Institute of Gerontology, Federal City College, 425 Second Street, N.W., Washington, DC 20001

ROBBINS, Deborah Ellen, 2120 Huidekoper Place, Washington, DC 20007

ROBINS, Edith G., Division of Long-Term Care, Department of Health, Education and Welfare, Room 11A-33, 5600 Fishers Lane, Rockville, Maryland 20852

ROBINSON, Marion, c/o Merck Sharp & Dohme Research Laboratories, Rahway, New Jersey 07065

ROSS, Dr Ian P., Women's College Hospital, 76 Grenville Street, Toronto, Ontario M5S 1B2, Canada

ROTT, Elizabeth G., National Association of Counties, 1735 New York Avenue, N.W., Washington, DC 20006

ROYE, Marcia, Associate Executive Director, American Geriatrics Society, 10 Columbus Circle, Room 1470, New York, New York 10019

RYAN, Nancy, Triage, Inc., 269 N. Washington Street, Plainville, Connecticut 06062

SANCHEZ, David J., Jr., M.D., Division of Ambulatory and Community Medicine, University of California at San Francisco, Building 9, Room 306, 1001 Potrero Avenue, San Francisco, California 94110

SCHRANK, Dr Harris T., The Equitable Life Assurance Society of the United States, 1285 Avenue of the Americas, New York, New York 10019

SCHULTZ, Phyllis R., R.N., Medical Care and Research Foundation, 1565 Clarkson Street, Denver, Colorado 80218

SENSE, Eleanora, 1009 1/2 Military Road, Columbus, Mississippi 39701

SHANAS, Ethel, University of Illinois at Chicago Circle, Box 4348, Chicago, Illinois 60680

SHOCKET, Barbara, M.Ed., Dade County Comprehensive Alcohol Program, 726 W. Dilido Drive, Miami Beach, Florida 33139

SHOCKET, Everett, M.D., Ten Hundred Building, Suite 210, 1000 Lincoln Road, Miami Beach, Florida 33139

SKELTON, Dr David, St. Boniface General Hospital, 409 Tache Avenue, St. Boniface, Manitoba, Canada

SLOBODA, Sharon B., Catholic University School of Nursing, 6119 Utah Avenue, N.W., Washington, DC 20015

SOLDE, Beth J., Assistant Director, Center for Demographic Studies, Duke University, 2117 Campus Drive, Durham, North Carolina 27706

SOLON, Jerry A., Ph.D., National Institute on Aging, NIH Building 31, Room $b-63, Bethesda, Maryland 20014

SPILANE, Michael, M.D., St. Paul-Ramsey Hospital, 640 Jackson Street, St. Paul, Minnesota 55101

SPRENGER, Gordon, Minneapolis Age and Opportunity Center, 1801 Nicolett Avenue South, Minneapolis, Minnesota 55403

STEEL, Knight, M.D., University of Rochester, Monroe Community Hospital, 435 E. Henrietta, Rochester, New York 14603

STERN, Elliot, Minority Staff, Subcommittee on Health and Long Term Care, U.S. House Select Committee on Aging, Room 715, 300 New Jersey Avenue, S.E., Washington, DC

SWEENEY, Sandra, 223 — 12th Street, S.E., Washington, DC 20003

TAVANI, Cleonice, Federal Council on the Aging, Donohoe Building, Room 4022, Washington, DC 20201

THOMSON, J. M., D.P.H., "Woodville," Haines Hill, Taunton, Somerset, England

VIGNOLA, Margo L., American Public Welfare Association, 1155 — 16th Street, N.W., Washington, DC 20036

WALKER, Marcus L., Johns Hopkins University School of Hygiene and Public Health, 533-A North Bond Street, Baltimore, Maryland 21205

WALTON, Sarah, Office of the Commissioner, Public Services Administration, Social and Rehabilitation Services, 330 C Street, S.W., Washington, DC 20201

WASHBURN, Howard W., Pacific Homes,

5250 Santa Monica Boulevard, Los Angeles, California 90029

WIESEN, Chuck, Minneapolis Age and Opportunity Center, 1801 Nicolett Avenue South, Minneapolis, Minnesota 55403

WILLIAMS, Jacquelyn, M.P.H., National Center on the Black Aged, 1730 M Street, N.W., Suite 811, Washington, DC 20036

WILLIAMS, T. Franklin, M.D., University of Rochester and Monroe Community Hospital, 435 E. Henrietta Road, Rochester, New York 14603

WINSTEN, Jay A., Ph.D., Office of the Dean, Harvard School of Public Health, Boston, Massachusetts 02115

WOODRUFF, Mrs Pamela J., George Washington University School of Sociology, 2515 K Street, N.W. 404, Washington, DC 20037

YEE, Lucio C., Jr., M.D., 12110 Grant Street, Crown Point, Indiana 46307

ZIMMER, Anne, American Public Health Association, c/o 168 South Clinton Avenue, RCA, Rochester, New York 14604

Index